Biostatistics with R
An Introductory Guide for Field Biologists

Biostatistics with R provides a straightforward introduction on how to analyse data from the wide field of biological research, including nature protection and global change monitoring. The book is centred around traditional statistical approaches, focusing on those prevailing in research publications. The authors cover *t* tests, ANOVA and regression models, but also the advanced methods of generalised linear models and classification and regression trees. Chapters usually start with several useful case examples, describing the structure of typical datasets and proposing research-related questions. All chapters are supplemented by example datasets and thoroughly explained, step-by-step R code demonstrating the analytical procedures and interpretation of results. The authors also provide examples of how to appropriately describe statistical procedures and results of analyses in research papers. This accessible textbook will serve a broad audience of interested readers, from students, researchers or professionals looking to improve their everyday statistical practice, to lecturers of introductory under-graduate courses. Additional resources are provided on www.cambridge.org/biostatistics.

Jan Lepš is Professor of Ecology in the Department of Botany, Faculty of Science, University of South Bohemia, České Budějovice, Czech Republic and senior researcher in the Biology Centre of the Czech Academy of Sciences in České Budějovice. His main research interests include plant functional ecology, particularly the mechanisms of species coexistence and stability, and ecological data analysis. He has taught many ecological and statistical courses and supervised more than 80 student theses, from undergraduate to PhD.

Petr Šmilauer is Associate Professor of Ecology in the Department of Ecosystem Biology, Faculty of Science, University of South Bohemia, České Budějovice, Czech Republic. His main research interests are multivariate statistical analysis, modern regression methods and the role of arbuscular mycorrhizal symbiosis in the functioning of plant communities. He is co-author of multivariate analysis software Canoco 5, CANOCO for Windows 4.5 and TWINSPAN for Windows.

'We will never have a textbook of statistics for biologists that satisfies everybody. However, this book may come closest. It is based on many years of field research and the teaching of statistical methods by both authors. All useful classic and advanced statistical concepts and methods are explained and illustrated with data examples and R programming procedures. Besides traditional topics that are covered in the premier textbooks of biometry/biostatistics (e.g. R. R. Sokal & F. J. Rohlf, J. H. Zar), two extensive chapters on multivariate methods in classification and ordination add to the strength of this book. The text was originally published in Czech in 2016. The English edition has been substantially updated and two new chapters 'Survival Analysis' and 'Classification and Regression Trees' have been added. The book will be essential reading for undergraduate and graduate students, professional researchers, and informed managers of natural resources.'

Marcel Rejmánek,
Department of Evolution and Ecology, University of California, Davis, CA, USA

Biostatistics with R

An Introductory Guide for Field Biologists

JAN LEPŠ
University of South Bohemia, Czech Republic

PETR ŠMILAUER
University of South Bohemia, Czech Republic

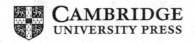

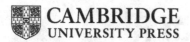

Shaftesbury Road, Cambridge CB2 8EA, United Kingdom

One Liberty Plaza, 20th Floor, New York, NY 10006, USA

477 Williamstown Road, Port Melbourne, VIC 3207, Australia

314–321, 3rd Floor, Plot 3, Splendor Forum, Jasola District Centre, New Delhi – 110025, India

103 Penang Road, #05–06/07, Visioncrest Commercial, Singapore 238467

Cambridge University Press is part of Cambridge University Press & Assessment, a department of the University of Cambridge.

We share the University's mission to contribute to society through the pursuit of education, learning and research at the highest international levels of excellence.

www.cambridge.org
Information on this title: www.cambridge.org/9781108727341

DOI: 10.1017/9781108616041

© Jan Lepš and Petr Šmilauer 2020

First published 2020

A catalogue record for this publication is available from the British Library

ISBN   978-1-108-48038-3   Hardback
ISBN   978-1-108-72734-1   Paperback

Additional resources for this publication at www.cambridge.org/biostatistics

Contents

Preface

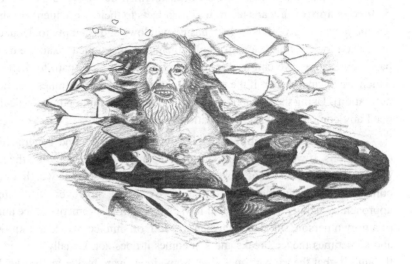

Modern biology is a quantitative science. A biologist weighs, measures and counts, whether she works with aphid or fish individuals, with plant communities or with nuclear DNA. Every number obtained in this way, however, is affected by random variation. Aphid counts repeatedly obtained from the same plant individual will differ. The counts of aphids obtained from different plants will differ more, even if those plants belong to the same species, and samples coming from plants of different species are likely to differ even more. Similar differences will be found in the nuclear DNA content of plants from the same population, in nitrogen content of soil samples taken from the same or different sites, or in the population densities of copepods across repeated samplings from the same lake. We say that our data contain a random component: the values we obtain are random quantities, with a part of their variation resulting from randomness.

But what actually is this randomness? In posing such a question, we move into the realm of philosophy or to axioms of probability theory. But what is probability? A biologist is usually happy with a pragmatic concept: we consider an event to be random if we do not have a causal explanation for it. Statistics is a research field which provides recipes for how to work with data containing random components, and how to distinguish deterministic patterns from random variation. Popular wisdom says that statistics is a branch of science where precise work is carried out with imprecise numbers. But the term **statistics** has multiple meanings. The layman sees it as an assorted collection of values (football league statistics of goals and points, statistics of MP voting, statistics of cars passing along a highway, etc.). Statistics is also a research field (often called mathematical statistics) providing tools for obtaining useful information from such datasets. It is a separate branch of science, to a certain extent representing an application of probability theory. The term statistic (often in singular form) is also used in another sense: a numerical characteristic computed from data. For example, the well-known arithmetic average is a statistic characterising a given data sample.

In scientific thinking, we can distinguish deductive and inductive approaches. The **deductive approach** leads us from known facts to their consequences. Sherlock Holmes may use the facts that a room is locked, has no windows and is empty to deduce that the room must have been locked from the outside. Mathematics is a typical example of a deductive system: based on axioms, we can use a purely logical (deductive) path to derive further statements, which are always correct if the initial axioms are also correct (unless we made a mistake in the derivation). Using the deductive approach, we proceed in a purely logical manner and do not need any comparison with the situation in real terms.

The **inductive approach** is different: we try to find general rules based on many observations. If we tread upon 1-cm-thick ice one hundred times and the ice breaks each time, we can conclude that ice of this thickness is unable to carry the weight of a grown person. We conclude this using inductive thinking. We could, however, also employ the deductive approach by using known physical laws, strength measurements of ice and the known weight of a grown person. But usually, when treading on thin ice, we do not know its exact thickness and sometimes the ice breaks and sometimes it does not. Usually we find, only after breaking through it, that the ice was quite thin. Sometimes even thicker ice breaks, but such an event is affected by many circumstances we are not able to quantify (ice structure, care in treading, etc.) and we therefore consider them as random. Using many observations, however, we can estimate the probability of breaking through ice based on its thickness by using the methods of mathematical statistics. Statistics is therefore a tool of inductive thinking in such cases, where the outcome of an experiment (or observation) is affected by random variability.

Thanks to advances in computer technology, statistics is now available to all biologists. Statistical analysis of data is a necessary prerequisite of manuscript acceptance in most biological journals. These days, it is impossible to fully understand most of the research papers in biological journals without understanding the basic principles of statistics. All biologists must plan their observations and experiments, as only correctly collected data can be useful when answering their questions with the aid of statistical methods. To collect your data correctly, you need to have a basic understanding of statistics.

A knowledge of statistics has therefore become essential for successful enquiry in almost all fields of biology. But statistics are also often misused. Some even say that there are three kinds of lies: a non-intentional lie, an intentional lie and statistics. We can 'adorn' bad data by employing a complex statistical method so that the result looks like a substantial contribution to our knowledge (even finding its way into prestigious journals). Another common case of statistical misuse is interpreting statistical ('correlational') dependency as causal. In this way, one can 'prove' almost anything. A knowledge of statistics also allows biologists to differentiate statements which provide new and useful information from those where statistics are used to simply mask a lack of information, or are misused to support incorrect statements.

The way statistics are used in the everyday practice of biology changed substantially with the increased availability of statistical software. Today, everyone can evaluate her/his data on a personal computer; the results are just a few mouse clicks away. While your computer will (almost) always offer some results, often in the form of a nice-looking graph, this rather convenient process is not without its dangers. There are users who present the results provided to them by statistical programs without ever understanding what was computed. Our book therefore tries not only to teach you how to analyse your data, but also how to understand what the results of statistical processing mean.

What is **biostatistics**? We do not think that this is a separate research field. In using this term, we simply imply a focus on the application of statistics to biological problems. Alternatively, the term **biometry** is sometimes used in a similar sense. In our book, we place an emphasis on understanding the principles of the methods presented and the rules of their use, not on the mathematical derivation of the methods. We present individual methods in a way that we believe is convenient for biologists: we first show a few examples of biological problems that can be solved by a given method, and only then do we present its principles and assumptions. In our explanations we assume that the reader has attended an introductory undergraduate mathematical course, including the basics of the theory of probability. Even so, we try to avoid complex mathematical explanations whenever possible.

This book provides only basic information. We recommend that all readers continue a more detailed exploration of those methods of interest to them. The three most recommended textbooks for this are Quinn & Keough (2002), Sokal & Rohlf (2012) and Zar (2010). The first and last of these more closely reflect the mind of the biologist, as their authors have themselves participated in ecological research. In this book, we adopt some ideas from Zar's textbook about the sequence in which to present selected topics. After every chapter, we give page ranges for the three referred textbooks, each containing additional information about the particular methods. Our book is only a slight extension of a one-term course (2 hours lectures + 2 hours practicals per week) in Biostatistics, and therefore sufficient detail is lacking on some of the statistical methods useful for biologists. This primarily concerns the use of multivariate statistical analysis, traditionally addressed in separate textbooks and courses.

We assume that our readers will evaluate their data using a personal computer and we illustrate the required steps and the format of results using two different types of software. The program R lacks some of the user-friendliness provided by alternative statistical packages, but offers practically all known statistical methods, including the most modern ones, for free (more details at cran.r-project.org), and so it became *de facto* a standard tool, prevailing in published biological research papers. We assume that the reader will have a basic working knowledge of R, including working with its user interface, importing data or exporting results. The knowledge required is, however, summarised in Appendix A of this book, which can be found after the last chapter. The program Statistica represents software for the less demanding user, with a convenient range of menu choices and extensive dialogue boxes, as well as an easily accessible and modifiable graphical presentation of results. Instructions for its use are available to the reader at the textbook's website: www.cambridge.org/biostatistics.

Example data used throughout this book are available at the same website, but also from our own university's web address: www.prf.jcu.cz/biostat-data-eng.xlsx.

Note that in most of our 'use case examples' (and often also in the example data), the actual (or suggested) number of replicates is very low, perhaps too low to provide reasonable support for a real-world study. This is just to make the data easily tractable while we demonstrate the computation of test statistics. For real-world studies, we recommend the reader strives to attain more extensive datasets. If there is no citation for our example dataset, such data are not real.

In each chapter, we also show how the results derived from statistical software can be presented in research papers and also how to describe the particular statistical methods there.

In this book, we will most frequently refer to the following three statistical textbooks providing more details about the methods:

- J. H. Zar (2010) *Biostatistical Analysis*, 5th edn. Pearson, San Francisco, CA.
- G. P. Quinn & M. J. Keough (2002) *Experimental Design and Data Analysis for Biologists*. Cambridge University Press, Cambridge.
- R. R. Sokal & E. J. Rohlf (2012) *Biometry*, 4th edn. W. H. Freeman, San Francisco, CA.

Other useful textbooks include:

- R. H. Green (1979) *Sampling Design and Statistical Methods for Environmental Biologists*. Wiley, New York.
- R. H. G. Jongmann, C. J. F. ter Braak & O. F. R. van Tongeren (1995) *Data Analysis in Community and Landscape Ecology*. Cambridge University Press, Cambridge.
- P. Šmilauer & J. Lepš (2014) *Multivariate Analysis of Ecological Data Using Canoco 5*, 2nd edn. Cambridge University Press, Cambridge.

More advanced readers will find the following textbook useful:

- R. Mead (1990) *The Design of Experiments. Statistical Principles for Practical Application*. Cambridge University Press, Cambridge.

Where appropriate, we cite additional books and papers at the end of the corresponding chapter.

Acknowledgements

Both authors are thankful to their wives Olina and Majka for their ceaseless support and understanding. Our particular thanks go to Petr's wife Majka (Marie Šmilauerová), who created all the drawings which start and enliven each chapter.

We are grateful to Conor Redmond for his careful and efficient work at improving our English grammar and style.

The feedback of our students was of great help when writing this book, particularly the in-depth review from a student point of view provided by Václava Hazuková. We appreciate the revision of Section 2.7, kindly provided by Cajo ter Braak.

1 Basic Statistical Terms, Sample Statistics

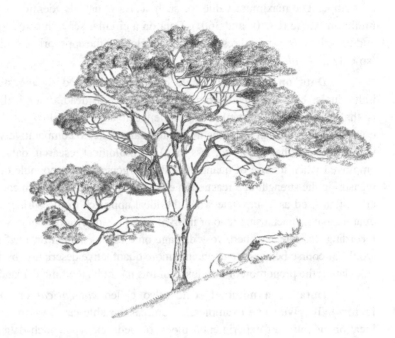

1.1 Cases, Variables and Data Types

In our research, we observe a set of objects (**cases**) of interest and record some information for each of them. We call all of this collected information the **data**. If plants are our cases, for example, then the data might contain information about flower colour, number of leaves, height of the plant stem or plant biomass. Each characteristic that is measured or estimated for our cases is called a **variable**. We can distinguish several data types, each differing in their properties and consequently in the way we handle the corresponding variables during statistical analysis.

Data on a ratio scale, such as plant height, number of leaves, animal weight, etc., are usually quantitative (numerical) data, representing some measurable amount – mass, length, energy. Such data have a constant distance between any adjacent unit values (e.g. the difference between lengths of 5 and 6 cm is the same as between 8 and 9 cm) and a naturally defined zero value. We can also think about such data as ratios, e.g. a length of 8 cm is twice the length of 4 cm. Usually, these data are non-negative (i.e. their value is either zero or positive).

Data on an interval scale, such as temperature readings in degrees Celsius, are again quantitative data with a constant distance (interval) between adjacent unit values, but there is no naturally defined zero. When we compare e.g. the temperature scales of Celsius and Fahrenheit, both have a zero value at different temperatures, which are defined rather arbitrarily. For such scales it makes no sense to consider ratios of their values: we cannot say that 8°C is twice as high a temperature as 4°C. These scales usually cover negative, zero, as well as positive values. On the contrary, temperature values in Kelvin (°K) can be considered a variable on a ratio scale.

A special case of data on an interval scale are **circular scale data**: time of day, days in a year, compass bearing – azimuth, used often in field ecology to describe the exposition of a slope. The maximum value for such scales is usually identical with (or adjacent to) the minimum value (e.g. 0° and 360°). Data on a circular scale must be treated in a specific way and thus there is a special research area developing the appropriate statistical methods to do so (so-called *circular statistics*).

Data on an ordinal scale can be exemplified by the state of health of some individuals: excellent health, lightly ill, heavily ill, dead. A typical property of such data is that there is no constant distance between adjacent values as this distance cannot be quantified. But we can order the individual values, i.e. to comparatively relate any two distinct values (greater than, equal to, less than). In biological research, data on an ordinal scale are employed when the use of quantitative data is generally not possible or meaningful, e.g. when measuring the strength of a reaction in ethological studies. Measurements on an ordinal scale are also often used as a surrogate when the ideal approach to measuring a characteristic (i.e. in a quantitative manner, using ratio or interval scale) is simply too laborious. This happens e.g. when recording the degree of herbivory damage on a leaf as none, low, medium, high. In this case it would of course be possible to attain a more quantitative description by scanning the leaves and calculating the proportion of area lost, but this might be too time-demanding.

Data on a nominal scale (also called *categorical* or *categorial variables*, or **factors**). To give some examples, a nominal variable can describe colour, species identity, location, identity of experimental block or bedrock type. Such data define membership of a particular case in a class, i.e. a qualitative characteristic of the object. For this scale, there are no constant (or even quantifiable) differences among categories, neither can we order the cases based on such a variable. Categorical data with just two possible values (very often *yes* and *no*) are often called **binary data**. Most often they represent the presence or absence of a character (leaves glabrous or hairy, males or females, organism is alive or dead, etc.).

Ordinal as well as categorical variables are often coded in statistical software as natural numbers. For example, if we are sampling in multiple locations, we would naturally code the first location as 1, the second as 2, the third as 3, etc. The software might not know that these values represent categorical data (if we do not tell it in some way) and be willing to compute e.g. an arithmetic average of the location identity, quite a nonsensical value. So beware, some operations can only be done with particular types of data.

Quantitative data (on an interval or a ratio scale) can be further distinguished into **discrete** vs. **continuous data**. For continuous data (such as weights), between any two measurement values there may typically lie another. In contrast we have discrete data, which are most often (but not always) counts (e.g. number of leaves per plant), that is non-negative integer numbers. In biological research, the distinction between discrete and continuous data is often blurred. For example, the counts of algal cells per 1 ml of water can be considered as a continuous variable (usually the measurement precision is less than 1 cell). In contrast, when we estimate tree height in the field using a hypsometer (an optical instrument for measuring tree height quickly), measurement precision is usually 0.5 m (modern devices using lasers may be more precise), despite the fact that tree height is a continuous variable. So even when the measured variable is continuous, the obtained values have a discrete nature. But this is an artefact of our measurement method, not a property of the measured characteristic: although the recorded values of tree height will be repeated across the dataset, the probability of finding two trees in a forest with identical height is close to zero.

1.2 Population and Random Sample

Our research usually refers to a large (potentially even infinitely large) group of cases, the **statistical population (or statistical universe)**, but our conclusions are based on a smaller group of cases, representing collected observations. This smaller group of observations is called the **random sample**, or often simply the **sample**. Even when we do not use the word *random*, we assume randomness in the choice of cases included in our sample. The term (statistical) *population* is often not related to what a biologist calls a population. In statistics this word has a more general meaning. The process of obtaining the sample is called **sampling**.

To obtain a random sample (as is generally assumed by statistical methods), we must follow certain rules during case selection: each member (e.g. an individual) in the statistical population must have the same and independent chance of being selected. The randomness of our choice should be assured by using random numbers. In the simplest (but often not workable) approach, we would label all cases in the sampled population with numbers from 1 to N. We then obtain the required sample of size n by choosing n random whole numbers from the interval $(1, N)$ in such a way that each number in that interval has the same chance of being selected and we reject the random numbers suggested by the software where the same choice is repeated. We then proceed by measuring the cases labelled with the selected n numbers.

In field studies estimating e.g. the aboveground biomass in an area, we would proceed by selecting several sample plots in the area in which the biomass is being collected. Those plots are chosen by defining a system of rectangular coordinates for the whole area and then generating random coordinates for the centres of individual plots. Here we assume that the sampled area has a rectangular shape[1] and is large enough so that we can ignore the possibility that the sample plots will overlap.

It is much more difficult to select e.g. the individuals from a population of freely living organisms, because it is not possible to number all existing individuals. For this, we typically sample in a way that is assumed to be close to random sampling, and subsequently work with the sample as if it were random, while often not appreciating the possible dangers of our results being affected by sampling bias. To give an example, we might want to study a dormouse population in a forest. We could sample them using traps without knowing the size of the sampled population. We can consider the individuals caught in traps as a random sample, but this is likely not a correct expectation. Older, more experienced individuals are probably better at avoiding traps and therefore will be less represented in our sample. To adequately account for the possible consequences of this bias, and/or to develop a better sampling strategy, we need to know a lot about the life history of the dormouse.

But even sampling sedentary organisms is not easy. Numbering all plant individuals in an area of five acres and then selecting a truly random sample, while certainly possible in principle, is often unmanageable in practical terms. We therefore require a sampling method

---

[1] But if not, we can still use a rectangular envelope enclosing the more complex area and simply reject the random coordinates falling outside the actual area.

suitable for the target objects and their spatial distribution. It is important to note that a frequently used sampling strategy in which we choose a random location in the study area (by generating point coordinates using random values) and then select an individual closest to this point is not truly random sampling. This is because solitary individuals have a higher chance of being sampled than those growing in a group. If individuals growing in groups are smaller (as is often the case due to competition), our estimates of plant characteristics based on this sampling procedure will be biased.

Stratified sampling represents a specific group of sampling strategies. In this approach, the statistical population is first split into multiple, more homogeneous subsets and then each subset is randomly sampled. For example, in a morphometric study of a spider species we can randomly sample males and females to achieve a balanced representation of both sexes. To take another example, in a study examining the effects of an invasive plant species on the richness of native communities, we can randomly sample within different climatic regions.

> **Subjectively choosing individuals, either considered typical for the subject or seemingly randomly chosen (e.g. following a line across a sampling location and occasionally picking an individual), is not random sampling and therefore is not recommended to define a dataset for subsequent statistical analysis.**

The sampled population can sometimes be defined solely in a hypothetical manner. For example, in a glasshouse experiment with 10 individuals of meadow sweetgrass (*Poa pratensis*), the reference population is a potential set of all possible individuals of this species, grown under comparable conditions, in the same season, etc.

1.3 Sample Statistics

Let us assume we want to describe the height for a set of 50 pine (*Pinus* sp.) trees. Fifty values of their height would represent a complete, albeit somewhat complex, view of the trees. We therefore need to simplify (summarise) this information, but with a minimal loss of detail. This type of summarisation can be achieved in two general ways: we can transform our numerical data into a graphical form (visualise them) or we can describe the set of values with a few **descriptive statistics** that summarise the most important properties of the whole dataset.

Among the choice of graphical summaries we have at our disposal, one of the most often used is the **frequency histogram** (see Fig. 1.2 later). We can construct a frequency histogram for a particular numerical variable by dividing the range of values into several classes (sub-ranges) of the same width and plotting (as the vertical height of each bar) the count of cases in each class. Sometimes we might want to plot the relative frequencies of cases rather than simple counts, e.g. as the percentage of the total number of cases in the whole sample (the histogram's shape or the information it portrays does not change, only the scale used on the vertical axis). When we have a sufficient number of cases and sufficiently narrow classes (intervals), the shape of the histogram approaches a characteristic of the variable's distribution called *probability density* (see Section 1.6 and Fig. 1.2 later). Further information about graphical summaries is provided in a separate section on graphical data summaries (Section 1.5).

Alternatively, we can summarise our data using descriptive statistics. Using our pine heights example, we are interested primarily in two aspects of our dataset: what is the typical ('mean') height of the trees and how much do the individual heights in our sample differ. The first aspect is quantified using the **characteristics of position** (also called central tendency), the second by the **characteristics of variability**. The characteristics of a finite set of values (of a random sample or a finite statistical population) can be determined precisely. In contrast, the characteristics of an infinitely large statistical population (or of a population for which we have not measured all the cases) must be **estimated** using a random sample. As a formal rule, the characteristics of a statistical population are labelled by Greek letters, while we label the characteristics of a random sample using standard (Latin) letters. The counts of cases represent an exception: N is the number of cases in a statistical population, while n is the number of cases (size) of a random sample.

1.3.1 Characteristics of Position

Example questions: What is the height of pine trees in a particular valley? What is the pH of water in the brooks of a particular region? For trees, we can either measure all of them or be happy with a random sample. For water pH, we must rely on a random sample, measuring its values at certain places within certain parts of the season.

Both examples demonstrate how important it is to have a well-defined statistical population (universe). In the case of our pine trees, we would probably be interested in mature individuals, because mixing the height of mature individuals with that of seedlings and saplings will not provide useful information. This means that in practice, we will need an operational definition of a 'mature individual' (e.g. at least 20 years old, as estimated by coring at a specific height).

Similarly, for water pH measurements, we would need to specify the type of streams we are interested in (and then, probably using a geographic information system – GIS, we select the sampling sites in a way that will correspond to random sampling). Further, because pH varies systematically during each day, and around the year, we will also need to specify some time window when we should perform our measurements. In each case, we need to think carefully about what we consider to be our statistical population with respect to the aims of study. Mixing pH of various water types might blur the information we want to obtain. It might be better to have a narrow time window to avoid circadian variability, but we must consider how informative is, say, the morning pH for the whole ecosystem. It is probably not reasonable to pool samples from various seasons. In any case, all these decisions must be specified when reporting the results. Saying that the average pH of streams in an area is 6.3 without further specification is not very informative, and might be misleading if we used a narrow subset of all possible streams or a narrow time window. Both of these examples also demonstrate the difficulty of obtaining a truly random sample; often we must simply try our best to select cases that will at least resemble a random sample.

Generally, we are interested in the 'mean' value of some characteristic, so we ask what the location of values on the chosen measurement scale is. Such an intuitively understood mean value can be described by multiple characteristics. We will discuss some of these next.

1.3.1.1 Arithmetic Mean (Average)

The arithmetic mean of the statistical population μ is

$$\mu = \frac{\sum_{i=1}^{N} X_i}{N} \tag{1.1}$$

while the arithmetic mean of a random sample $\overline{X}$ is

$$\overline{X} = \frac{\sum_{i=1}^{n} X_i}{n} \tag{1.2}$$

Example calculation: The height of five pine trees (in centimetres, measured with a precision of 10 cm) was 950, 1120, 830, 990, 1060. The arithmetic average is then $(950 + 1120 + 830 + 990 + 1060)/5 = 990$ cm. The mean is calculated in exactly the same way whether the five individuals represent our entire *population* (i.e. all individuals which we are interested in, say for example if we planted these five individuals 20 years ago and wish to examine their success) or whether these five individuals form our *random sample* representing all of the individuals in the study area, this being our statistical *population*. In the first case, we will denote the mean by μ, and this is an exact value. In the second scenario (much more typical in biological sciences), we will never know the exact value of μ, i.e. the mean height of all the individuals in the area, but we use the sample mean $\overline{X}$ to estimate its value (i.e. $\overline{X}$ is the estimate of μ).

Be aware that the arithmetic mean (or any other characteristics of location) cannot be used for raw data measured on a circular scale. Imagine we are measuring the geographic exposition of tree trunks bearing a particular lichen species. We obtain the following values in degrees (where both 0 and 360 degrees represent north): 5, 10, 355, 350, 15, 145. Applying Eq. (1.2), we obtain an average value of 180, suggesting that the mean orientation is facing south, but actually most trees have a northward orientation. The correct approach to working with circular data is outlined e.g. in Zar (2010, pp. 605–668).

1.3.1.2 Median and Other Quantiles

The median is defined as a value which has an identical number of cases, both above and below this particular value. Or we can say (for an infinitely large set) that the probability of the value for a randomly chosen case being larger than the median (but also smaller than the median) is identical, i.e. equal to 0.5. For theoretical data distributions (see Section 1.6 later in this chapter), the median is the value of a random variable with a corresponding distribution function value equal to 0.5. We can use the median statistic for data on ratio, interval or ordinal scales. There is no generally accepted symbol for the median statistic.

Besides the median, we can also use other **quantiles**. The most frequently used are the two **quartiles** – the **upper quartile**, defined as the value that separates one-quarter of the highest-value cases and the **lower quartile**, defined as the value that separates one-quarter of the lowest-value cases. The other quantiles can be defined similarly, and we will return to this topic when describing the properties of distributions.

In our pine heights example (see Section 1.3.1.1), the median value is equal to 990 cm (which is equal to the mean, just by chance). We estimate the median by first sorting the values according to their size. When the sample size (n) is odd, the median is equal to $X_{(n+1)/2}$, i.e. to the value in the centre of the list of sorted cases. When n is even, the median is estimated as the centre of the interval between the two middle observations, i.e. as $(X_{n/2} + X_{n/2+1})/2$. For example, if we are dealing with animal weights equal to 50, 52, 60, 63, 70, 94 g, the median estimate is 61.5 g. The median is sometimes calculated in a special way when its location falls among multiple cases with identical values (tied observations), see Zar (2010, p. 26).

As we will see later, the population median value is identical to the value of the arithmetic mean if the data have a symmetrical distribution. The manner in which the arithmetic mean and median differ in asymmetrical distributions (see also Fig. 1.1) is shown

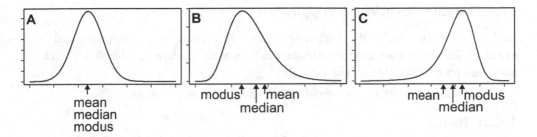

Figure 1.1 Frequency histograms idealised into probability density curves, with marked locations indicating different characteristics of position. Data values are plotted along the horizontal axis and frequency (probability) on the vertical axis. The distribution in plot A is symmetrical, while in plot B it is positively skewed and in plot C it is negatively skewed.

below. In this example we are comparing two groups of organisms which differ in the way they obtain their food, with each group comprising 11 individuals. The amount of food (transformed into grams of organic C per day) obtained by each individual was as follows:

      Group 1: 15, 16, 16, 17, 17, 18, 18, 19, 19, 20, 21
      Group 2: 5, 5, 6, 6, 7, 8, 9, 15, 35, 80, 120

In the first group, the arithmetic average of consumed C is 17.8 g, while the average for the second group is 26.9 g. The average consumption is therefore higher in the second group. But if we use medians, the value for the first group is 18, but just 8 in the second group. A typical individual (characterised by the fact that half of the individuals consume more and the other half less) consumes much more in the first group.

1.3.1.3 Mode
The mode is defined as the most frequent value. For data with a continuous distribution, this is the variable value corresponding to the local maximum (or local maxima) of the probability density. There might be more than one mode value for a particular variable, as a distribution can also be bimodal (with two mode values) or even polymodal. The mode is defined for all data types. For continuous data it is usually estimated as the centre of the value interval for the highest bar in a frequency histogram. If this is a polymodal distribution, we can use the bars with heights exceeding the height of surrounding bars. It is worth noting that such an estimate depends on our choice of intervals in the frequency histogram. The fact that we can obtain a sample histogram that has multiple modes (given the choice of intervals) is not sufficient evidence of a polymodal distribution for our sampled population values.

1.3.1.4 Geometric Mean
The geometric mean is defined as the n-th root of a multiple (Π operator represents the multiplication) of n values in our sample:

$$ GM = \sqrt[n]{\prod_{i=1}^{n} X_i} = \left(\prod_{i=1}^{n} X_i\right)^{1/n} \tag{1.3} $$

The geometric mean of our five pines example will be $(950 \times 1120 \times 830 \times 990 \times 1060)^{1/5} = 984.9$. The geometric mean is generally used for data on a ratio scale which do not contain zeros and its value is smaller than the arithmetic mean.

1.3.2 Characteristics of Variability (Spread)

Besides the 'mean value' of the characteristic under observation, we are often interested in the extent of differences among individual values in the sample, i.e. how variable they are. This is addressed by the characteristics of variability.

Example question: How variable is the height of our pine trees?

1.3.2.1 Range

The range is the difference between the largest (maximum) and the smallest (minimum) values in our dataset. In the tree height example the range is 290 cm. Please note that the range of values grows with increasing sample size. Therefore, the range estimated from a random sample is not a good estimate of the range in the sampled statistical population.

1.3.2.2 Variance

The variance and the statistics derived from it are the most often used characteristics of variability. The variance is defined as an average value of the second powers (squares) of the deviations of individual observed values from their arithmetic average. For a statistical population, the variance is defined as follows:

$$\sigma^2 = \frac{\sum_{i=1}^{N}(X_i - \mu)^2}{N} \tag{1.4}$$

For a sample, the variance is defined as

$$s^2 = \frac{\sum_{i=1}^{n}(X_i - \bar{X})^2}{n-1} \tag{1.5}$$

The s^2 term is sometimes replaced with *var* or *VAR*. The variance of a sample is the best (unbiased) estimate of the variance of the sampled population.

Example calculation: For our pine trees, the variance is defined (if we consider the five trees as the whole population) as $((950 - 990)^2 + (1120 - 990)^2 + (830 - 990)^2 + (990 - 990)^2 + (1060 - 990)^2)/5 = 9800$. However, it is more likely that these values would represent a random sample, so the proper estimate of variance is calculated as $((950 - 990)^2 + (1120 - 990)^2 + (830 - 990)^2 + (990 - 990)^2 + (1060 - 990)^2)/4 = 12{,}250$. Comparing Eqs (1.4) and (1.5), we can see that the difference between these two estimates diminishes with increasing n: for five specimens the difference is relatively large, but it is more or less negligible for large n. The denominator value, i.e. $n - 1$ and not n, is used in the sample because we do not know the real mean and thus must estimate it. Naturally, the larger our n is, the smaller the difference is between the estimate $\bar{X}$ and an (unknown) real value of the mean μ.

1.3.2.3 Standard Deviation

The standard deviation is the square root of the variance (for both a sample and a population). Besides being denoted by an s, it is often marked as *s.d.*, *S.D.* or *SD*. The standard deviation of a statistical population is defined as

$$\sigma = \sqrt{\sigma^2} \tag{1.6}$$

The standard deviation of a sample is defined as

$$s = \sqrt{s^2} \tag{1.7}$$

When we consider the five tree heights as a random sample, $s = \sqrt{12{,}250}$ cm^2 = 110.70 cm.

1.3.2.4 Coefficient of Variation

In many variables measured on a ratio scale, the standard deviation is scaled with the mean (sizes of individuals are a typical example). We can ask whether the height of individuals is more variable in a population of the plant species *Impatiens glandulifera* (with a typical height of about 2 m) or in a population of *Impatiens noli-tangere* (with a typical height of about 30 cm). We must therefore relate the variation with the average height of both groups. In other similar cases, we characterise variability by the coefficient of variation (*CV*, sometimes also *CoV*), which is a standard deviation estimate divided by the arithmetic mean:

$$CV = \frac{s}{\overline{X}} \tag{1.8}$$

The coefficient of variation is meaningful for data on a ratio scale. It is used when we want to compare the variability of two or more groups of objects differing in their mean values.

In contrast, it is not possible to use this coefficient for data on an interval scale, such as comparing the variation in temperature among groups differing in their average temperature. There is no natural zero value and hence the coefficient of variation gives different results depending on the chosen temperature scale (e.g. degrees Celsius vs. degrees Fahrenheit). Similarly, it does not make sense to use the *CV* for log-transformed data (including pH). In many cases the standard deviation of log-transformed data provides information similar to *CV*.

1.3.2.5 Interquartile Range

The interquartile range – calculated as the difference between the upper and lower quartiles – is also a measure of variation. It is a better characteristic of variation than the range, as it is not systematically related to the size of our sample. The interquartile range as a measure of variation (spread) is a natural counterpart to the median as a measure of position (location).

1.4 Precision of Mean Estimate, Standard Error of Mean

The sample arithmetic mean is also a random variable (while the arithmetic mean of a statistical population is not). So this estimate also has its own variation: if we sample a statistical population repeatedly, the means calculated from individual samples will differ. Their variation can be estimated using the variance of the statistical population (or of its estimate, as the true value is usually not available). The variance of the arithmetic average is

$$s_{\overline{X}}^2 = s_X^2 / n \tag{1.9}$$

The square root of this variance is the standard deviation of the mean's estimate and is typically called the **standard error of the mean**. It is often labelled as $s_{\bar{x}}$, *SEM* or *s.e.m.*, and is the most commonly employed characteristic of precision for an estimate of the arithmetic mean. Another often-used statistic is the confidence interval, calculated from the standard error and discussed later in Chapter 5. Based on Eq. (1.9), we can obtain a formula for directly computing the standard error of the mean:

$$s_{\bar{x}} = \frac{s_X}{\sqrt{n}} \tag{1.10}$$

Do not confuse the standard deviation and the standard error of the mean: the standard deviation describes the variation in sampled data and its estimate is not systematically dependent on the sample size; the standard error of the mean characterises the precision of our estimate and its value decreases with increasing sample size – the larger the sample, the greater the precision of the mean's estimate.

1.5 Graphical Summary of Individual Variables

Most research papers present the characteristics under investigation using the arithmetic mean and standard deviation, and/or the standard error of the mean estimate. In this way, however, we lose a great deal of information about our data, e.g. about their distribution. In general, a properly chosen graph summarising our data can provide much more information than just one or a couple of numerical statistics.

To summarise the shape of our data distribution, it is easiest to plot a frequency histogram (see Figs 1.2 and 1.3 below). Another type of graph summarising variable distribution is the **box-and-whisker plot** (see Fig. 1.4 explaining individual components of this plot type and Fig. 1.5 providing an example of its use). Some statistical software packages (this does not concern R) use the box-and-whisker plot (by default) to present an arithmetic mean and standard deviation. Such an approach is suitable only if we can assume that the statistical population for the visualised variable's values has a normal (Gaussian) distribution (see Chapter 4). But generally, it is more informative to plot such a graph based on median and quartiles, as this shows clearly any existing peculiarities of the data distribution and possibly also identifies unusual values included in our sample.

1.6 Random Variables, Distribution, Distribution Function, Density Distribution

All the equations provided so far can be used only for datasets and samples of finite size. As an example, to calculate the mean for a set of values, we must measure all cases in that set and this is possible only for a set of finite size. Imagine now, however, that our sampled statistical population is infinite, or we are observing some random process which can be repeated any number of times and which results in producing a particular value – a particular random entity. For example, when studying the distribution of plant seeds, we can release each seed using a tube at a particular height above the soil surface and subsequently measure its speed at the end of the tube.[2] Such a measurement process can be repeated an infinite number of times.[3] Measured speed can be considered a random variable and the measured times are the **realisations** of that random variable. Observed values of a random variable are actually a random sample from a potentially infinite set of values – in this case all possible speeds of the seeds. This is true for almost all variables we measure in our research, whether in the field or in the lab.

---

[2] So-called *terminal velocity*, considered to be a good characteristic of a seed's ability to disperse in the wind.

[3] In practice this is not so simple. When we aim to characterise the dispersal ability of a plant species we should vary the identity of the seeds, with the tested seeds being a random sample from all the seeds of given species.

A random variable can be characterised by the probabilities of having particular values, and the complete set of such probabilities is called the **probability distribution** (often simply referred to as a **distribution**). In this section, we focus exclusively on the distribution of quantitative data (on a ratio or interval scale), but distinguish discrete and continuous variables in two separate subsections. In practice, however, many methods targeting continuous variables are also applied to discrete variables, particularly when the discrete variable has many possible values.

1.6.1 Probability Distributions and Distribution Functions of Discrete Random Variables

For a **discrete** random variable, its individual possible values can be numbered (it must have a denumerable set of values). The **probability distribution** of a discrete variable X is an enumeration of possible values x_i and the corresponding probabilities of X having a particular value, i.e. $p_i = P(X = x_i)$. The probability distribution can therefore be specified by a table (see Table 1.1) or formula.

It is logical that the sum of all probabilities p_i must be equal to 1:

$$\sum_{i=1}^{n} p_i = 1 \tag{1.11}$$

We can also define the function $F(x)$ equal to the probability $P(X < x)$, i.e. the probability that a random variable will be smaller than a chosen value x. This function is called the **distribution function**, sometimes also a *cumulative distribution function*, of the random variable X. We can say that

$$F(x) = \sum_{x_i < x} p_i \tag{1.12}$$

with the summation performed over all values of i for which $x_i < x$. For example, the probability that x is smaller than 5 is equal to the sum of probabilities belonging to x-values smaller than 5.

For a discrete random variable, we can calculate its mean value using

$$\mu = \sum_{i=1}^{n} x_i p_i \tag{1.13}$$

and its variance using

$$\sigma^2 = \sum_{i=1}^{n} (x_i - \mu)^2 p_i \tag{1.14}$$

The standard deviation σ is then a square root of the variance.

Table 1.1 *Specifications of a probability distribution for a discrete random variable*

x_i	x_1	x_2	$\cdots$	x_n
p_i	p_1	p_2	$\cdots$	p_n

1.6.2 Distribution Functions and Probability Density of Continuous Random Variables

A random variable X which may attain any numerical value from a given interval is called a **continuous random variable**. Given that the set of possible values of X is potentially infinite (although in practice we are limited by the precision of our measurement method), we must define its probability distribution function as a so-called **probability density function** $f(x)$ using the following formula:

$$f(x) = \lim_{\Delta x \to 0} \frac{P(x < X \leq x + \Delta x)}{\Delta x} \tag{1.15}$$

What does a graph of a probability density function tell us? Recall how a frequency histogram is constructed. If we set Δx in Eq. (1.15) to one and plot the value $P(x < X \leq x + \Delta x)/\Delta x$ against x, we obtain a histogram of relative frequencies, with each plotted value corresponding to the probability that the value of random variable X lies in the interval $(x, x + 1)$. This is illustrated in Fig. 1.2A for a histogram based on 30 randomly sampled values of a continuous variable.[4] As we narrow the interval (see Fig. 1.2B with a step of 0.2, based on 15,000 randomly sampled observations), the probability of having the value in such a range will decrease proportionally (the narrower the interval, the less likely it is that a value will fall into it). That is why the denominator in Eq. (1.15) contains the Δx-value, which corrects for the dependency of the probability on the interval width. As Δx approaches zero, we obtain the probability density function, illustrated in Fig. 1.2C. It can therefore be understood as an idealised histogram of relative frequencies for an infinitely large statistical population.

A continuous random variable can also be specified using a (cumulative) **distribution function** $F(x) = P(X < x)$, where x is any real number. The distribution function thus represents the probability of a random variable value being less than x.

We can use the distribution function to define quantiles. A statistic X_p defined as $F(X_p) = p$ is called a **quantile**, with its reference value (p) often being expressed on a percentage scale.

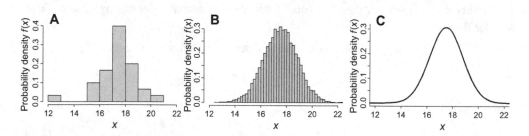

Figure 1.2 The genesis of a probability density function from a histogram of relative frequencies. Plot A represents a histogram based on 30 observations of a variable with a mean of 17.5 and a standard deviation of 1.3. Plot B represents a similarly constructed histogram for 15,000 observations coming from the same sampled statistical population (universe), using narrower intervals for the plotted bars. Both histograms use probability density scaling, so that the total area of their bars is equal to 1. Plot C represents the probability density function of the infinite sampled population.

---

[4] We admit we have cheated here; the histograms in parts A and B are not based on data measured in the field but were generated as random draws from a theoretical statistical distribution called the normal distribution (to be discussed in Chapter 4) with specified parameters (mean and standard deviation).

For example, $X_{0.95}$ is often called the 95% quantile. It represents the value for which the distribution function is equal to 0.95. This means that a random variable value exceeds this quantile with probability p = 0.05.[5] The $X_{0.5}$ quantile is called the median, and $X_{0.25}$ and $X_{0.75}$ are the lower and upper quartiles, respectively. If the probability density function has a maximum, then the corresponding x-value is called the mode.

For a continuous random variable X, the mean value is defined as

$$\mu = \int_{-\infty}^{+\infty} x f(x)\, dx \tag{1.16}$$

and the variance as

$$\sigma^2 = \int_{-\infty}^{+\infty} (x - \mu)^2 f(x) dx \tag{1.17}$$

where the $\int$ symbol represents integration over the full range of real values that the variable X can eventually have.

Some of the distributions can be theoretically derived and it is possible to define a formula for their probability density function and distribution function. Such distributions have specific names (e.g. normal, F, t, binomial or χ^2) and their values can be computed in statistical programs (as described in Chapter 4).

The random process which leads us to the realisation of a random variable will itself generate the random nature of any summary statistic calculated from that variable. For example, a sample arithmetic mean is a random variable.

1.7 Example Data

The data in the *Chap1* sheet of the *biostat-data-eng.xlsx* file contain observations from 24 experimental meadow plots in a field experiment studying the effect of mowing (variable *Mown* records whether a particular plot was mown or not) on the count of plant seedlings that germinated during a single season on the plot (variable *Seedlings*). Because the researcher assumed that the mowing can influence the seedling count through a change in the amount of plant litter on the soil surface, the percentage litter cover was also recorded (variable *LitterCov*).

Our task (within the context of this chapter) is to calculate the basic sample statistics of the *Seedlings* and *LitterCov* variables both for the entire dataset and also separately for the mown and unmown plots, as well as to create a graphical summary of the data.

1.8 How to Proceed in R

We can import the data from the sheet *Chap1* into a data frame called *chap1*. The basic descriptive statistics can be obtained for numerical variables in a data frame using the *summary* function:

---

[5] Sometimes also described as 'with 5% probability', although formally it is not correct to present probabilities on the percentage scale.

```
summary( chap1)
  Seedlings        Mown      LitterCov
Min.    :   6.00   no :12   Min.    : 0.00
1st Qu.: 18.75    yes:12   1st Qu.: 2.00
Median : 31.50             Median :11.50
Mean    : 49.42            Mean    :18.58
3rd Qu.: 75.25            3rd Qu.:35.00
Max.    :168.00           Max.    :50.00
```

1st Qu. and *3rd Qu.* represent the lower and upper quartile, respectively. The meaning of the other labels is hopefully clear. If you need to calculate other statistics that are not included in the *summary* output, you can do so with the function *sapply*. Here you will specify not only the data, but also the function calculating the summary statistics, e.g. function *var* for calculating the sample variance estimate:

```
sapply( chap1, var)
  Seedlings          Mown      LitterCov
1969.2971014    0.2608696   354.3405797
```

Of course, calculating the variance for a factor (variable *Mown*) is not a good idea and the value shown for this variable represents the variance for factor levels transformed into numbers (0 for *no* and 1 for *yes*). We can calculate the variance for a specific variable e.g. as

```
with( chap1, var( Seedlings))
[1] 1969.297
```

Further modification of existing functions is also possible, e.g. to calculate the coefficient of variation we can proceed by passing an inline function as follows:

```
sapply( chap1[,c(1,3)], function(x) sd(x)/mean(x))
Seedlings LitterCov
0.8980121 1.0129472
```

We used column selection in the *chap1* data frame to omit the calculation on the second variable.

When we need to calculate sample statistics for individual groups of data, the *split* function is our friend. This function splits the values of a variable given in its first parameter into groups defined by the second parameter (using the function *with* makes the names of variables present in the data frame *chap1* accessible, so we do not need to refer to it repeatedly):

```
X <- with( chap1, split( Seedlings, Mown))
X
$no
[1]   18   10  168   29   34   30    6    8   61   33   19   27
$yes
[1]  144   14   70   40   31   91   32  103    9   93   94   22
```

```
sapply( X, mean)
      no      yes
36.91667 61.91667
```

```
sapply( X, var)
      no      yes
1926.447 1850.265
```

1.8.1 Graphical Summary of Quantitative Variables

Although the basic installation of R contains functions for creating the standard summarising graphs (e.g. *hist* or *boxplot*), we recommend that the reader uses functions offered in more developed graphing packages (e.g. *lattice* or *ggplot2*), as they allow further extension when we need to create more complex layouts (such as separated plots for groups of observations, but plotted using a shared scale). Here we will use the *lattice* package, starting with a frequency histogram for the count of seedlings:

```
library( lattice)
histogram( ~Seedlings, data=chap1, col="gray")
```

The resulting graph (see Fig. 1.3) has the range of possible seedling count values on the horizontal *x*-axis divided into six intervals of the same width, and the height of each grey bar represents (on the vertical *y*-axis) the percentage of the sample size (*n*). The raw counts of cases can be used instead of percentage values, but for this you must explicitly specify the parameter *type* with the value set to 'count'. The *histogram* function has many more options that allow you e.g. to change the labels for axes, set the range of variable values, explicitly set the number of intervals or even the values of the breaks among the intervals, etc. When setting the width of intervals, be careful not to set it too narrow. For example, if we wish to measure

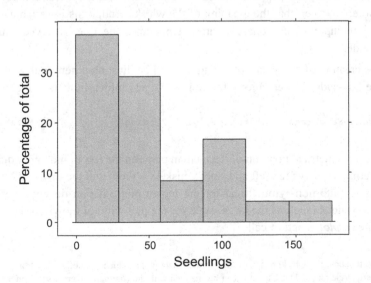

Figure 1.3 Frequency histogram of seedling counts in individual experimental plots (*n* = 24).

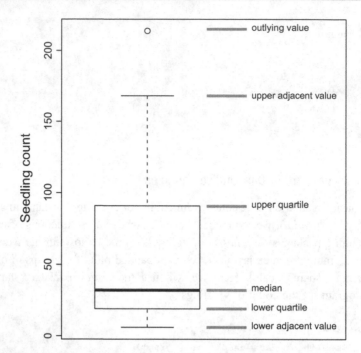

Figure 1.4 Explanation of box-and-whisker plot components: see Section 1.3.1.2 for an explanation of median and quartiles; lower and upper adjacent values are the positions of the smallest and largest observations that are still within the range (median − 1.5 IQR, median + 1.5 IQR), where IQR is the interquartile range (see Section 1.3.2.5); outlying values are all individual observations outside the range of adjacent values.

tree heights with a precision of 1 m, the chosen interval width must be at least 1 m. Otherwise, some of the intervals cannot contain measurements.

Box-and-whisker plot diagrams can be created in the *lattice* package with the function *bwplot*. Figure 1.4 explains the meaning of individual graphical components of this plot type. Note, however, that the meaning of the whisker endpoints is variable – sometimes they mean a multiple of interquartile range, sometimes the true observed minimum and maximum value.[6]

The creation of a whisker-plot diagram will be illustrated here with a graph plotting two separate box-and-whisker objects for non-mown and mown plots (see Fig. 1.5).

```
bwplot( Mown~Seedlings, data=chap1, ylab="Mowing")
```

The asymmetrical position of the median between the lower and upper quartiles – but also the differing length of the left and right whiskers – show that the distribution of seedling count values is quite non-symmetrical for the mown plots. If you do not want to plot the outlying observations (such as the large value for the plot without mowing), you can add *do. out* = *F* to the *bwplot* function call.

---

[6] In the *bwplot* function, the whiskers span to the furthest data points which are not further from the box than 1.5 times the interquartile range. The 1.5 value can be changed with the *coef* parameter; if you prefer the whiskers to span from minimum to maximum value, you can set *coef* = 0 in the *bwplot* call.

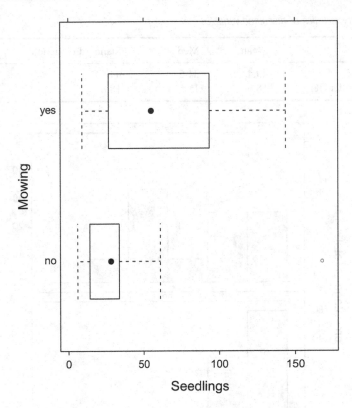

Figure 1.5 Two box-and-whisker plots in the same graph, allowing one to compare the distribution of seedling count values between the mown and unmown experimental plots. See Fig. 1.4 for an explanation of the plot components (the medians are plotted here as filled black circles and the plots are rotated by 90 degrees).

To create separate frequency histograms for the seedling count in the mown and non-mown plots, we can use the following command (with the results illustrated in Fig. 1.6):

```
histogram( ~Seedlings|Mown, data=chap1, col="gray")
```

1.9 Reporting Analyses

Presenting statistical summaries of variables is rare in standard research papers. They do, however, offer the reader a chance to compare observed values and their variations with other datasets he/she might be acquainted with. Statistical summaries are usually limited to just a single characteristic of position (mean) and one characteristic of variation (spread) per variable. For our example, we have extended these traditionally reported characteristics (arithmetic mean and standard deviation) with the very useful median statistic.

1.9.1 Methods

Measured quantitative variables were summarised using mean, median and sample standard deviation.

Table X *Summary statistics of measured variables*

	Mean	Median	Standard deviation	Sample size
Seedling count	49.4	31.5	44.4	24
Cover of plant litter (%)	18.6	11.5	18.8	24

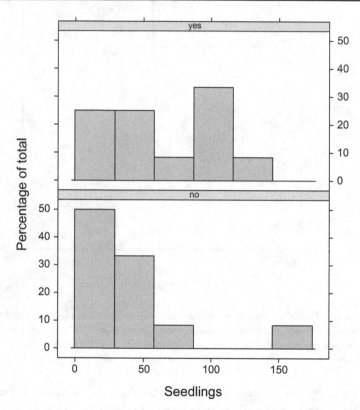

Figure 1.6 Frequency histograms (on percentage scale) for seedling counts in the experimental plots, comparing the mown (top) and unmown (bottom) plot types. Title bars for each panel specify the corresponding level of factor *Mown* for a particular group of cases.

Note that the above sentence would be present in your methods only if requested during a review process – the use of such simple statistics is usually skipped in the Methods section.

1.9.2 Results

We recorded seedling counts and estimated percentage cover of plant litter on all 24 experimental plots (see Table X for statistical summaries).

1.10 Recommended Reading

Zar (2010), pp. 1–48.
Quinn & Keough (2002), pp. 7–17 and pp. 58–61 for graphical summaries.
Sokal & Rohlf (2012), pp. 9–22 (data types and samples), pp. 39–58 (descriptive statistics), pp. 59–68 (distributions and probability).

2 Testing Hypotheses, Goodness-of-Fit Test

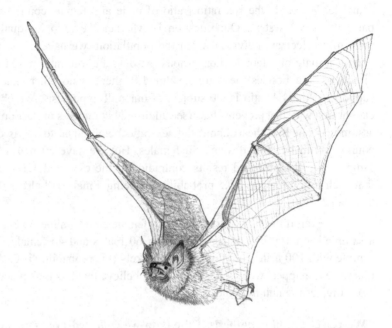

2.1 Principles of Hypothesis Testing

Two archetypal statistical procedures are the **estimation** of parameters and the **testing** of hypotheses. In Chapter 1, we introduced the estimation of parameters for a statistical population and in this chapter we will handle the basics of hypothesis testing. One of the ground tenets of scientific research is that an agreement of our data with a hypothesis does not necessarily imply that the hypothesis is correct. In contrast, if the collected data contradict our hypothesis, this suggests that the hypothesis cannot be correct. In other words, we cannot prove a hypothesis using the data we have collected, but based on such data, we may eventually reject it. This is the main principle of statistical hypothesis testing. We will illustrate it using tests on nominal (categorical) data, because we feel this example is easiest to understand. Before that, however, we summarise the procedure:

- We formulate a **null hypothesis, labelled as** H_0. This formulation must be done in a way that allows our data to disprove the hypothesis if it is not correct. Usually, our null hypothesis is formulated so that it complements the idea that we want to support with our data. So a typical null hypothesis says something like 'there is no difference ...', 'there is no dependency of X on Y', etc.

- Next we try to prove that the collected data are not compatible with (i.e. contradict) the null hypothesis, and this is usually based on a test statistic, as described below.
- If we demonstrate a sufficient discrepancy between our data and the null hypothesis, we reject it and instead accept the **alternative hypothesis** (H_A), which negates (complements) the null hypothesis (H_0).

To illustrate hypothesis testing in more detail, let us move to a specific biological example. We study the sex ratio (ratio of male and female counts) of long-eared bats in a particular cave system. Our question is whether the ratio is equal to 1.0, i.e. when we randomly select an individual from the population, we have the same probability (0.5) of getting a male or a female. For various reasons, the true ratio might differ from 1.0 in both directions, but besides the neutral value 1.0, there is no other exact ratio a theory would support, so the 1:1 ratio is the subject of our null hypothesis. We observed 100 individuals caught in a way that prevents bias (see additional comments in Section 2.2). Hence, we would assume (if our hypothesis about the sex ratio being equal to 1.0 is correct) that the 'ideal' counts would be 50 males and 50 females. But we have 60 males and 40 females in our sample. Are the observed results contradicting the expected 1:1 ratio, i.e. our assumption that each individual has a 0.5 probability of being a male and also a 0.5 probability of being a female?

Even if the true ratio of male and female counts in the cave is 1:1, we can still obtain a sample with 100 individuals containing 60 males and 40 females. We can even obtain a sample with 100 males, but this is very unlikely (the probability is 0.5^{100}, i.e. about 10^{-30}). If this were to happen, we would certainly not believe that this took place just by chance and we would reject the null hypothesis.

> **We reject a null hypothesis if the data we collected are very unlikely given the null hypothesis.**

But what does 'very unlikely' mean for a particular dataset and specific null hypothesis? The general statistical recipe for drawing a conclusion about the null hypothesis is the following:

- We first decide how 'unlikely' the outcome of our trial must be for us to conclude that the null hypothesis can be rejected. In other words, we choose the maximum probability that the data will be as much or more different from the null hypothesis expectation (under the assumption that our null hypothesis is correct) that will lead to rejecting the null hypothesis. This is the so-called **test significance level** (α) and we usually choose a value of 0.05 or 0.01 (alternatively, some users express the values on the percentage scale, i.e. 5% or 1%).
- Then we calculate the value of a **test statistic**. Test statistics are constructed in such a way that the more the observed data differ from the null hypothesis expectation, the higher is the value of the test statistic (in some cases this applies to the absolute value of the test statistic). We must know the distribution of values of this test statistic when the null hypothesis is correct. This means that we also know the test statistic value that is exceeded with a probability of 0.05 (or 0.01). Such values are called **critical values** of the test statistic's distribution.
- So if the test statistic value calculated for our data exceeds the critical value for a chosen significance level (α), we reject the null hypothesis. We usually characterise this situation by

saying that the result (or the discrepancy with the null hypothesis) is significant at the particular significance level.

In our example of male and female bat counts we are using categorical data, and so we will use the **goodness-of-fit** test. The test statistic is called the χ^2 statistic and is calculated as follows:

$$\chi^2 = \sum_{i=1}^{k} \frac{\left(f_i - \hat{f}_i\right)^2}{\hat{f}_i} \tag{2.1}$$

where k is the total number of categories ($k = 2$ in our example), f_i is the observed frequency for the i-th category (sometimes labelled O_i, referring to the word *observed*) and $\hat{f}_i$ is the expected frequency for the i-th category (sometimes labelled E_i, referring to the word *expected*).

So if we use this test statistic formula for our example data, both of the expected frequency values are 50 and so the test statistic will be

$$\chi^2 = \frac{(60 - 50)^2}{50} + \frac{(40 - 50)^2}{50} = 4.0$$

We then compare this value of 4.0 with a critical value of the χ^2 distribution for the chosen significance level α and given degrees of freedom. The **degrees of freedom** (usually labelled as df or DF) represent the number of categories minus one ($k - 1$) used in the test. It is the number of frequencies we need to know to fully describe our data. The frequency for the last category is not required, because we can calculate its value from the preceding $k - 1$ frequencies and the total number of observations (n, here equal to 100), which is considered as *a priori* knowledge in our test. For our two-category example (males and females), $DF = 1$. If we know that out of 100 individuals, 60 were males, we know the result of the whole sampling. The test statistic value 4.0 is larger than the critical value $\chi^2_{0.05,1}$ (i.e. α set to 0.05 and with one degree of freedom), which is equal to 3.84, and so we know that the estimated significance level (p) is less than 0.05 (actually $p = 0.0455$). Our conclusion will therefore be that the observed frequencies differ significantly from the frequencies expected for a sex ratio equal to 1.

2.2 Possible Errors in Statistical Tests of Hypotheses

We will now use the bat example to explain two possible errors we might commit when testing statistical hypotheses. For this, however, we must pretend that we know the true state of the phenomenon about which we hypothesise,[1] i.e. for our example we must pretend that we know the true value of the sex ratio of bats in the cave system we're studying.

1. Let us first assume that the true sex ratio is really equal to 1.0, and we collected just 100 individuals as in our earlier example. Naturally we could repeat the sampling a second or third time if we have the resources to do so. We might find that the results differ across individual samplings.

   1a. Let's imagine that the first sampling of 100 bats yields the same results as those seen in our earlier example: 60 males and 40 females. As we have seen above, these observed

---

[1] If we knew the truth, there would be no need to hypothesise and to perform statistical tests of hypotheses. But this is just an 'if' game that we need to play to discuss possible errors in our decisions in more definitive terms.

frequencies lead to a rejection of our null hypothesis. But here we know this decision about the null hypothesis is not correct – we have committed a so-called **Type I error** (by rejecting a correct null hypothesis). When we work with real data we do not know whether this error has occurred or not. We do, however, know how likely this error is: this is given by the *a priori* chosen significance level α (0.05 in our case). In other words, the significance level of our test is the conditional probability of rejecting a null hypothesis which in fact should not be rejected.

1b. Next we take another sample of 100 bats, collecting them again from a cave system in which the real sex ratio is equal to 1.0. But this time, we obtain 55 males and 45 females. So the value of the test statistic will be different, $\chi^2 = (55 - 50)^2/50 + (45 - 50)^2/50 = 1.0$. This value is clearly smaller than the critical value of $\chi^2_{0.05,1}$ (3.84), so the probability of committing an error by rejecting the null hypothesis is larger than the chosen α. Consequently, we do not reject the null hypothesis, and as we are pretending to know the true sex ratio, we know that not rejecting the null hypothesis was the correct decision.

2. Let us imagine that the true ratio is different in our cave system: in fact, there are more males than females. For the sake of specificity, let us pretend the true sex ratio is 1.5, with 60% of individuals in the caves being male. And again, with repeated sampling of 100 individuals, we will get varying results depending on chance.

2a. We can again obtain 60 males and 40 females in our sample. Remember, however, that in real research we do not know the truth, so our null hypothesis still represents the simple assumption that the sex ratio is equal to 1.0, with the expected frequencies being 50 and 50 for our 100-individual sample. As we have already seen above (1a), the test statistic has a value of 4.0 and so we reject the null hypothesis. This time, however, our decision is correct, as the sex ratio is not 1.0 but 1.5.

2b. Now let us check what happens if our sample contains 55 males and 45 females. Our test statistic's value will again be 1.0, as in (1b) above, and so we cannot reject the null hypothesis. Although in this case this is an incorrect decision, as the true sex ratio is 1.5. We have committed a **Type II error**. Its probability is labelled β, but we usually do not know its value (unlike the probability of Type I error). But the two types of error are – for a given sample size – inversely related: the larger α we choose, the smaller β we get, and vice versa. This is why we should not be too 'ambitious' when setting the value of α – limiting the probability of one kind of error will increase the frequency of the other. An important characteristic of statistical tests is their **power**, calculated as $1 - \beta$. Clearly the power of different (alternative) tests must be compared with the same chosen α. As we do not know the probability of Type II error (β), an appropriate statement about our decision is that – **based on our data, we cannot reject the null hypothesis**. It is **not correct** to say that we have proven the null hypothesis!

So we can summarise the four cases discussed above. We have two possibilities about the truth (the null hypothesis is correct or it is not) and in either case, we can make two alternative decisions (we reject the null hypothesis or we do not reject it). These four combinations can be summarised in a two-by-two table (Table 2.1).

The two types of error are inherent in statistical decision-making and are a consequence of the stochastic (random) nature of the processes under study. Consequently, there is

Table 2.1 *Type I and Type II errors in statistical testing*

		The truth	
		H_0 is correct	H_0 is not correct
Our decision	**We reject H_0**	Type I error committed (happens with probability α)	Correct decision
	H_0 not rejected	Correct decision	Type II error committed (happens with probability β)

no way to eliminate them entirely from our decisions. The smaller the Type I error probability (α) we set, the larger the expected Type II error probability. Returning to our bat example, we might want to minimise Type I error even more and so we set $\alpha = 0.01$. The corresponding critical value ($\chi^2_{0.01,1}$) is then larger, namely 6.63. What are the consequences of this change? In example 1a above, we do not commit a Type I error thanks to stricter criteria. But in example 2a, we cannot reject the null hypothesis and hence we make a Type II error.

However, imagine that (for some reason) we want to keep the Type I error rate low and thus insist on the requirement of $\alpha = 0.01$. Then the chance that we will be able to reject the null hypothesis is rather low, even in the case that the true sex ratio is 1.5 (60:40). What can we do about this? The most general recommendation is to increase the sample size. We can collect e.g. 1000 individuals and expect that, as in example 2a, the counts will exactly reflect the true ratio in the whole population. In this case, we find 600 males and 400 females, with the test statistic $\chi^2 = 40.0$ greatly exceeding the critical value for $\alpha = 0.01$.

In contrast, if we increase the sample size in example 1a (i.e. when the sex ratio in the population is 1.0), it is very unlikely that we will find 600 males and 400 females; the same relative deviation from the null hypothesis is much more likely in small than in large samples. Thus, although decreasing α increases β **at a fixed sample size,** we can keep both α and β low if we have a large enough sample size. This is a general rule: having everything else fixed, β decreases and thus the test power increases with increasing sample size.

Beware: **We must use the observed frequencies (counts) in the goodness-of-fit test. We cannot transform them into percentage values for the calculation of our test statistic!**

Further, should the real sex ratio in the cave be 3:1, we can expect that among 100 sampled individuals, we will find a ratio of 75:25. In this case, the test statistic will be $\chi^2 = 25.0$, and we can easily reject the null hypothesis at any feasible significance level. This is another general rule – the test power increases not only with sample size, but also with the size of the deviation from the null hypothesis. However, as we are not able to manipulate reality, the only way to increase our test power is to increase our sample size.

Our bat example can also be used to illustrate a quite different set of errors – those not related to statistical decisions, but affecting them nevertheless. In the discussion above, we consider the 100 sampled individuals to be a random sample from the population of bats in that cave system, i.e. each individual in the cave has the same probability of being sampled, and this probability is independent of whether any other individual is sampled. Let us imagine that our sampling is carried out during the winter hibernation period when most bats are hanging from the cave ceilings. It might happen that the females select less accessible locations on the ceiling (e.g. deeper inside crevices) or that the males respond to an intruder more quickly and fly off with a higher probability than the females. Either way, we get a biased sex ratio from our sampling, because the probability of being sampled differs among individuals, depending on their sex.

Further, the bats may form groups of predominantly the same sex as a result of ceiling preference. Then, when we manage to climb to a particular part of the ceiling and sample all of the available individuals there, we create yet another bias: the selection of an individual in our sample should be independent of the selection of other individuals in the sample. All of the sampling difficulties we have described may lead to a sample that is not completely random, and this might lead to a large deviation from the state assumed under the null hypothesis. Depending on our sampling approach, therefore, we can reject the null hypothesis for three quite different reasons:

1. the null hypothesis **is not** correct;
2. the null hypothesis **is** correct, but we commit a Type I error;
3. the null hypothesis **is** correct, but not all of the assumptions of our chosen test were fulfilled.

The example illustrates another aspect of statistical testing in biology – we take the statements that (1) the sex ratio in the cave is 1:1 and (2) each individual has a probability of being male equal to 0.5, as equivalent (and, naturally, we do not return each individual after being sampled). This means that we consider the number of individuals to be infinitely high. As a matter of fact, the number of bats in the cave system is finite. Thus, at least in theory, we are able to sample them all and find the real number of males and females, and very probably those counts will not be exactly equal. Even though this is rarely stated, we are often not interested in the finite set of individuals that are actually present in the cave at the time of sampling, but rather in a potential (and this might be infinitely large) set of individuals that might be present there. So, in many cases, we somehow pretend that our statistical population (statistical universe) is a potentially infinite set.

The goodness-of-fit test and its formula in Eq. (2.1) can be used for any number of categories. The following example illustrates an experiment in insect behaviour, in which bees were entering a test space with yellow, red and blue discs. For each individual bee, we recorded the colour of the disc that the bee lands on for the first time. Our null hypothesis (H_0) states that the probability of choosing a particular disc does not depend on its colour. The alternative hypothesis (H_A) therefore states that the probability of landing on a disc is affected by its colour. In this way, we can explore whether the bees might use the object's colour as a visual cue. We observed 100 bees. The frequencies of first-choice colours were: yellow 47 times, red 38 times, blue 15 times. Is it possible to detect any colour preference among the bees? According to our null hypothesis there is no effect of colour on choosing a disc, so all three discs have the same probability of being chosen, namely 1/3. Consequently, the expected frequencies for our sample of 100 bees are (with some rounding) 33.33 for each of the three colours of disc.

The value of the χ^2_2 statistic is 16.3416, which is larger than the critical value for $\alpha = 0.05$ and $DF = 2$ (equal to 5.991), and we must therefore reject the null hypothesis (with $p = 0.00028$). If we look at the contributions of individual colours to the test statistic value (last row of Table 2.2), we can see that the largest effect was in the avoidance of the blue disc, followed by the higher-than-expected frequency of landings on the yellow disc.

Table 2.2 *Applying the goodness-of-fit test to data from the bee experiment*

Disc colour	Yellow	Red	Blue	Sum
Observed (O) frequencies	47	38	15	100
Expected (E) frequencies	33.33	33.33	33.33	99.99
(O − E)	13.67	4.67	−18.33	
(O − E)^2/E	5.6066	0.6543	10.0807	**16.3416**

We can use the bee experiment to illustrate some additional criteria for the correct use of the goodness-of-fit test:

> **Observed frequencies originate from independent trials**. This is why we need to make sure each bee moves alone in the experimental space, without the presence of other bees. If we allow all 100 bees to enter the space together and then count the number of bees sitting on each disc, the (possibly significant) deviation from our null hypothesis might be caused by the aggregative behaviour of the bees. In addition to testing bees separately, we must also make sure that the bees do not mark the disc in some way (for example by a chemical compound) that would affect subsequent bees. One possible solution is to replace the three discs for each individual bee.
>
> **The sample size is fixed before the experiment starts**. An approach unfortunately used by some researchers, whereby they increase the sample size after they find that the differences for the first say 100 bees are not significant, is incorrect. This is because we have seriously inflated the Type I error probability by repeatedly testing H$_0$ using a gradually extending sample.

Another issue which arises when we do not adequately fulfil the test requirements is the interpretability of our results. In our example experiment, we must make sure that the effect of colour is not confounded – for example with an effect of some light gradient. If the yellow disc is always nearest to a window in our experimental space, the preference for that disc may not be due to its yellow colour, but due to the effect of light from the window. To prevent this or other spatially structured artefacts, it is advisable to repeatedly randomise the order of discs during the trial.

In our next example we leave behind field research for a while, moving instead to the experimental garden of Gregor Johann Mendel, a nineteenth-century monk who initiated the ideas behind the laws of Mendelian inheritance. He studied the heritability of plant traits using pea plants by employing a hybridisation approach. In our example we focus on two traits: the shape of peas (round vs. wrinkled) and their colour (green vs. yellow). Here a round shape and yellow colour are considered the dominant forms of each trait. We followed the properties of seeds from 250 plants in our experiment, expecting the ratio between the frequencies of the four possible trait combinations in F2 generation to be 9:3:3:1 for round/yellow, wrinkled/yellow, round/green and wrinkled/green seeds, respectively. So this ratio (with corresponding probabilities 0.5625, 0.1875, 0.1875, 0.0625, respectively) represents our null hypothesis. Among the 250 plants in our experiment, the observed frequencies were 126, 55, 60, 9. We can calculate the expected frequencies by multiplying the above probabilities with the total sample size ($n = 250$), and we obtain the following values (rounded): 140.625, 46.875, 46.875, 15.625. Using Eq. (2.1), we calculate the value of the χ^2 statistic as 9.413 and because the critical value $\chi^2_{0.05,3}$ is 7.815, we reject the null hypothesis at $\alpha = 0.05$.

Surely we could also test other proportions for our data (e.g. 4:2:2:1), but there are no theoretical grounds justifying this choice. On the contrary, the ratio 9:3:3:1 follows from a logical extension of the standard Mendelian ratio of 3:1 between dominant and recessive forms of a trait, after we combine two independent traits. Obviously, the formulation of a null hypothesis is – similar to the experimental design – affected not only by statistical principles, but primarily by our understanding of the research topic. Whereas rejecting the null hypothesis about the 9:3:3:1 ratio is a good foundation of further research investigating e.g. whether individual genotypes have a different viability, or whether some alleles are mutually dependent, the rejection of a null hypothesis about the 4:2:2:1 ratio is simply useless.

The null hypothesis is given in mathematical terms – in the examples above we use probabilities or expected frequencies. All other considerations about the experiment or its results are non-statistical ones. In our bee experiment, we can undoubtedly claim that when we reject the null hypothesis that the probability of landing is independent of disc colour, the bees must be able to distinguish colours. Nevertheless, a hypothesis that 'bees do not distinguish colours' is not a null hypothesis of a statistical test.

2.3 Null Models with Parameters Estimated from the Data: Testing Hardy–Weinberg Equilibrium

In all of the previous examples, the null models were stated *a priori* and were thus completely independent of the data used in the test. However, there are occasions when a part of the data is used for the formulation of the null model; testing the Hardy–Weinberg equilibrium in population genetics is a typical example. When we test whether an observed population is in a Hardy–Weinberg equilibrium we use the goodness-of-fit test, but in the context whereby the collected data are used to calculate the frequencies expected under the assumptions of Hardy–Weinberg equilibrium.

The model of Hardy–Weinberg equilibrium focuses (in its bare minimum presented here) on the frequency of genotypes in a population of diploid organisms classified by their allele combination for a particular gene locus. Each locus has two alleles, labelled A and a, with their relative frequencies in the population being p and q, respectively. If a population is in a Hardy–Weinberg equilibrium, the proportion of the two alleles does not change (much) across generations and the proportion of genotypes is p^2, $2pq$, q^2 for, respectively, the AA, Aa, aa genotypes. To estimate the genotype frequencies, we must first estimate p (the estimate of q is then $1 - p$) as (2 times the observed count of AA genotypes + the count of Aa genotypes)/ (2 times the count of all specimens). Then we proceed as we would in a standard goodness-of-fit test, but instead of comparing our test statistic with a χ^2 distribution with two degrees of freedom, we compare it against a χ^2 distribution with just one degree of freedom, because we estimated the parameter p of the null model (the model representing the null hypothesis) from the collected data. In general, the degrees of freedom for null models where we estimated d parameters of the model from the data are calculated as $df = k - d - 1$.

2.4 Sample Size

The goodness-of-fit test is only approximate in its assumption that the test statistic comes from a χ^2 distribution if the null hypothesis is correct. The approximation is very good if our sample is large: it is recommended that none of the expected frequencies is smaller than 1 and no more than 20% of the frequencies are smaller than 5. If this does not apply to our data then it is advisable to pool categories with low frequencies if possible (i.e. if it makes sense).

2.5 Critical Values and Significance Level

Most statistical tests can be characterised by the following general procedure. We first calculate a **test statistic** (for example the χ^2 statistic in the goodness-of-fit test). We know the distribution a particular test statistic should have if the null hypothesis is correct and the test assumptions are met. For example, we know that the χ^2 test statistic calculated using Eq. (2.1) comes from a particular distribution with a known distribution function (if the null hypothesis generating the expected frequencies is correct). This distribution is given the same name as the test statistic (χ^2). This is a distribution of continuous variables but our test statistic is calculated from counts of cases, so it is obviously a discrete entity. This is why a sufficient sample size is important, as its large value limits the extent of 'discontinuity' of the test statistic's distribution. The χ^2 distribution belongs to a set of distributions referred to as sampling distributions and so its shape is affected by the data properties, expressed here by the degrees of freedom. We can calculate the 95% (or 0.95) quantile of this and similar distributions.

By definition, a 95% quantile is a value that a random variable exceeds with probability 0.05. For our goodness-of-fit test and the χ^2 distribution, the 95% quantile is therefore the critical value at a 5% significance level (i.e. at $\alpha = 0.05$). At the same time we know that the value of the χ^2 test statistic increases when the deviation of our data from the expectations of the null hypothesis also increases (this is a general property of most test statistics).

If the value of the test statistic calculated for our data exceeds the critical value at the 5% significance level, we can say that if the null hypothesis is correct, then the probability of obtaining data that deviates this much (or even more) from the H_0 expectation is less than 5%.

Statistical programs display test results that not only show the value of the test statistics, but also a probability value, most often called *Probability* or just *P* or *p*, and sometimes also the *achieved significance level*. This probability can be calculated as 1 − the value of the distribution function for the test statistic value, so this is the same as an integral of the probability density function from the test statistic value up to $+\infty$. We can see this probability as the grey area in the graph of the probability density function in Fig. 2.1, covering the extreme area ('tail') under the density function curve. This area represents the probability that a sample drawn from the population will deviate from the expectations based on our null hypothesis to the same extent[2] as (or even more than) the sample we have actually obtained. This probability is the *p*-value. If this *p*-value is smaller than the *a priori* chosen α (usually with a value of 0.05), the difference is significant at $\alpha = 0.05$.

---

[2] The extent of this deviation from the expectations of the null hypothesis is measured by the value of our test statistic.

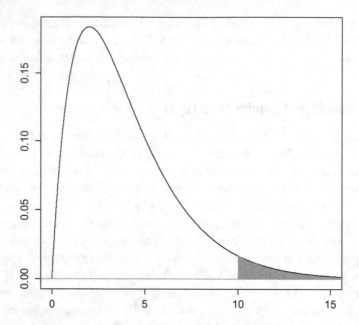

Figure 2.1 Probability density function for a χ^2 distribution with four degrees of freedom. The full area below the curve is equal to 1, the size of the grey area corresponds to the probability that the variable (test statistic) plotted on the horizontal axis will have a value greater than 10.0. If our test produces a test statistic value equal to 10.0, the grey area then represents the achieved significance level of the test (here $p = 0.0404$).

In research papers we most often present the results of statistical testing in the following way (using the goodness-of-fit test in the bee experiment example, detailed in Table 2.2 above): *The observed frequencies of bees landing on certain colours of disc* (47:38:15) *deviated significantly from the expectation of showing no preference* ($\chi^2_2 = 16.34$, $p < 0.05$). As the achieved significance level was much lower ($p = 0.00028$) than the *a priori* chosen α, we can either use a lower α-value (like $p < 0.001$) or even specify the achieved significance level ($p = 0.00028$) directly, as discussed below.

We recommend the reader takes the following advice into account when presenting the results of statistical tests. We use the letter α for an *a priori* chosen significance level (above which we are not prepared to reject the null hypothesis), so we can for example report that 'the test is significant at $\alpha = 0.05$'. In contrast, we use P (or p) for the achieved significance level, so that in the same context as before, we would write '$p < 0.05$'. If your statistical software reports that $p = 0$ (or, more often, something like $p = 0.0000$), this only means that the achieved (positive) significance level value is smaller than the display precision adopted by that software. If this happens then you should not report in your papers that $p = 0$, but rather something like $p < 10^{-4}$. However, we usually report the actual significance value unless it is too low. When we report, for example, that $p = 0.049$, this gives an indication to our readers that we found the difference to be significant at the 5% level, but barely so. Similarly, by reporting that $p = 0.052$, we suggest that we cannot reject the null hypothesis, but that we missed the target 'by just a small margin'. The significance level is a most valuable piece of information and therefore we recommend taking this approach when reporting the results of any statistical test (see also Section 2.8).

In the dawn of hypothesis testing, the procedure which was strictly recommended was to first set the α-value and then – depending on the test outcome – give a clear conclusion:

rejecting or not rejecting the null hypothesis. Nowadays the prevailing approach is to present the significance level (p-value) and then use it to judge the reliability of our results. For most statistical tests performed on the results of field research, this is an entirely satisfactory approach – for example when we try to determine the sex ratio of bats in a cave system, we must be ready to accept some ambiguity. On the contrary, we must stick to the original procedure if we are, for instance, deciding whether to replace an old drug with a new one, based on a test comparing drug efficiencies in clinical trials. The pharmaceutical company involved in such research must decide how much risk it is prepared to bear and compare it with the outcome of the statistical test.

2.6 Too Good to Be True

We start with a fictitious example. Company X is producing a new type of chewing gum which has been blamed for causing increased mortality in consumer sperm cells bearing the Y chromosome (therefore daughters will prevail among their offspring). To dispel such accusations, the company hired a guy who spent two years of his life chewing their product intensively. After this exposure period, his sperm cells were examined using a sample of 10,000 cells. In the company's press release, they say that they found the Y chromosome in 5001 cells, while it was missing in 4999 cells. The company then concluded that this aligns sufficiently with the expected 1:1 ratio and so their chewing gum is entirely harmless. As statisticians, what can we say about the reported results?

Ignoring the fact that their experimental design is not particularly good (there is no control and the effects are measured on just a single individual), we can still try to evaluate the results using the χ^2 goodness-of-fit test. Comparing the observed and expected frequencies (5000 for both categories of sperm cells), we get $\chi^2_1 = 0.0004$, $p = 0.984$. So the difference from the null hypothesis is non-significant, but the achieved significance level approaches 1 (certainty). This is quite suspicious. It tells us that if the true ratio of the two cell types is indeed 1:1, the probability that we find a larger discrepancy in our cell counts than what we have observed is more than 98%. Or, in other words, observing this close a match across a sample of 10,000 cells is very improbable (less than 2% probability). So either the company had damn good luck with their experimental subject or, more likely, they falsified the experimental results to match their needs. We believe that their results are too good to be true.

This example is of course a fictitious one (no one tries to deceive their customers, right?). Nevertheless, it illustrates that statistical methodology can be used to spot falsified results. A similar case is very well known in the world of science: if we look at the results of the original experiments done by Gregor Mendel in the nineteenth century, we find that the agreement of the hypothesised ratios is 'too good', as pointed out in 1936 by the famous statistician R. A. Fisher. Gregor Mendel was operating without a knowledge of statistics. The principles of statistical testing were not known at that time, let alone the requirements for a goodness-of-fit statistical test. He never claimed to create a random, unbiased sample of observations – on the contrary, he wrote that when the sample was too small, he added new individuals.[3] This story is still popular in the statistical realm (see e.g. the Wikipedia article

---

[3] If you sequentially add new individuals, you can expect that the results will fluctuate around the true ratio, which in this case is 3:1. But if you stop adding new cases at the moment when the results are sufficiently close to your null hypothesis, then the agreement with this hypothesis will be much better than you can expect using a fixed sample size.

about Gregor Mendel) and nicely illustrates two points: (a) when publishing your results, be sure to describe how the data were collected in detail; and (b) when using historical data, do not assume they were collected with statistical principles in mind.

2.7 Bayesian Statistics: What is It?

Testing research hypotheses with the aid of rejectable null hypotheses forms the core methodology of classical inferential statistics. It has been widely applied in the field of natural sciences (and elsewhere) since the first half of the twentieth century. But this is not the only methodological framework supporting research involving statistical analyses. In the past 30 years, the use of **Bayesian statistics** has expanded widely into many research fields and now represents a viable alternative to classical statistics. In this section, we will briefly summarise this methodological framework and recommend a couple of introductory textbooks to the interested reader. Our book stays focused solely on the classical statistical framework, as it still dominates the territory of natural sciences.

While the core of classical inferential statistics is rooted in hypothesis testing (while parameter estimation and confidence intervals are often-neglected cousins), Bayesian statistics are centred around estimating parameters of statistical models.[4] While the population parameters (which we attempt to estimate) in classical statistics are always seen as constant yet unknown values, the Bayesian statistic accepts the possibility that such a parameter (we will call it θ) is a random variable. The primary outcome of a Bayesian analysis is a probability density function $P(\theta|\text{data})$, which describes how likely all possible values are for the statistical parameter θ based on the data sample we collected.

The Bayesian statistical framework represents a consistent methodology, which covers the same range of questions as the classical statistical framework, even surpassing it in the area of complex statistical modelling. Another advantage of the Bayesian framework is its ability to account for previous knowledge about the investigated parameters, based on the use of *priors* (see below).[5] The general framework of Bayesian statistics is usually introduced by a single formula representing the so-called Bayes' theorem. This theorem is closely related to a formula in probability theory, which does not involve parameters or data, but instead describes the relationship between probabilities of various events. The formula is given here:

$$P(A|B) = \frac{P(B|A).P(A)}{P(B)} \tag{2.2}$$

and its simplest description would say that the probability of event A happening under the condition that event B took place (conditional probability of A given B) is equal to a multiple[6]

---

[4] But this does not mean that you cannot test hypotheses with Bayesian statistics, as we mention later.

[5] This is also one of the aspects of classical statistics which sometimes comes under criticism – the answers to our research questions provided by statistical models are based solely on the data we have collected, while the information provided by earlier studies only comes into play in research papers during the discussion of the results (with the exception of so-called meta-analyses, not presented in this book).

[6] Note that the multiple in the numerator equals $P(A \text{ and } B)$, i.e. the probability that both events occur. Equation (2.2) therefore follows from the definition of conditional probability.

of the conditional probability of B given A and the (unconditional) probability of event A divided by the unconditional probability of event B.

But the P symbols do not need to refer to just single probability values (estimates), but also to probability density functions, leading us to Bayes' theorem in Bayesian statistics:

$$P(\theta|\text{data}) = \frac{P(\text{data}|\theta).P(\theta)}{P(\text{data})} \qquad (2.3)$$

In the above equation, θ is the parameter we're investigating, $P(\theta)$ represents our *a priori* idea about the probability of possible values for the parameter – i.e. the *prior* – and $P(\text{data}|\theta)$ is the likelihood function. The likelihood function describes the probability of observing the data for various possible values of parameter θ. The denominator value is of lesser interest,[7] but it ensures that the area under the probability density curve produced by the above equation (i.e. $P(\theta|\text{data})$) – usually called the **posterior probability of θ** – is equal to 1, as we are used to for density distribution functions (see Section 1.6.2). We do not need to have any *a priori* knowledge of the parameter we are studying (or we might not wish for our knowledge to affect the results) and in such a case, we can use what are known as *non-informative priors* which typically claim that all possible values of θ are equally probable.

We must also mention that the primary result of a Bayesian method – the posterior probability $P(\theta|\text{data})$ – can be used (among others) to construct the **Bayesian credible interval** of θ. If you imagine the posterior probability represented by a curve with a single peak (at the most likely or most frequently occurring value of the parameter θ), you can imagine (for example) the 95% credible interval covering the area around that peak, with a size of 0.95 (with the total area under the curve being 1.0). The resulting Bayesian credible interval might then present a path for testing hypotheses – see our comment about the equivalence of the coverage of a confidence interval for an average with a single-sample t test (see Section 5.5).

We will conclude our short excursion into Bayesian statistics with a practical view of its use in natural sciences. Generally, it is a mathematically elegant framework for statistical analysis of any type of research problem, powerful enough to match the standard methods of classical statistics and to provide solutions for new, unique problems that occasionally occur, particularly in quickly developing research fields (such as bioinformatics). The price to pay for its use is a learning curve probably even more steep than that of classical statistics.[8] Another fact to consider is that with non-informative priors and classical assumptions (e.g. with θ being a mean, the $P(\text{data}|\theta)$ function might be represented by a density distribution curve of normal distribution), the resulting estimates or credible intervals might be identical or very close to the estimates or confidence intervals of classical statistics. Beyond the simplest models, Bayesian data analysis is more computer-intensive, typically requiring Markov Chain Monte Carlo simulation for their estimation. These three aspects are, we feel, responsible for the rather slow uptake of Bayesian statistics among practicing researchers. Another factor might be the 'mass effect', i.e. the expectation that more readers will understand how you

---

[7] $P(\text{data})$ is computed as a mean value of the likelihood function $P(\text{data}|\theta)$ to standardise the numerator.
[8] If you would ever believe that is possible...

have analysed data in your paper if you present results of classical statistical methods rather than Bayesian statistics, but this context might change in future.

To readers wishing to learn more about the Bayesian framework, we would recommend either Kéry (2010) or (if you get on well with formal mathematical notation) Marin & Robert (2014), both providing practical examples in R statistical software.

2.8 The Dark Side of Significance Testing

Statistical hypothesis testing has provided natural and social sciences with an important research tool for more than 100 years. Its widespread use has, however, inevitably led to its misuse, often caused by mere ignorance, but sometimes resulting from less well-intentioned efforts. As the demonstration of novel patterns beyond that of known relationships between entities and processes became firmly interrelated with a presentation of 'significant' outcomes of statistical tests, researchers are placed under increasing pressure to present as many 'significant' test results as possible to ensure the success of their submitted manuscripts (and thus also of their careers).

It is no wonder that some statisticians started to express strong objections against the way the methodology of hypothesis testing is used, with the first voices heard in the second half of the twentieth century (Rozeboom, 1960). A powerful wave of dissatisfaction with the current state of affairs emerged more recently, however, and resulted in the publication of consensual views of the misuse of the statistical significance concept and of p-values, assembled by the professional organisation of American statisticians (Wasserstein & Lazar, 2016). This manifest was followed by a special issue of *The American Statistician* journal, in which statisticians elaborated their ideas on how to progress beyond the '$p < 0.05$' era (Wasserstein et al., 2019).

This critical view originates chiefly from two areas: misinterpreting the meaning of the p-value, and an overly narrow focus on the null hypothesis and its rejection/non-rejection. We handle these two areas in the following two subsections.

2.8.1 Misinterpretation of p-Values

Estimated p-values are often thought to measure the correctness of null hypotheses, or even (in a negatively proportional relationship) the correctness of alternative (research) hypotheses. But this is an overly simplistic way of interpreting Type I error probability. The best way to look at the estimated p-value is as a measure of the incompatibility between the dataset we have collected and the stated null hypothesis, but only when the underlying assumptions of the method estimating the p-value are fulfilled (Wasserstein & Lazar, 2016). This means that a blind rejection of the null hypothesis whenever we arrive at $p < 0.05$ – without paying attention to method assumptions, the quality of our dataset[9] or the findings of other researchers in earlier studies – is clearly an ignorant use of the hypothesis testing approach.

We can learn more about the deceptive nature of p-values by using a little piece of Bayesian methodology (see Section 2.7). We start by assuming that our *a priori* expectations

---

[9] Which includes not just its size, but also its general representativeness for the sampled population.

about the correctness of the null (H_0) and alternative (H_A) hypotheses have the same strength. When we then collect a dataset in a way to reflect our research questions, and if the test of H_0 against the data leads to a significant p-value ($p < \alpha$), we can re-evaluate the probability of the alternative hypothesis (i.e. we estimate its posterior probability).[10] We hope that this posterior probability of H_A will be high, because our p-value for the test was below say 0.05. But surprisingly, for a test yielding $p = 0.05$, the posterior probability of H_A is at most 0.71[11] and for $p = 0.01$ at most 0.89. This is also why Benjamin & Berger (2019) recommended labelling only test results with $p < 0.005$ as 'significant', and calling the outcomes with p-values between 0.005 and 0.05 simply 'suggestive'. It should also be noted that the 1-complement of the posterior probability of H_A (e.g. 0.29 for $p = 0.05$ when the prior probabilities were 0.5 for both H_0 and H_A) is an estimate of how probable it is that the claimed effect (i.e. a claim of H_A validity) is incorrect. This probability is also called the *false positive risk* (FPR), see Colquhoun (2019).

We must stress, however, that our *a priori* expectations about the correctness of null and alternative hypotheses usually do not have the same strength. Most of the time we carry out our experiments after we are confident enough about the merits of the alternative (research) hypothesis, so our trust in the null hypothesis is quite low. Consequently, the probability of false positive risk would be lower than suggested in the preceding paragraph. We design our experiments to confirm our expectation that the treatment will have an effect. For example, we carry out a removal experiment (removing neighbouring individuals around the focal ones) to examine the existence of competitive (negative) or facilitative (positive) effects. We seldom believe that there are no effects among the individuals, which would be the claim of our null hypothesis. We are thus not using p-values for ourselves, but instead just as a way of communicating the results to the readers of our papers (and before this, to the reviewers and editors). By presenting the low p-value we are simply saying – you can trust these results, the probability that such results can be obtained by chance is very low. Similarly, in observational studies, we often design our sampling plan to confirm some of our subjective, non-quantitative, superficial observations.

The p-values are also often erroneously used to measure the importance or size of the studied effects. But this is generally incorrect, as for a particular effect size its significance grows (p-value decreases) when we increase the sample size.

2.8.2 Too Much Attention on p-Values

A related problem, and one that occurs all too frequently, is the excessive simplification of how we deal with hypothesis tests and statistical models underlying the hypotheses. The statistical significance is (partly due to the commonsense meaning of the word 'significance') directly interpreted as scientifically important. But if we are to correctly attribute importance to our findings, then we must judge much more than the p-value. Can we really radically change our judgement when we obtain $p = 0.049$ instead of $p = 0.051$? In our research reports we must fully disclose not only the questions we are addressing, but also our sampling design

---

[10] This is done with the help of the Bayesian factor (*BF*) representing the ratio between the likelihood of the observed data under the alternative hypothesis (H_A) and the likelihood of the same data under the null hypothesis (H_0).

[11] This is based on estimating the upper bound of the Bayesian factor (*BFB*) as $1.0/(-e\ p\ \ln(p))$ and then using it to estimate the upper limit of the conditional probability $Pr(H_A|p) = BFB/(1 + BFB)$, see Benjamin & Berger (2019).

(allowing the reader to judge the representativeness of our data) and the statistical procedures in sufficient detail for their full reproduction by the interested reader. While this looks like the usual demand of any decent research journal, in reality many authors tend to filter their descriptions to sweep less successful aspects of their study under the carpet.

If our study is not the first one to address a particular question, we must also appropriately discuss the results of other authors, as they can provide better estimates of prior probabilities for the hypotheses we are testing and suggest what a biologically reasonable size of the studied effects might be. Thorough quantification and a research-related discussion of effect size, rather than its mere testing, are other aspects of scientific investigation which are not sufficiently covered by the present-day applications of statistics. Ideally, we should estimate the minimum size of a biologically important effect before collecting our data, and use it when interpreting the importance of our findings.

2.8.3 Suggested Solutions

These criticisms of current practice are mostly agreed upon by statisticians, yet the way this practice must be (or, more practically, can be) changed brings controversies among the critics. Some authors suggest that the word 'significant' or 'non-significant', when speaking about the outcomes of statistical tests, should be completely banned (using the estimated p-values on a continuous scale just as we do with any number of important characteristics coming from our studies; see Wasserstein et al., 2019), but most authors also agree that binary decisions for our tested hypotheses cannot be completely abandoned in specific situations (Wasserstein et al., 2019).

We have already mentioned the importance of stating a minimum meaningful effect size. Further, when the estimated effects are tested against their null hypothesis value (typically 0 for the parameters of statistical models), we should also compare those estimates against the meaningful minimum effect values. The estimated effect sizes should be presented as interval estimates (typically producing confidence intervals, see Section 5.5) and we should discuss the biological implications of both estimated interval boundaries. As a matter of fact, these approaches have already been put forward. For example, Steidl & Thomas (2001) have argued that we should distinguish statistically and biologically significant results on the basis of comparing the range of the estimated confidence interval with the minimum meaningful ecological effect. Whereas we consider this approach highly relevant, even after many years we do not see it being generally adopted by researchers. One of the reasons probably lies in the subjectivity of assessment – what is a minimum biologically meaningful effect? In applied studies (e.g. agricultural research), the effects of fertilisers or pesticides on the final yield can be considered meaningful if the profit exceeds the expenses, so we can reliably estimate it. On the contrary, determining a biologically meaningful increase in the biomass of an individual after some addition of nutrients or after removal of its competitors can be hotly debated, and the determination of such limits might need an independent study.

Another important suggestion concerns researchers' openness. We should report all of the tests we performed on the data, rather than 'cherry-picking' the results which achieved low p-values. Although this might seem like a simple, straightforward suggestion, we believe that many researchers will struggle to keep within such a rule on a voluntary basis. Moreover, the feasibility of such an approach will depend on substantial changes in editorial policies in research journals.

In conclusion, we advise our readers to remember that the classical hypothesis testing has its own limits and should not be carried out in a mechanical, mindless way. Reporting the actual *p*-values rather than just relating them to 0.05 (or any other level) is certainly a move in the right direction. But as a tool to communicate your results to readers, deeply rooted in the present-day scientific methodology, classical hypothesis testing will dominate in empirical research journals for many years to come.

2.9 Example Data

All data for this chapter are in the *Chap2* sheet of the example data file. We will illustrate the standard goodness-of-fit test with two examples. The first one was already described above and concerns the genetic experiment of the round vs. wrinkled and yellow vs. green peas. The observed frequencies for each of the four trait combinations are in the *Observed* column, while the expected counts are already calculated in the *Expected* column.

The second example also refers to a genetic experiment: in the first filial (F1) generation of a cross between *AA* and *aa* diploid individuals, we expect that all of the individuals will be of the dominant allele (*A*) phenotype. Among 2000 offspring, we observed three with a recessive phenotype. Does the observed result differ from the expected? Observed frequencies are present in the *Obs_ind* column (with values 1997 and 3); expected ones (2000 and 0) are in the *Exp_ind* column.

To illustrate how we might use the goodness-of-fit test for testing Hardy–Weinberg equilibrium, we will use the following example. In a population of diploid mammals, we found 15 individuals of the genotype *AA*, 20 individuals of the genotype *Aa* and 77 individuals of the genotype *aa*. Is the population in a Hardy–Weinberg equilibrium? The observed counts of individuals are in the *Individuals* column, while the expected counts (their calculation is illustrated in a separate sheet named *Chap2-HW*) are in the *Exp_indiv* column.

2.10 How to Proceed in R

We recommend that you import each pair of columns (representing individual examples) as a separate data frame in R (e.g. *chap2.a*, *chap2.b*, *chap2.c*), as these pairs of variables differ in the number of rows. As a matter of fact, we will be ignoring the second variable in each frame, because in R software, our expectations (implied by the null hypothesis) are specified not as expected frequencies, but rather as the probabilities for individual categories.

We will handle the test for the first example as follows (the first command just displays the contents of the *Observed* variable):

```
chap2.a$Observed
[1] 126 55 60 9
```

```
with( chap2.a, chisq.test( Observed, p=c(9,3,3,1)/16))
        Chi-squared test for given probabilities
data: Observed
X-squared = 9.4133, df = 3, p-value = 0.02427
```

We will analyse the second example in a similar way:

```
chap2.b$Obs_ind
[1] 1997 3
```

```
with( chap2.b, chisq.test( Obs_ind, p=c(1,0)))
        Chi-squared test for given probabilities
data: Obs_ind
X-squared = Inf, df = 1, p-value < 2.2e-16
...
```

Note that dividing by the expected frequency of the recessive phenotypes, which in this case is equal to 0, wreaks havoc with the application of the χ^2 statistic formula, so the test statistic value is estimated as infinitely large and hence infinitely improbable (and it is therefore shown as the smallest positive value R is able to display, namely 2.2×10^{-16}). In simpler terms, given that the probability of observing recessive phenotypes is set to 0, we can reject the null hypothesis as soon as we observe even a single individual with a recessive phenotype, and so nobody would really perform the above test.

While we stated at the start of this section that expected frequencies cannot be submitted to the *chisq.test* function, this is not entirely true. You can pass them as a vector to the *p* parameter, but then you must specify an additional argument, namely *rescale. p = TRUE*, which standardises the *p*-values so that they sum up to 1.0.

Finally, we will illustrate how to analyse the example testing the Hardy–Weinberg equilibrium of the mammal population. This time we will use the *rescale.p* parameter and also store the test result as a variable. We store the test result like this so that the value of the test statistic can be used later and also so that the incorrect *p*-value (based on the χ^2 distribution with two degrees of freedom) is not shown:

```
hw <- with( chap2.c, chisq.test( Individuals, p=Exp_indiv,
                                  rescale.p=T))
hw$statistic
X-squared
  26.3543
```

We need to subtract one from the count of degrees of freedom implied by the three categories we are comparing, so we need to compare with a χ^2 distribution with $df = 1$:

```
pchisq( hw$statistic, df=1, lower.tail=F)
   X-squared
 2.841857e-07
```

Instead of calculating the 1-complement from the distribution function value, we used the *lower.tail* argument with its non-default value *FALSE* in order to obtain the upper tail area probability.

If we need to calculate the corresponding critical value for a known probability, we can use the *qchisq* function (here we pass the more 'natural' 0.95 value to the distribution function, but we also illustrate the alternative use of 0.05 and the *lower.tail* = *F*) in the alternative command:

```
qchisq( 0.95, df=5)
[1] 11.0705

qchisq( 0.05, df=5, lower.tail=F)
[1] 11.0705
```

Similar pairs of functions also exist for the other types of distribution, such as the normal distribution (functions *pnorm* and *qnorm*), *t* distribution (*pt* and *qt*) or *F* distribution (*pf* and *qf*), but the required parameters for them differ (e.g. the normal distribution is not a sampling distribution, so does not use *df*, but it is parameterised by its mean and standard deviation).

2.11 Reporting Analyses

Here we provide examples of how to report our analyses using the pea appearance example (with analyses using the *chap2.a* data frame in Section 2.10).

2.11.1 Methods

The difference between the observed frequency of the four phenotypes and the expected 9:3:3:1 ratio was tested using a goodness-of-fit test based on the χ^2 statistic.

2.11.2 Results

The frequencies of the four phenotypes differed significantly ($\chi^2_3 = 9.41, p = 0.0243$) from the expected ratio.

(As authors, we would likely expand on this statement by describing which categories are more frequent, and which are less frequent, compared with the null model.)

2.12 Recommended Reading

Zar (2010), pp. 74–85 (testing hypotheses), pp. 466–489 (goodness-of-fit test).

Quinn & Keough (2002), pp. 32–57 (testing hypotheses) and p. 381 (goodness-of-fit test).

Sokal & Rohlf (2012), pp. 119–131 (testing hypotheses), pp. 703–738 (goodness-of-fit test).

D. J. Benjamin & J. O. Berger (2019) Three recommendations for improving the use of *p*-values. *The American Statistician*, **73**(S1): 186–191.

D. Colquhoun (2019) The false positive risk: a proposal concerning what to do about *p*-values. *The American Statistician*, **73**(S1): 192–201.

M. Kéry (2010) *Introduction to WinBUGS for Ecologists. A Bayesian Approach to Regression, ANOVA, Mixed Models and Related Analyses*. Academic Press, Amsterdam, 302 pp.

J. M. Marin & C. P. Robert (2014) *Bayesian Essentials with R*, 2nd edn. Springer, New York, 296 pp.

W. M. Rozeboom (1960) The fallacy of the null-hypothesis significance test. *Psychological Bulletin*, **57**: 416–428.

R. J. Steidl & L. Thomas (2001) Power analysis and experimental design, in S. M. Scheiner & J. Gurevitch (eds), *Design and Analysis of Ecological Experiments*, 2nd edn. Oxford University Press, Oxford, pp. 14–36.

R. L. Wasserstein & N. A. Lazar (2016) The ASA's statement p-values: context, process, and purpose. *The American Statistician*, **70**: 129–133.

R. L. Wasserstein, A. L. Schirm & N. A. Lazar (2019) Moving to a world beyond '$p < 0.05$'. *The American Statistician*, **73**(S1): 1–19.

3 Contingency Tables

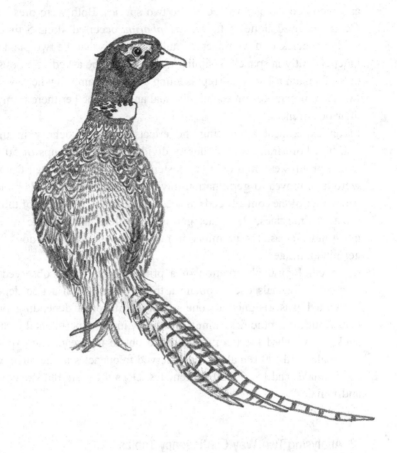

Contingency tables are a useful tool to summarise the relationship between two or more categorical variables (i.e. variables measured on a nominal scale). Most of the time we will focus on the relationship between two variables, leading to two-way contingency tables. We will therefore begin with these.

3.1 Two-Way Contingency Tables

3.1.1 Use Case Examples

1. The occurrence of a moth species under various management regimes in temperate grasslands was investigated on 45 experimental sites known to host healthy moth populations in the past: 15 sites are mown in summer; 15 sites are mown in autumn; 15 sites are abandoned meadows. The moth species was present in: 12 sites mown in summer; 13 sites mown in autumn; 6 sites where mowing has ceased. Does the presence of the moth differ across sites under different management regimes? Or, more precisely, can we reject the null

hypothesis that the probability of the moth species persisting in a site does not depend on the management regime?

2. The spatial separation of two plant species (*Carex rostrata* and *Eriophorum angustifolium*) was investigated across a site. We placed 100 plots of identical size at random positions and recorded the occurrence of the two species. Both were present together in 45 plots, *Carex* occurred alone 15 times, *Eriophorum* occurred alone 5 times, while 35 plots had neither species. Can we reject the null hypothesis that the two plant species are distributed independently in space? A similar question may be asked of an observation of n individuals of a mammal species (representing a random sample) where we record the presence of two taxa of parasites on each individual and ask whether there is any relationship between their occurrences.

3. In an experiment simulating the effects of endozoochory in the field, a sample of 100 hawthorn fruits was randomly divided into two groups of 50 fruits each. The fruits in one group were then fed to a rooster and the seeds collected from his excrement. These were then moved to germination trays, together with the seeds removed from the control fruits. Out of the control seeds, 8 seeds germinated, while out of those passing through the rooster's intestines, 28 seeds germinated. Does the passage of seeds through animal intestines increase the germination rate? Or, more precisely, does the passage change the germination rate?

4. In an ethological observation of a primate species, we observed whether the strategy primate individuals use to obtain a treat hanging from a tree depends on gender. Each individual was assigned to one of three categories depending on its problem-solving behaviour during the first minute of its stay in the experimental area: (a) used an available stick; (b) climbed the tree; (c) failed to obtain the treat. The experiment was done with 100 males and 100 females. The observed frequencies in the three categories were 32, 43, 25 for males and 15, 65, 20 for females. Does the preferred strategy differ between males and females?

3.1.2 Analysing Two-Way Contingency Tables

We will illustrate the general procedure using example 4 above. One of the two categorical variables (also called *factors*) has two categories (primate gender), while the other has three (problem-solving strategy). We will first illustrate the general symbols used for a 2×3 two-way contingency table in Table 3.1.

Here we assigned the two-level factor to the rows, but the actual assignment of rows and columns is an entirely arbitrary choice and does not affect the results.

Table 3.1 *Symbols used for a 2 × 3 contingency table*

		Factor 2			
		Category 1	Category 2	Category 3	Row sums
Factor 1	**Category 1**	f_{11}	f_{12}	f_{13}	R_1
	Category 2	f_{21}	f_{22}	f_{23}	R_2
	Column sums	C_1	C_2	C_3	n

Table 3.2 *The observed frequencies in the primate behavioural experiment with row and column totals*

		Solution			
		Stick	Tree	Failed	Row sums
Gender	Male	32	43	25	100
	Female	15	65	20	100
	Column sums	47	108	45	200

The number of rows is usually denoted by r and the number of columns by c; f_{ij} is the observed frequency of events (or individuals) in the i-th row and the j-th column, representing therefore the count of cases belonging to the i-th class in the first classification (i-th level of the first factor) and at the same time to the j-th class in the second classification (j-th level of the second factor). The sums of frequencies for individual classes are marked as R_i or C_j, depending on the factor's assignment to rows or columns. These sums are often called *marginal frequencies*. The total number of independent observations in the sample is n.

The observed frequencies and related summary statistics for example 4's data are given in Table 3.2.

The expected frequencies for contingency tables are calculated from the marginal frequencies for individual factor categories. We can estimate the probability that an individual (individual in our dataset, but more typically a case) will belong to category i of the first factor as $P_{i+} = R_i/n$. Similarly, the probability of an individual belonging to category j of the second factor can be estimated for our data as $P_{+j} = C_j/n$. Now, if we assume that the two factors are independent (the probability of belonging to a category of the first factor does not depend on the case's membership in categories of the second factor), we can use a basic rule of probability theory, where the probability of a joint occurrence of two independent events is the multiple of their independently estimated probabilities, i.e. $P_{ij} = P_{i+}P_{+j}$. The expected frequency is then estimated as the co-occurrence probability multiplied by sample size:

$$\hat{f}_{ij} = P_{ij}n = \frac{R_i C_j}{n} \tag{3.1}$$

The χ^2 test statistic is calculated in the same way as we have seen for a standard goodness-of-fit test introduced in Chapter 2 (Eq. (2.1)). Given the fact that we look at the observed and expected frequencies spread across multiple rows and columns of a two-way contingency table, we can rewrite the formula (without changing its meaning) in the following way:

$$\chi^2 = \sum_{i=1}^{r} \sum_{j=1}^{c} \frac{\left(f_{ij} - \hat{f}_{ij}\right)^2}{\hat{f}_{ij}} \tag{3.2}$$

This χ^2 statistic is often called Pearson's χ^2 (or even Pearson's X^2) statistic in this context. If the assumptions of the χ^2 test are met and the null hypothesis is correct, then the test statistic value comes from a χ^2 distribution with $(r - 1)(c - 1)$ degrees of freedom.

Example 3.1 Evaluating the contingency table from example 4 using a classical χ^2 test.

The results of the behavioural experiment 4 (Section 3.1.1) are summarised in Table 3.2. Using Eq. (3.1), we can calculate the expected frequencies for individual row and column combinations, with the results shown in the following table:

		Solution		
		Stick	Tree	Failed
Gender	Male	23.5	54.0	22.5
	Female	23.5	54.0	22.5

Null and alternative hypotheses for the statistical population characterised by our data are:

H_0: Success rate and problem-solving strategy are not dependent on gender.

H_A: Success rate and problem-solving strategy depend on individual's gender.

Now we apply the formula for the χ^2 statistic as given by Eq. (3.2):

$$(32 - 23.5)^2/23.5 + (43 - 54.0)^2/54.0 + (25 - 22.5)^2/22.5 + (15 - 23.5)^2/$$
$$23.5 + (65 - 54.0)^2/54.0 + (20 - 22.5)^2/$$
$$22.5 = 3.074 + 2.241 + 0.278 + 3.074 + 2.241 + 0.278 = \mathbf{11.186}$$

$$DF = (r - 1)(c - 1) = (2 - 1)(3 - 1) = 2, \ p = 0.0037$$

So we reject H_0.

3.1.3 Correction for Continuity

Some authors recommend continuity correction if the expected frequencies are low. This is a concern for any use of the χ^2 statistic, and also when we analyse contingency tables. The distribution of the standard χ^2 statistic is only approximately described by the χ^2 distribution (when the null hypothesis is true and the test requirements are fulfilled). This is because the χ^2 distribution is derived for continuous random variables,[1] while we are using discrete counts here. If we use high count values or we sum over many categories, the approximation is quite good, but not so for small sample sizes.

The general formula (directly comparable to Eq. (2.1)), with a so-called **Yates correction**, looks as follows:

$$\chi^2 = \sum_{i=1}^{k} \frac{\left(|f_i - \hat{f}_i| - 0.5\right)^2}{\hat{f}_i} \tag{3.3}$$

---

[1] Actually, the sums of squares of random variables with a normal distribution are assumed to have a χ^2 distribution.

This test statistic leads to a very conservative test. This means that the real Type I error probability is actually lower than the set α, and as a consequence the correction inflates the Type II error probability. The Yates correction is worth considering if any of the expected frequencies are lower than 5, but the authors of statistical textbooks tend to have different views regarding its use.

3.1.4 G Test

Instead of the classical χ^2 goodness-of-fit test, we can use an alternative G test (also known as the log-likelihood ratio test) to test the same type of hypothesis. Although the test statistic is based on different assumptions and consequently its formula is different from a standard χ^2 statistic, the G statistic is also assumed to come from a χ^2 distribution when the null hypothesis is correct. The following formula is appropriate when using natural logarithms (i.e. logarithms to the base e):

$$G = 2 \left(\sum_i \sum_j f_{ij} \ln f_{ij} - \sum_i R_i \ln R_i - \sum_j C_j \ln C_j + n \ln n \right) \qquad (3.4)$$

When we decide to use the decadic (base-10) logarithms, the appropriate formula is as follows:

$$G = 4.60517 \left(\sum_i \sum_j f_{ij} \log f_{ij} - \sum_i R_i \log R_i - \sum_j C_j \log C_j + n \log n \right) \qquad (3.5)$$

The study of primate behaviour in example 4 is analysed in Example 3.2 below. We can see that we obtain results quite similar to those using a standard χ^2 test.

Example 3.2 Evaluating the contingency table from example 4 using a G test.

The results of the behavioural experiment 4 (Section 3.1.1) are summarised in Table 3.2, including row and column totals.

The null and alternative hypotheses for the statistical population characterised by our data are:

H_0: Success rate and problem-solving strategy are not dependent on gender.
H_A: Success rate and problem-solving strategy depend on an individual's gender.

Now we apply the formula for the G statistic as given by Eq. (3.5):

$G = 4.60517 \times [32 \times 1.50515 + 43 \times 1.63347 + 25 \times 1.39794 + \ldots + 20 \times 1.30103 - (100 \times 2.0 + 100 \times 2.0) - (47 \times 1.6721 + 108 \times 2.0334 + 45 \times 1.65321) + 200 \times 2.30103] = 4.60517 \times [2.46685] = \mathbf{11.360}$

$$DF = 2, p = 0.0034$$

We therefore reject the null hypothesis.

3.1.5 Two-By-Two Tables

The simplest possible example of a two-way contingency table is a 2×2 table, which can be used for our examples 2 and 3 (Section 3.1.1). The general formula from Eq. (3.2) can then be simplified into an alternative formula used to conveniently compute the χ^2 statistic:

$$\chi^2 = \frac{n(f_{11}f_{22} - f_{12}f_{21})^2}{C_1 C_2 R_1 R_2} \tag{3.6}$$

Many statistical textbooks use different, more traditional symbols for 2×2 tables, namely a, b, c, d instead of $f_{11}, f_{12}, f_{21}, f_{22}$ and m, n, r, s for the marginal frequencies C_1, C_2, R_1, R_2. The χ^2 statistic computed for a 2×2 contingency table is compared with the χ^2 distribution with one degree of freedom. Its test of independence is therefore most affected by the non-continuous nature of the frequencies, particularly if (some of) the expected frequencies are low. But for a 2×2 table, it is possible to use the **Fisher's exact test**, which is based on combinatorics, allowing one to compute the exact probabilities of getting 2×2 tables with the same or larger deviation than the table in question (with particular a, b, c, d values) has, if the null hypothesis is correct.

3.2 Measures of Association Strength

So far, we have tested the null hypothesis of independence between two categorical variables, with the test either rejecting the null hypothesis or not. But we might also be interested in the strength of the relationship between two categorical variables. We will illustrate the difference between these two questions by taking an example evaluating interspecies relationships with a 2×2 contingency table. The sampling design used to collect the data will be similar to that described for example 2 (spatial separation of two plant species; Section 3.1.1). But here, we will work with different sample sizes. First (as shown in Table 3.3) we will work with a hypothetical sample of 1300 plots in which we have recorded the presence of two plant species. We will then compare our results with another study, where just 130 plots were used (see Table 3.4).

The χ^2 statistic calculated for this table has a value of 23.11 and so $p < 0.0001$. We can therefore clearly reject the null hypothesis. The expected frequency of shared occurrence is $300 \times 300/1300 = 69.23$. However, the two species occur together in 100 plots, and thus more frequently than we would expect if there is no dependency among their occurrences. We therefore characterise their dependency as a **positive association**. Similarly, when a count of joint occurrence is lower than expected under the null hypothesis, we would call this a **negative association**. It is probably useful to remind our readers that a positive association

Table 3.3 *Results of a hypothetical study recording the presence of two species in a set of 1300 plots*

		Species 1		
		Present	Absent	Sum
Species 2	**Present**	100	200	**300**
	Absent	200	800	**1000**
	Sum	**300**	**1000**	**1300**

Table 3.4 *Results of a hypothetical study recording the presence of two species in a set of 130 plots*

		Species 1		
		Present	Absent	Sum
Species 2	Present	10	20	30
	Absent	20	80	100
	Sum	30	100	130

does not necessarily imply an active positive effect of one species on the other – this will be discussed later in Section 3.4.

We now compare the above table with one where data were collected from just 130 plots (Table 3.4).

This table has identical relative frequencies as Table 3.3, but the total sample size is 10 times lower. The value of the test statistic ($\chi^2 = 2.311$) is therefore also 10 times smaller and with a corresponding $p = 0.128$ we can't reject the null hypothesis. But both tables could easily be obtained from a study of the same species in the same area,[2] and differ only in their sampling effort. The size of the χ^2 test statistic (and thus the significance level) obviously changes with the total sample size (n), even when the intensity of the relationship between two variables stays identical. This is quite reasonable: the more observations we have, the smaller the probability that the same relative deviation from the expected frequencies can be reached by chance. And the more observations we have, the stronger the evidence against the null hypothesis.[3] This again illustrates that the power of a test increases with the number of observations.

But the value of the χ^2 statistic tells us nothing of the intensity (and even less of the direction) of an association between pairs of species. For this we must use a statistic that does not change its value when the number of observations (n) changes but the relative deviation from randomness stays the same. As is often the case, multiple statistics of association have been proposed, and these have been quite popular in studies of 'species associations' (e.g. in example 2 at the start of this chapter).

One group of such statistics is based on the ratio $f_{11}.f_{22}/f_{21}.f_{12}$. This ratio is sometimes called Y. If $f_{11}.f_{22} > f_{21}.f_{12}$ the relationship between the categorical variables (usually representing species occurrences) is positive, while if $f_{11}.f_{22} < f_{21}.f_{12}$ the relationship is negative. The most often used coefficient (which is a function of Y) is the Q coefficient, also known as the Yule coefficient of association, calculated as

$$Q = \frac{f_{11}f_{22} - f_{21}f_{12}}{f_{11}f_{22} + f_{21}f_{12}} \tag{3.7}$$

The Q coefficient value varies from -1 to $+1$. For our two example tables (Tables 3.3 and 3.4 above), the value of Q is identical, namely $+0.333$.

---

[2] Although it is extremely unlikely to obtain exactly the same proportions from repeated samplings in a real-world study.

[3] For Table 3.4 the expected number of joint occurrences is 6.9. There is quite a high chance that we might observe 10 joint occurrences instead of the expected 6.9. But the probability that we observe – by chance – 100 joint occurrences instead of 69 is nearly zero.

An alternative coefficient is V, again with its possible values ranging from -1 to $+1$ and calculated as

$$V = \frac{(f_{11}f_{22} - f_{12}f_{21})}{\sqrt{C_1 C_2 R_1 R_2}} \tag{3.8}$$

If you compare the formula in Eq. (3.8) with the computational formula in Eq. (3.6), you can see that the value of V is actually

$$V = \sqrt{\frac{\chi^2}{n}} \tag{3.9}$$

together with the addition of a sign indicating direction (i.e. '+' for a positive association and '−' for a negative association). In this context, the V coefficient is also sometimes denoted using the Greek letter ϕ ('phi'), and is sometimes called the point correlation coefficient. Even the coefficient V has identical values for both Tables 3.3 and 3.4, namely $+0.1333$. This V coefficient is, in fact, a special case of Cramér's V, which does not have a sign (varies from 0 to +1) but can be applied as an association measure for contingency tables larger than the 2×2 tables.

3.3 Multidimensional Contingency Tables

Sometimes we need to study the relationships between more than two categorical variables. As an example, we want to study the relationship between two species, but across multiple years. In this way, we obtain a table (or rather a rectangular cuboid) as illustrated in Fig. 3.1.

The following null hypothesis is central for this type of contingency table: *The three investigated categorical variables are mutually independent*. This means that the frequency of

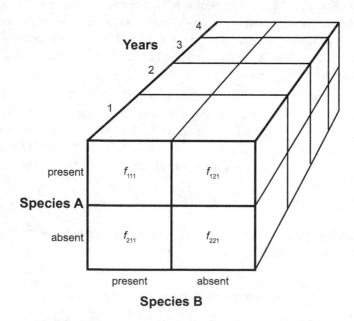

Figure 3.1 Example of a three-dimensional contingency table recording (co-)occurrence of two species across four years.

neither species changes with years, and the two species are mutually independent. The expected frequencies (implied by the null hypothesis) can be calculated as an n-multiple of the probability of joint co-occurrence of three independent events, namely

$$\hat{f}_{ijl} = P_i P_j P_l n = R_i C_j T_l / n^2 \tag{3.10}$$

where R_i is the total number of units with level i in the first variable (e.g. the first species), C_j is the number of units with level j in the second variable (e.g. the second species) and T_l is the number of units with level l in the third variable (e.g. in the year l). For instance, the expected value of f_{111} (number of plots in the first year of observation, containing both species 1 and 2) can be calculated as a multiple of the count of plots sampled in the first year, the total count of plots that contained species 1 and the total count of plots that contained species 2, divided by the second power of the total count of plots followed across all the years.

But we can also test different – more specific – hypotheses, such as an assumption that the frequency of both species changes with time, but the two species are mutually independent.

Besides the first-order interactions (involving pairs of categorical variables), we can also expect interactions of higher orders. In our example, such an interaction would describe a situation where the two studied species were statistically mutually dependent, but the strength of the relationship changed with time (perhaps even beginning as a positive relationship before becoming negative towards the end of the observation period). To test such complex hypotheses, we can use what are known as **log-linear models** (see Agresti, 2007), which represent a specific type of generalised linear model (see Section 15.5). A log-linear model describes the structure of dependency among units. We try to find a model which is as simple as possible, but sufficiently describes the observed data. The name 'log-linear model' comes from the fact that we must carry out a log-transformation: the dependency shown in the latter part of Eq. (3.10) can be expressed on a logarithmic scale as

$$\log \hat{f}_{ijl} = \log R_i + \log C_j + \log T_l - 2 \log n \tag{3.11}$$

In practice, we proceed by testing the data against a null hypothesis implied by the simplest model of Eq. (3.11): if we cannot reject this model, we cannot demonstrate any dependency among the categorical variables. If we can reject the model of total independency then we can start to gradually test more complex models. In the end, we accept and interpret the simplest of the models that we failed to reject (in favour of a more complex model). There are various strategies for selecting the simplest possible model when comparing multiple categorical variables.

3.4 Statistical and Causal Relationship

As the example problems listed in Section 3.1.1 demonstrate, two-way contingency tables (but also multidimensional tables) can be used to study dependency among categorical variables, whether we manipulate one of the variables with the aim of demonstrating its effect upon the other categorical variable or whether all data come from an observational study with no parts of the system being manipulated. Even in the latter case, we still assume that one of the variables might be the *cause* and the other the *consequence*. But we can also study the relationship between two categorical variables of similar standing (e.g. the relationship between the occurrence of two species). While the computational procedure and results of statistical testing can be identical in different scenarios, the way we interpret the results can differ substantially.

Let us take an example. We compare the study from example 3 (feeding hawthorn seeds to a rooster; Section 3.1.1) with another, seemingly very similar one. In the original example 3, we had 100 hawthorn seeds and half of them were selected for passage through the rooster's intestines, while the other half were left as control seeds. Germination success characterised the outcome of the experiment. In our alternative study we collected 50 hawthorn seeds in the field that were lying under shrubs and obviously not eaten, while the other 50 seeds were collected from the excrement of pheasants, for which they are a natural food.

What is the take-home message we get from the significant test results in these two experiments (i.e. demonstrating a significant relationship between seed passage through intestines and seed germinability)? In the original example the results came from a manipulative experiment: the 50 seeds that passed through the rooster's guts were selected randomly from an original pool of 100 seeds. If the germination rate differs between the two groups of seed, the only possible **cause** can be the passage through the rooster's intestines (how well a single rooster kept in captivity can represent the passage through pheasants' guts in nature is of course a matter for discussion in that study's report).

In the other study, the seeds left lying under the hawthorn shrubs by the pheasants may not be a random selection from the statistical population of all available seeds. On the contrary, we might reasonably expect that well-ripened fruits will be much more attractive to the pheasants, while underdeveloped fruits will fall to the ground and not receive much attention. It is therefore likely that the two groups of seeds differed even before the effect of the pheasants' guts could act upon one of them. Therefore, if we get a statistically significant result from this alternative study, we can conclude that the germinability of seeds found in excrement differs from the germinability of seeds from non-eaten fruits, but the hypothesis about the direct effect of the passage through intestines is just one of many possible explanations.

This example well illustrates the importance of manipulative experiments – in which the experimenter intentionally manipulates the value of one (or more) of the variables and follows the induced changes in other variable(s). This is the only way we can prove a causal relationship. In contrast, joint occurrence of two attributes of the same objects (here the germinability and the passage through the pheasants' intestines) only demonstrates a statistical dependency, which may or may not reflect a causal relationship. Very often the two variables are affected by a third variable which was not observed in the study (a **confounding variable**). In the study of spatial dependence of two species (our example 2), the two species (*Eriophorum angustifolium* and *Carex rostrata*) are not in a mutualistic relationship, but both respond concordantly to variation in soil moisture – both are found in wetter places. Finding the correct setup for a manipulative experiment is often challenging, particularly in field research where often unwieldy spatial and/or temporal scales are involved. So the matter of proving a causal relationship and its distinctiveness from a mere statistical dependency is a contentious issue in many research projects.

3.5 Visualising Contingency Tables

The simplest way to visualise the contents of a contingency table is by a **mosaic plot**. This is made by splitting an area of constant size into blocks which match the relative group sizes of the levels of categorical variables defining the table. This is illustrated by a mosaic plot in Fig. 3.2. The primate gender is represented by the two rows of the plot and as the same number of males and females were participating in the experiment, both rows have an identical height. But each row is also split into three blocks representing the three categories of problem-solving method (or not solving, for the *failed* category). The width of the blocks matches the proportional frequencies for the three categories within each gender. We can clearly see that females showed a strong preference for climbing the tree, and also had a lower failure rate than males. The mosaic plot can be created not only for two-way contingency tables, but also with multiple categorical variables. But with an increasing count of variables, it becomes more difficult to grasp the pattern and to judge the relative importance of individual deviations from a null model.

The deviations from the null model of independency among categorical variables can be plotted more directly (as so-called Pearson residuals, see Section 3.7 for their definition), as illustrated in Fig. 3.3. This time the graph can represent both positive and negative deviations of observed counts from frequencies expected by the null model by using the relative position of the bars to a dotted zero line. The height of each bar is proportional to the relative contribution of each deviation to the final χ^2 test statistic. This graph nicely identifies the use of the stick as the choice most distinguishing males and females, closely followed by the tree-climbing category.

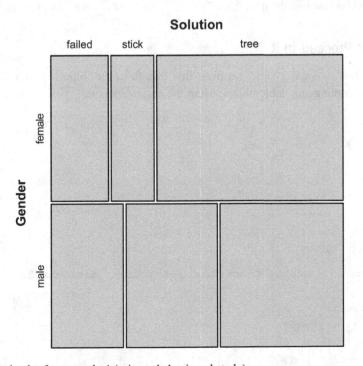

Figure 3.2 Mosaic plot for example 4 (primate behavioural study).

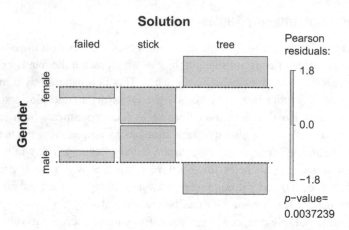

Figure 3.3 Association plot for example 4 (primate behavioural study), plotting the Pearson's residuals based on the null hypothesis expectations.

3.6 Example Data

The analysis of contingency tables will be demonstrated using example 4 (see Examples 3.1 and 3.2 above). The data are stored in the *Chap3* sheet of the spreadsheet file with examples. Data are not arranged into a two-dimensional table but have a linear arrangement, with the assignment of rows and columns in the desired contingency table determined by the values of two categorical variables (*Gender* and *Solution*). The counts of cases for individual combinations of gender and problem-solving are coded in the *Count* column. To illustrate the work with 2 × 2 tables, we use the data from Table 3.3, but they are not stored in the spreadsheet.

3.7 How to Proceed in R

To calculate the classical χ^2 test, we must first transform the imported data frame (named *chap3*) into a contingency table object, using the *xtabs* function:

```
chap3
    Gender   Solution   Count
1    male       stick       32
2  female       stick       15
3    male        tree       43
4  female        tree       65
5    male      failed       25
6  female      failed       20

> chap3.tab <- xtabs( Count~Gender+Solution, data=chap3)
> chap3.tab
          Solution
Gender    failed    stick    tree
  female      20       15      65
  male        25       32      43
```

The χ^2 test is then performed by the *chisq.test* function:

```
sol.chisq <- chisq.test( chap3.tab)
sol.chisq
        Pearson's Chi-squared test
data: chap3.tab
X-squared = 11.186, df = 2, p-value = 0.003724
```

The object returned by the *chisq.test* function (e.g. *sol.chisq* in our example above) contains additional information. We can, for example, check the residual values:

```
sol.chisq$residuals
        Solution
Gender     failed        stick        tree
female -0.5270463 -1.7534161   1.4969104
  male  0.5270463  1.7534161  -1.4969104
```

These are so-called **Pearson residuals**, i.e. the values $(O_i - E_i)/\sqrt{E_i}$, where O_i is the observed frequency in the i-th cell, while E_i is the expected frequency of the same cell. In this scaling, the sum of squared residuals is equal to the test statistic, i.e. to 11.186 in our example. The Yates correction is performed by the *chisq.test* function for 2×2 tables only (it is performed by default in this event). We may block it, however, by adding an optional parameter *correct = FALSE*.

The *chisq.test* function also offers an alternative test of the hypothesis regarding the independence of categorical variables by way of a Monte Carlo simulation (see Section 7.4 for another example of simulation testing). This approach is similar in some respects to Fisher's exact test, but does not obtain exact probabilities of the Type I error, but rather performs a random selection of possible combinations. The result becomes more precise with an increasing number of random trials (parameter *B*). For 1000 trials we get

```
chisq.test( chap3.tab, simulate.p.value=T, B=1000)
    Pearson's Chi-squared test with simulated p-value
    (based on 1000 replicates)
data: chap3.tab
X-squared = 11.186, df = NA, p-value = 0.002997
```

When we repeat the function call with 1 million trials, we get a different estimate:

```
chisq.test( chap3.tab, simulate.p.value=T, B=1000000)
    Pearson's Chi-squared test with simulated p-value
    (based on 1e+06 replicates)
data: chap3.tab
X-squared = 11.186, df = NA, p-value = 0.003852
```

Most importantly, we must remember that this is a Monte Carlo test, where a random subset of possible trials is chosen on each execution of the function. So the *p*-values you obtain from the above commands will almost certainly differ on your computer (to a small extent). This can be demonstrated by repeating the same function call with the same parameters as before:

```
chisq.test( chap3.tab, simulate.p.value=T, B=1000000)
    Pearson's Chi-squared test with simulated p-value
  (based on 1e+06 replicates)
data: chap3.tab
X-squared = 11.186, df = NA, p-value = 0.003806
```

We are well aware that the uncertainty in the answers provided by statistical software can sometimes undermine a user's trust in it. However, we should recall that we are estimating a probability by selecting a random subset of the possible assignments of trials into table cells, and when we use a random sampling in any other context (such as measuring the height of 10 shrubs to estimate their mean height) we also tend to get different answers.

To calculate the *G* test, it is best to use a log-linear model for a contingency table, i.e. a generalised linear model with assumed Poisson distribution (see Chapter 15 for additional information). We first estimate ('fit') a model of complete independence between the two categorical variables:

```
chap3.glm0 <- glm( Count~Gender+Solution, data=chap3,
                     family=poisson)
```

We then estimate an alternative model with an added interaction between the two factors. The interaction is marked by a colon (':') in the model formula:

```
chap3.glm <- update( chap3.glm0, .~.+Gender:Solution)
```

Finally, we compare these two models using the χ^2 (actually *G*) statistic:

```
anova( chap3.glm0, chap3.glm, test="Chisq")
Analysis of Deviance Table
Model 1: Count ~ Gender + Solution
Model 2: Count ~ Gender + Solution + Gender:Solution
  Resid. Df Resid. Dev Df Deviance Pr(>Chi)
1         2      11.36
2         0       0.00  2    11.36 0.003413 **
```

Please note the variation in terminology used in the table above. Here the χ^2 test statistic is labelled *Deviance* (and *Df* labels the degrees of freedom), while the χ^2 statistic is referred to directly in the achieved significance level (*Pr(>Chi)*).

Contingency tables can also be created directly by using the *rbind* function (or using the *cbind* function, as these two differ in direction only, whereby numeric vectors are grouped by either rows or columns). The following commands use this procedure in combination with the *chisq.test* function and they also illustrate the selective use of the Yates correction:

```
tab3.3 <- rbind( c( 100, 200), c( 200, 800))
tab3.3
     [ ,1] [ ,2]
[ 1,]  100  200
[ 2,]  200  800
```

```
chisq.test( tab3.3, correct=F)
    Pearson's Chi-squared test
data: tab3.3
X-squared = 23.111, df = 1, p-value = 1.529e-06
```

```
chisq.test( tab3.3, correct=T)
    Pearson's Chi-squared test with Yates' continuity correction
data: tab3.3
X-squared = 22.366, df = 1, p-value = 2.253e-06
```

Fisher's exact test is available in the *fisher.test* function and we illustrate its use on the 2×2 table we have created above:

```
fisher.test( tab3.3)
    Fisher's Exact Test for Count Data
data: tab3.3
p-value = 3.514e-06
alternative hypothesis: true odds ratio is not equal to 1
95 percent confidence interval:
 1.484557 2.684159
sample estimates:
odds ratio
  1.998839
```

But this function can also be used for tables larger than 2×2, as illustrated by our earlier example:

```
fisher.test( chap3.tab)
    Fisher's Exact Test for Count Data
data: chap3.tab
p-value = 0.003766
alternative hypothesis: two.sided
```

The usability of the *fisher.test* function depends on the size of the table: this includes not only the number of rows and columns, but also the size of frequency values in the table cells.

Cramér's V coefficient of association is available for contingency tables in the package *vcd* (Friendly & Meyer, 2015), with the function *assocstats*. Incidentally, this function also computes the classical Pearson's χ^2 test and the likelihood-based test, as seen in its output below:

```
library( vcd)
assocstats( tab3.3)
                      X^2 df    P(> X^2)
Likelihood Ratio 21.817  1 2.9986e-06
Pearson          23.111  1 1.5290e-06

Phi-Coefficient    : 0.133
Contingency Coeff.: 0.132
Cramer's V         : 0.133
```

The *vcd* package also provides support for the most frequently used methods of visualising the relationship between categorical variables – the mosaic plots and the association plots introduced in Section 3.5. The mosaic plot in Fig. 3.2 was created by the following call to the *mosaic* function:

```
mosaic( ~Gender+Solution, data=chap3.tab)
```

while the association plot in Fig. 3.3 was created using the *assoc* function as follows:

```
assoc( chap3.tab, shade=T)
```

3.8 Reporting Analyses

3.8.1 Methods

The dependency between the problem-solving strategy and ape gender was tested using Pearson's χ^2 test for contingency tables

    or

    The dependency between two factors was tested using a likelihood ratio test (using a log-linear model).

3.8.2 Results

The method of problem-solving and failure rates differed between males and females ($\chi^2_2 = 11.186$, $p = 0.0037$). Residuals of the contingency table model suggest there is little difference between both genders in their failure rate, but males prefer to use a stick, while females prefer to climb up the tree.

3.9 Recommended Reading

Zar (2010), pp. 490–517.
Quinn & Keough (2002), pp. 381–393 (contingency tables) and pp. 393–400 (log-linear models).
Sokal & Rohlf (2012), pp. 739–773.
A. Agresti (2007) *An Introduction to Categorical Data Analysis*, 2nd edn. Wiley, Hoboken, NJ.
M. Friendly & D. Meyer (2015) *Discrete Analysis with R: Visualization and Modeling Techniques for Categorical and Count Data*. Chapman & Hall/CRC, Boca Raton, FL, 562 pp.

4 Normal Distribution

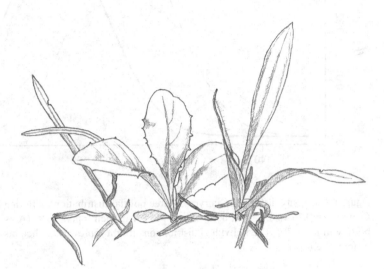

4.1 Main Properties of a Normal Distribution

With this chapter we start to focus on quantitative data. In statistical methods, a **normal distribution** (sometimes also called a Gaussian distribution) is the most frequently considered distribution type when describing the values of a quantitative random variable. As we explain below, the normal distribution has an exceptional position among the range of distributions available to us. In theory, the normal distribution is only applicable to data on an interval scale, but in practice we happily use it for continuous data on a ratio scale (if the variable's mean is at least several standard deviation units above zero), and sometimes even for discrete data types when there is a reasonably high number of distinct discrete values.

The probability density function of a normal distribution is described by a symmetrical, bell-shaped curve (see e.g. Fig. 4.1) and its values can be calculated using the following formula:

$$f(x) = \frac{1}{\sigma\sqrt{2\pi}} \cdot e^{\frac{-(x-\mu)^2}{2\sigma^2}} \tag{4.1}$$

This function contains two constant values: π and e (the latter is referred to as Euler's number, which is also the base of natural logarithms) and two normal distribution parameters: μ and σ.[1]

---

[1] Beware that there is some imprecision in our use of these two symbols, as we use them with two partly different meanings: here we use them as two parameters of the normal distribution, but we also use them elsewhere as the statistical population's parameters of the mean (μ) and standard deviation (σ), whether the corresponding variable has a normal distribution or not.

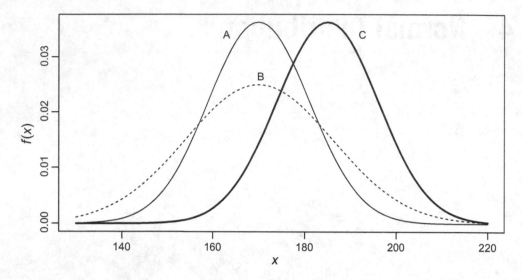

Figure 4.1 Density distribution curves of three normal distributions differing in their μ parameter (A vs. C, with $\mu = 170$ vs. $\mu = 185$, both with $\sigma = 11$) or in their σ parameter (A vs. B, with $\sigma = 11$ vs. $\sigma = 16$, both with $\mu = 170$). The individual distributions might represent the heights of people from three different regions.

It is possible to demonstrate that μ is the mean value and σ^2 is the variance of a random variable with a normal distribution. More specifically, we can use the function $f(x)$ from Eq. (4.1) to calculate the population mean as given in Eq. (1.16) and the population variance as given in Eq. (1.17).

The role of both parameters (μ and σ^2) is shown in Fig. 4.1, where the parameters are varied to produce different density distribution curves. Parameter μ determines the bell curve's position along the scale of x-values, while the σ parameter determines the perceived 'width' of a bell-shaped curve.

The exceptional standing of the normal distribution within the field of statistical analysis follows, to some extent, from the *central limit theorem*. While this theorem has a wider scope, it also implies that the mean value of a 'very large' random sample is a random variable with an approximately normal distribution. This is true even when the sampled statistical population has a distribution other than the normal distribution.[2]

4.2 Skewness and Kurtosis

As we have seen in Chapter 1, *variance* (which is the average value of the squared deviations from the mean) is a measure of data variation.[3] The mean value of the third powers of deviations from the mean (i.e. third central moment, κ_3) is a measure of distribution **skewness**.

---

[2] From this it follows that a violation of assumed normality is a more acute problem for small samples than for larger samples.

[3] More generally, the average value of the i-th powers of the deviations from the mean is called the i-th central moment, often labelled κ_i (using the Greek letter 'kappa'); the variance is therefore κ_2, the second central moment.

The sum of the (plain) differences from the mean is (by definition) equal to zero. Let us imagine a set of values in which a single large positive deviation is compensated by several negative deviations of a lesser extent. The third power of the large positive deviation is a positive value of a greater extent, while the third powers of the small negative deviations are still negative, yet their extent is negligible compared with that of the large positive deviation. The corresponding distribution is **positively skewed**, and a complementarily shaped distribution is **negatively skewed** (see subplots B and C in Fig. 1.1). The values of the κ_3 statistic are in cubed units (if we measure our variable e.g. in cm, then κ_3 is in cm^3). The value of κ_3 also changes with the overall data variability and with the chosen units: if we change our measurement e.g. from metres to centimetres, the value of κ_3 increases 10^6 times. We therefore use an alternative parameter of skewness γ_1, with the κ_3 value divided by the third power of the standard deviation, i.e. $\gamma_1 = \kappa_3/\sigma^3$. The γ_1 parameter is dimensionless and simply reflects the shape of the probability density function. All normal distributions have $\gamma_1 = \kappa_3 = 0$.

Apart from the symmetrical shape of the distribution curve, we can also explore how much the values are aggregated around the mean vs. spread in a way that makes the distribution flatter than a normal distribution. We describe this by the **kurtosis** of the distribution. A 'spiky' distribution is called *leptokurtic*, while a distribution which is too flat is *platykurtic*. A standard, normal distribution is *mesokurtic*. For a normal distribution, $\kappa_4/\sigma^4 = 3$, so that the standard measure of kurtosis has a value $\gamma_2 = \kappa_4/\sigma^4 - 3$. Consequently, leptokurtic distributions have $\gamma_2 > 0$, while platykurtic distributions have $\gamma_2 < 0$.

4.3 Standardised Normal Distribution

If a variable X has a normal distribution with parameters μ and σ^2 (we usually write this formally as $X \sim N(\mu, \sigma^2)$), then after a transformation

$$Z_i = \frac{X_i - \mu}{\sigma} \tag{4.2}$$

the variable Z has a normal distribution with mean equal to 0 and variance equal to 1 (so the standard deviation is also equal to 1). This is called the **standardised normal distribution** (or *standard score* or *normal deviate*). In the good old days, the standardisation of a general normal distribution was used to determine the probability that the observation values lie in a particular interval. This was the case because, back then, the values of the distribution function $F(x)$ for a standardised normal distribution were tabulated. Nowadays we can calculate these probabilities (or their complementary quantiles, matching the chosen probabilities) for a normal distribution with any parameters using statistical software.

But some quantiles of a standardised normal distribution are well known and frequently used. The values -1.96 and $+1.96$ are, respectively, the 2.5% and 97.5% quantiles of the $N(0, 1)$ distribution. This means that 95% of the population values lie between those values if a variable has a standardised normal distribution. These quantiles also lead to the often-advised decision to plot the arithmetic average $\pm$ two standard deviations to summarise a group of observations. If these statistics represent population parameters (although they are typically just sample estimates) for a normal distribution, approximately 95% of all observations would lie within this defined interval. It might also be useful to remember that in the range from -1 to $+1$ of a standardised normal distribution (or in the range of $\mu - \sigma, \mu + \sigma$

of a general normal distribution) lie approximately 68.2% of all observations, as those limits represent the 15.9% and 84.1% quantiles, respectively.

4.4 Verifying the Normality of a Data Distribution

Sometimes we need to determine whether the data in our sample were taken from a statistical population with a normal distribution. There are multiple alternative approaches for addressing this task, ranging from an inspection of descriptive graphs to formal statistical tests.

The following points introduce two graphical methods and three ways of testing the null hypothesis that the data are a random sample from a population characterised by a normal distribution.

1. The simplest way, and one which is often employed, is an inspection of the shape of a frequency histogram created from our data. We should focus primarily on the symmetry of our histogram. The sample-based histogram can be compared with a theoretical curve of the probability density function of a normal distribution with its mean and variance estimated from our sample. Such an enhanced histogram is illustrated in Fig. 4.2. The lack of correspondence between the bars and the curve suggests that the plotted data have certainly not come from a normal distribution. Moreover, the theoretical curve would imply that negative counts of seedlings should be relatively common, again showing how far the data are from normality.

2. Alternatively, we can draw a **normal probability plot**. We plot the variable values along the horizontal axis, while the relative fraction of cases smaller than the given value is plotted on the vertical axis. In this way, the points representing individual cases approximate a (cumulative) distribution function. But such a function has a sigmoidal shape for a normal distribution. Therefore, the fractions are often plotted on a *probability scale*, with the scale being gradually shrunk towards $p = 0.5$. As a consequence, the plotted points should – for a normal distribution – lie on a straight line, usually plotted as a reference guide in the graph. Possible deviations from normality are seen as a non-linear pattern of the points.

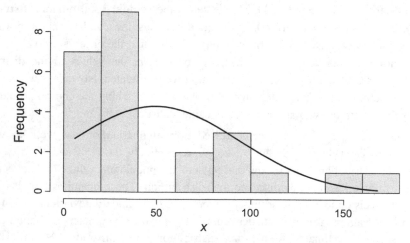

Figure 4.2 A frequency histogram using our example data (seedling counts in 24 plots), where the distribution across the count intervals is supplemented with the curve of a fitted normal distribution.

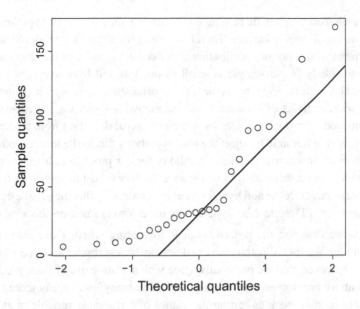

Figure 4.3 A normal probability plot for our example data (seedling counts in 24 plots).

Nowadays the preferred method is to use a **normal QQ (quantile–quantile) diagram**. It differs from a normal probability plot simply by the units which are employed, with the quantiles of a matching normal distribution plotted for individual observations on the vertical axis, which can then be compared with the observed values. This diagram is often plotted with the meaning of its axes swapped, as illustrated in Fig. 4.3. We must be aware that there is never perfect agreement with the reference line for a random sample, but the deviation of points from the line should not be too large or have a systematic pattern. So the information provided by Fig. 4.3 suggests that the distribution of the seedling counts is not very well described by a normal distribution.

3. We can evaluate how well our data fit a normal distribution using a χ^2 test of goodness-of-fit. We start by estimating the mean and variance from our data, and then use those estimates as the assumed parameters of a normal distribution. The range of observed values must be divided into a certain number of intervals (classes), with their count depending on the sample size (n). We can calculate the estimated observation frequency for a normal distribution for each interval, and compare these frequencies, using a goodness-of-fit test, with the real observation counts in the intervals. In this test, the number of degrees of freedom is equal to the *number of intervals* – 1 – *number of estimated parameters*, so for a normal distribution this is the *number of intervals* – 3.

4. The so-called **Kolmogorov–Smirnov test** allows us to compare our data with the normal distribution and focuses on the maximum difference between the observed and expected relative cumulative frequency of observations, using it to calculate a test statistic with a χ^2 distribution assuming the null hypothesis is correct (this hypothesis states that the sampled population has a particular distribution – here the normal one).

5. There is also the **Shapiro–Wilk test**, which specifically tests the normality and has a larger power than the Kolmogorov–Smirnov test.

6. Finally, we can calculate the skewness (γ_1) and/or kurtosis (γ_2) of our data and test whether the values differ significantly from 0.

We remind our readers that a non-significant outcome for a null hypothesis test is not proving that the hypothesis is correct. Therefore, when we obtain a non-significant result for a test of agreement with a normal distribution, this does not prove that our data have a normal distribution, particularly if our sample is small as our test will have very low power. When verifying normality before applying some of the parametric tests which assume a normal distribution (*t* tests, analysis of variance – see the following chapters), we encounter a rather paradoxical situation. For small samples (where the eventual deviation from a normal distribution is critical), we are not able to reject the null hypothesis due to the low test power, but this outcome gives us an unwarranted feeling of validity for our procedure. In contrast, with large samples (for which the *t* tests or analysis of variance are very robust to deviations from a normal distribution), we often reject the null hypothesis even for a small, often negligible deviation from the normal distribution. Despite this, some editors or reviewers insist on this kind of testing.

Below we describe the procedure in R for testing whether our data agree with a normal distribution. We then illustrate how to describe the test results in a research paper. This does not mean, however, that we personally agree with a routine use of these procedures. The reasons given above are not the only ones – in addition many users apply these tests in quite an inappropriate context, such as testing the values of a response variable in an analysis of variance (or linear regression or two-sample *t* test) for normality. It might be useful to compare the residuals of such models with a normal distribution, i.e. the variability left after subtracting the systematic effects described by the models. Regardless, it is more appropriate to focus on the unchanging extent of variability of those residuals, rather than on a precise distribution of their values. Additional information and practical hints can be found in Sections 8.8 and 10.1.

The χ^2 goodness-of-fit test and the Kolmogorov–Smirnov test can also be used to compare the distribution of data values with theoretical distributions other than a normal distribution.

4.5 Example Data

We assume that the height of university students follows a normal distribution with a mean value of 175 cm and a standard deviation of 14 cm. We ask: (a) How large is the fraction of all students with height greater than 190 cm? (b) How large is the fraction of students with height between 160 and 180 cm? (c) How many students, out of a group of 380, are expected to have height over 200 cm? (d) What range will be covered by the heights of the smallest 10% of students?

The data for seedling counts of grassland plants and plant litter cover in 24 experimental plots can be found in the *Chap4* sheet of the example data file (see Chapter 1 for a more detailed description). Compare the distribution of the values for our *Seedlings* variable with a normal distribution. If you find a large deviation, then try to compare the log-transformed values of this variable.

4.6 How to Proceed in R

4.6.1 Finding the Values of a Distribution Function and Quantiles

Like the examples in Chapter 2, here we will also use two functions for calculating the quantiles of a normal distribution and for calculating the cumulative probability of a normal variate value. Their names are *qnorm* and *pnorm*, respectively, and their first parameter gives the probability or normal variate value, while the following two parameters give the mean value and standard deviation of the reference normal distribution. With the help of these two functions, we can easily answer the above questions.

(a) About 14% of students will have height greater than 190 cm and consequently 86% will have height smaller than 190 cm:

```
1 - pnorm( 190, 175, 14)
```
```
[1]  0.1419884
```

(b) To answer the second question, we must first calculate the fraction of students with height up to 180 cm and then subtract the fraction of students with height up to 160 cm:

```
pnorm( 180, 175, 14) - pnorm( 160, 175, 14)
```
```
[1]  0.4975192
```

The proportion of students with height between 160 and 180 cm is therefore c. 49.8%.

(c) The solution is similar to that of question (a), but we must multiply the estimated probability of students with height above 200 cm by the size of the sample:

```
380 * (1 - pnorm( 200, 175, 14))
```
```
[1]  14.08765
```

The expected count of students taller than 200 cm is therefore 14.

(d) The shortest 10% of students will have height lower than the 0.10 quantile of the normal distribution under consideration, i.e. their height will be up to 157 cm:

```
qnorm( 0.10, 175, 14)
```
```
[1]  157.0583
```

4.6.2 Testing for an Agreement with a Normal Distribution

To visually compare a frequency histogram with a normal distribution, we can define and use the following function *hist.norm*:

```
hist.norm <- function( x, nbins=10)
{
  hist.x <- hist( x, breaks=nbins, col="light blue", main="")
  x.val <- seq( min(x), max(x), length=50)
  x.fit <- dnorm( x.val, mean=mean(x), sd=sqrt(var(x)))
  x.fit <- x.fit * diff( hist.x$mids[1:2]) * length( x)
  lines( x.val, x.fit, col="red", lwd=2)
}
hist.norm( chap4$Seedlings)
```

This function allows you to change the number of histogram intervals using the *nbins* parameter; other choices (curve smoothness and colours) are fixed. The resulting diagram is shown in Fig. 4.2.

A normal QQ plot can be created using the following two commands (diagram is shown in Fig. 4.3):

```
qqnorm( chap4$Seedlings)
qqline( chap4$Seedlings, distribution=qnorm, lwd=2)
```

The Pearson's χ^2 test can specifically compare your quantitative data with a normal distribution. The optional package *nortest* (not installed by default, you must install it explicitly in your R environment) offers the *pearson.test* function, which may be used as follows:

```
library( nortest)
pearson.test( chap4$Seedlings)
        Pearson chi-square normality test
data: chap4$Seedlings
P = 20.667, p-value = 0.0009363
```

It is slightly inconvenient that a function which calculates the test based on a χ^2 statistic does not display the degrees of freedom. But their value is calculated and can be obtained by extracting it directly from the function's return value:

```
pearson.test( chap4$Seedlings)$df
[1] 5
```

The *pearson.test* function automatically subtracts two degrees of freedom when estimating the mean and variance (the two parameters of the reference normal distribution, see Section 4.4).[4] So, based on the return value ($df = 5$), we can determine that the test was based on comparing observed and expected frequencies in eight intervals. The function unfortunately does not merge intervals with insufficient expected frequencies, but we can achieve this in an approximate way by selecting the number of intervals using the *n.classes* parameter:

```
pearson.test( chap4$Seedlings, n.classes=4)
        Pearson chi-square normality test
data: chap4$Seedlings
P = 4.3333, p-value = 0.03737
```

If you prefer to use the Kolmogorov–Smirnov test for comparing our data to a normal distribution, then it can be done as follows:

---

[4] You can use an optional parameter *adjust* = F in the function call if you do not wish to adjust the degrees of freedom when estimating the two parameters of the normal distribution.

```
with( chap4, ks.test( Seedlings, "pnorm", mean( Seedlings),
      sqrt( var( Seedlings))))

        One-sample Kolmogorov-Smirnov test
data: Seedlings
D = 0.26086, p-value = 0.06268
alternative hypothesis: two-sided
```

Another popular test is the Shapiro–Wilk test, which is available in the function *shapiro.test*:

```
shapiro.test( chap4$Seedlings)

        Shapiro-Wilk normality test
data: chap4$Seedlings
W = 0.8305, p-value = 0.0009702
```

Overall, our tests suggest (with a possible mild deviation of the Kolmogorov–Smirnov test) that the seedling count data do not come from a population with a normal distribution. For an alternative view, recall that the mean number of seedlings is 49.4 and the standard deviation is 44.4 (see Section 1.8). We can then find out that a corresponding normal distribution should have more than 13% of its values smaller than zero:

```
pnorm( 0, 49.4, 44.4)
[1] 0.1329374
```

This is clearly impossible for seedling counts. As such, this can be enough to suggest that it is not a good idea to approximate these data (in fact, any data on a ratio scale where mean and standard deviation are of a similar size) by the normal distribution. We will therefore check whether a log-transformation might increase the 'normality' of the distribution:

```
shapiro.test( log(chap4$Seedlings))

        Shapiro-Wilk normality test
data: log(chap4$Seedlings)
W = 0.96591, p-value = 0.5678
```

And apparently, it does! As none of the counts has a zero value, we can directly apply the *log* function to the variable. Often, however, count data contain zeros, and in that case the variable X must be transformed using $\log(X + 1)$.

4.7 Reporting Analyses

4.7.1 Methods

We tested the consistency of the distribution of observed seedling counts with a normal distribution using Pearson's χ^2 test with adjusted degrees of freedom (*or* using the Kolmogorov–Smirnov test; *or* using the Shapiro–Wilk test of normality).

4.7.2 Results

The distribution of the seedling counts was found to deviate significantly from a normal distribution ($\chi^2_1 = 4.33$, $p = 0.037$) and this discrepancy was fixed by log-transforming the variable values.

In case the deviation from a normal distribution is substantially reduced after applying log-transformation, but is still significant (particularly if we have a large sample, where such a deviation is not likely to matter), we can opt to use the following statement in the Methods section: 'Data were log-transformed to improve their normality.'

4.8 Recommended Reading

Zar (2010), pp. 66–96.
Quinn & Keough (2002), pp. 17–18.
Sokal & Rohlf (2012), pp. 93–117.

5 Student's *t* Distribution

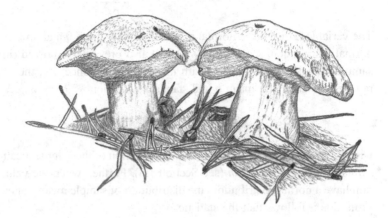

5.1 Use Case Examples

The following three example tasks represent the questions we will learn to address by the methods introduced in this chapter. Note, however, that we will continue with tests based on the *t* distribution in Chapter 6 also.

1. We know the concentration of the stable carbon isotope ^{13}C in air and we consider this concentration as a fixed value. We measure the concentration of ^{13}C in 10 experimental plants (this value is expected to differ among the plants). We can then ask whether the carbon isotope concentration in plants (its mean value) is identical to its concentration in air. If not, it may suggest that the plants discriminate among the various carbon isotopes when they fix carbon during the photosynthetic process.
2. To examine the effects of upper soil layer depth (composed mostly of dry needles) on the fructification of the mycorrhizal fungus *Suillus variegatus*, 10 pairs of 5 × 5 m plots were established in a pine forest. Within each pair, one plot was left non-manipulated (a control plot), while in the other plot the surface layer was removed up to a depth of 5 cm in autumn. Fructification was monitored on all 20 plots during the following two years. We ask whether there is a significant difference in the total count of sporocarps within the pairs of plots with different soil layer manipulations, i.e. presence or absence of the top 5 cm. This question can be reformulated to instead ask whether the average difference between plot pairings (when subtracting e.g. the count in a control plot from the count in a disturbed plot) is significantly different from zero.
3. We measured the concentration of lead (Pb) in the muscles of a common fish species across some chosen geographic area. We need to know an interval which includes, with a certain probability (usually 0.95), the unknown mean value of Pb concentration for all fish individuals of that species in the area.

5.2 *t* Distribution and its Relation to the Normal Distribution

We discussed in Chapter 4 that a variable X with a normal distribution, mean μ and variance σ^2_X can be transformed into a variable Z so that

$$Z = \frac{X - \mu}{\sigma_X} \tag{5.1}$$

The variable Z then has a normal distribution with mean 0 and unit variance (the standardised normal distribution, see Section 4.3). We also previously showed (in Section 1.4) that if we sample a statistical population with mean μ and variance σ^2_X, then the sample mean $\overline{X}$ is a random variable with mean μ and standard deviation[1]

$$\sigma_{\overline{X}} = \frac{\sigma_X}{\sqrt{n}} \tag{5.2}$$

where n is the sample size. The standard deviation of the sample mean is more often called the *standard error of the mean* (see Section 1.4). Further, when the values of a sampled population have a normal distribution, the distribution of sample means taken from it is also normal.[2] From this it follows that the statistic

$$Z = \frac{\overline{X} - \mu}{\sigma_{\overline{X}}} \tag{5.3}$$

has a standardised normal distribution. This could be used to test various hypotheses about the sample mean, such as whether an estimate of our sample mean differs significantly from a particular value. This is because, for a standardised normal distribution of Z, we can say what the probability of occurrence is for a given Z value. However, there is an issue with using the standardised normal distribution for such purposes. In the vast majority of cases we do not know the value of $\sigma_{\overline{X}}$, we only have its estimate $s_{\overline{X}}$, and this estimate is also subject to random variation.

So, a similarly computed statistic

$$t = \frac{\overline{X} - \mu}{s_{\overline{X}}} \tag{5.4}$$

follows a distribution different from the standardised normal distribution, namely the **t distribution** (also known as Student's *t* distribution),[3] which deviates (usually mildly) from the standardised normal distribution. Similar to a χ^2 distribution, it is a sampling distribution dependent on the degrees of freedom (here $df = n - 1$, where n is the sample size). The larger the sample, the more closely the t distribution resembles the normal distribution (see Fig. 5.1) – a standardised normal distribution corresponds to a t distribution with $df = \infty$.

---

[1] **Sampling a population of finite size**: in the field of natural sciences, our random sample is usually taken from a (potentially) infinite population of values, or this population is at least substantially larger than our sample. But if our sample represents a larger part of the sampled population (say at least 5%), then the mean estimate will be more precise than indicated by the formulas given in this section. There are formulas that estimate the standard error of the mean and correct for the finite nature of the sampled population, but they are seldom used.

[2] In fact, we can claim that the distribution of a sample mean is closer to a normal distribution than the distribution of the sampled statistical population (as a consequence of the *central limit theorem*, see Section 4.1).

[3] Student was the pseudonym of a statistician and chemist working in the Guinness brewery in Dublin, William S. Gosset, who described the *t* distribution.

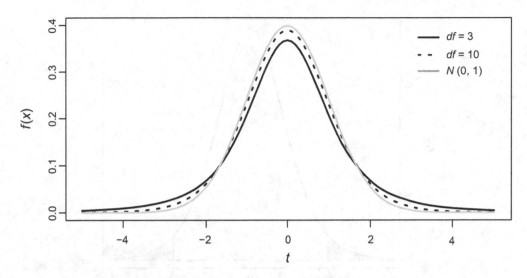

Figure 5.1 Probability density curves for two examples of a *t* distribution with varying degrees of freedom (*df*), together with a standardised normal distribution, $N(0, 1)$.

5.3 Single Sample Test and Paired *t* Test

The *t* distribution belongs to one of the most frequently used distributions in statistical practice. Its simplest use concerns the testing of hypotheses about a single sample: we can ask whether an estimated mean differs significantly from a particular theoretical (hypothetical) value. We can use our understanding of the *t* distribution in order to calculate its quantiles. The *t* distribution is always symmetrically spread around the zero value, which is therefore its mean. The probability that the value of a test statistic will be either smaller than a 2.5% quantile or larger than a 97.5% quantile of the matching *t* distribution is equal to 5% (see Fig. 5.2) – the usual α level for statistical tests.

As Fig. 5.2 shows, the 2.5% quantile is a negative value and the 97.5% quantile is a positive value, but their absolute values are identical (due to distribution symmetry around the zero point). We reject the null hypothesis at $\alpha = 0.05$ if the *t* statistic has a value smaller than the 2.5% quantile or larger than the 97.5% quantile. Alternatively, we may say that we reject the null hypothesis when $|t| > 97.5\%$ quantile. So the 97.5% quantile is the critical value for a **two-tailed test** at $\alpha = 0.05$ (at 5% significance level). More generally, we can say that the critical value for a two-tailed test at the significance level α is equal to the $((1 - \alpha/2) \times 100)\%$ quantile of the distribution. It is usually labelled as $t_{\alpha(2),df}$. The value '2' in the parentheses refers to using a two-tailed test; *df* represents the degrees of freedom. The use of the words 'two-tailed' (or 'two-sided') implies that we reject the null hypothesis if the value of the test statistic falls into one of the two extreme areas (tail areas) of the distribution curve (i.e. when the deviation from a null hypothesis can be in one of two opposite directions, see Fig. 5.2).

We will use example 1 from Section 5.1 to illustrate a single-sample (also called one-sample) *t* test. The concentration of the stable carbon isotope ^{13}C is given by the deviation of the observed $^{13}C/^{12}C$ ratio from the same ratio in a standard sample, and this measure is denoted by $\delta^{13}C$. In this example we will consider its value in air to be equal to -8 and unchanging (which is, for sure, a very simplistic view). We collected 10 plants of a particular

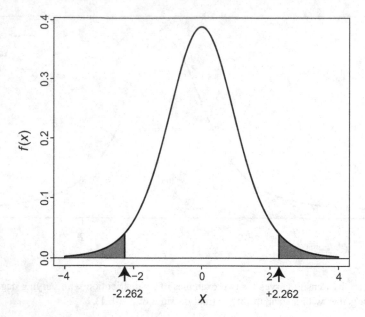

Figure 5.2 The probability density curve of a t_9 distribution, with the shaded parts representing the critical regions for a two-tailed (symmetrical) test with α set to 0.05; the critical value $t_{0.05(2),9}$ is shown with the associated positive and negative signs and represents the inner borders of the two shaded areas.

species (representing a random sample from all possible plants of that species in the area of interest) and we ask whether the mean $\delta^{13}C$ value in that species' biomass differs from the concentration in air (i.e. from -8). The null hypothesis can therefore be formulated as: The mean value (μ) of $\delta^{13}C$ in the biomass of our plant species is equal to the value of $\delta^{13}C$ in air (i.e. -8). In more general terms, we can write the null hypothesis as $H_0: \mu = \mu_0$ ($\mu_0 = -8$ for our example). The alternative hypothesis then states $H_A: \mu \neq \mu_0$. The value of the t statistic can be calculated using Eq. (5.4), with the μ value replaced by μ_0. The computation is illustrated in Example 5.1.

When presenting t test results these days, we usually do not compare our t statistic with a critical value, but we (or rather the software) compute how likely it is that we obtain a deviation from the null hypothesis so distant or even more distant from zero than the (absolute) value of the computed test statistic (i.e. 6.287 in our example). The probability computed in this way ($p = 0.000143$ in our example, see Example 5.1) is then the (achieved) significance of a two-sided t test (reported usually as p, P or *Probability* by statistical software). The transformation of the test statistic into the significance level p is further illustrated by Fig. 5.3.

One of the most frequent uses of this test is to compare two values measured on each of our subjects under investigation. Let's say, for example, that we want to demonstrate the effect of cross-pollination compared with self-pollination. We first select 30 individuals of an entomogamous flowering plant. On each plant, two flowers are selected – one as a control and in the other, we prevent insects from accessing the flower.[4] At the time of fruiting we

---

[4] In a real experiment we would have to check whether our method of preventing insects from pollinating our flowers does not have any other effect on the seed set and that self-pollination takes place.

Example 5.1 Two-sided *t* test of the agreement (significant difference) of a sample average with a hypothesised average of the sampled population ($\mu_0 = -8$).

The $\delta^{13}C$ values for 10 plants of the same species (representing C_4 plants with their specific type of photosynthesis) were $-10, -12, -13, -11, -15, -13, -16, -19, -11, -14$.

$H_0: \mu = -8$ $H_A: \mu \neq -8$ $\alpha = 0.05$

Estimated sample mean $\overline{X} = -13.4$

Estimated sample standard deviation $s_X = 2.716$

Standard error of the mean $s_{\overline{X}} = \frac{2.716}{\sqrt{10}} = 0.8589$

Test statistic $t = \frac{\overline{X} - \mu}{s_{\overline{X}}} = \frac{-13.4 - (-8)}{0.8589} = -6.287$ $df = n - 1 = 10 - 1 = 9$

The significance level is $p = 0.000143$ (see commentary below this example and Fig. 5.3), so we reject H_0 and state that our sample of 10 plants originates from a statistical population with mean different from -8.

$t_{0.975,\ 9}$ (i.e. the 97.5% quantile of the *t* distribution with $df = 9$) = 2.262 (see Fig. 5.2).

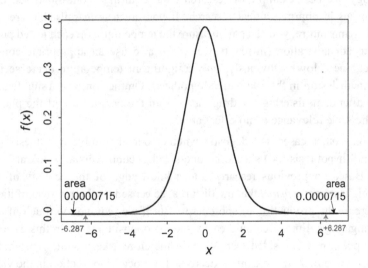

Figure 5.3 Two-sided single-sample *t* test of the difference between the mean and the expected value (-8.0). The calculated test statistic (see Example 5.1) is -6.287. The probability that we obtain this or a more extreme value (in both directions, i.e. <-6.287 or $>+6.287$) can be calculated using the probability density function of the t_9 distribution, shown here as the black curve. The total area under the density curve is equal to 1 (for a range of *x*-values from minus to plus infinity). The probability we seek is therefore equal to the sum of areas under the curve to the left from -6.287 and to the right from $+6.287$, i.e. $2 \times 0.0000715 = 0.000143$.

determine the seed set (i.e. the number of seeds per flower) for each preselected pair of flowers of each plant. We then test the difference between seed set in the control and treated flowers of each plant. We will therefore have a set of 30 differences and we ask whether their mean value is significantly different from zero. Our null hypothesis therefore states that the mean value of the difference between treated and control flowers is equal to 0. Testing this type of H_0 is usually called a **paired *t* test** (or *paired samples t test*).

A paired *t* test is often employed to evaluate field experiments such as that described in example 2 in Section 5.1. There we ask whether the removal of the upper soil layer changes the frequency of fungal sporocarps. Because there is a substantial spatial variability in the abiotic and biotic conditions across the experimental area, it is advantageous to establish the experiment using pairs of plots (with two plots located nearby and differing in the presence or absence of the soil manipulation treatment) and consequently test the differences between two plots within each pair. If we decide to place the control and modified plots independently at random locations, we cannot use the paired *t* test and we need to use the two-sample *t* test as described in Chapter 6.

5.4 One-Sided Tests

In the *t* tests discussed so far, we assumed H_0: $\mu = \mu_0$ as our null hypothesis and rejected it when the deviation from the null hypothesis, be it positive or negative, was improbably large. Thus in these cases the alternative hypothesis was H_A: $\mu \neq \mu_0$. But sometimes we are interested in a deviation which operates in a single direction. Although it is outside the realm of field biology, the best example of research data requiring a one-sided test comes from testing new drugs in pharmaceutical research. If you are testing pills that are designed to decrease body temperature, you can e.g. measure the temperature on each tested person before and after drug administration (in reality we would also use an appropriate control for the placebo effect, see below). Obviously, only a significant temperature decrease is a pattern which warrants inclusion in the alternative hypothesis. On the contrary, a significant temperature increase after administering the drug has – from the perspective of the pharmaceutical company – the same relevance as no effect at all.

In some other cases, the decision whether our alternative hypothesis (and consequently the null hypothesis too) should be one-sided is controversial. Look at example 2 in Section 5.1. Based on previous research and a knowledge of the ecology of this fungus species, we might expect *a priori* that the disturbance caused by the removal of the upper soil layer will increase the production of sporocarps. But if we remove too much of the soil and disturb the fungal mycelium, we could easily see the opposite effect. In this case it might be dangerous to perform a one-sided test. We will therefore take a somewhat similar experimental approach where we try to explain decreased sporocarp production in the vicinity of air pollution sources and test a working hypothesis that the increased amount of nutrients (such as the nitrogen entering the forest ecosystem in rain water) will reduce the production of sporocarps. We again have 10 pairs of plots – one is watered in monthly intervals with a solution of NH_4NO_3, thus providing a source of inorganic nitrogen ions, while the other is treated with identical amounts of pure water.[5] Again we observe the total number of sporocarps produced in the 20 plots in the following two years, with this being our response variable. Our research hypothesis – converted into an alternative hypothesis for our one-sided paired *t* test – is that the change in sporocarp count due to nitrogen addition is negative, i.e. H_A: $\mu_{Ctrl-N} > 0$. Consequently, the null hypothesis states that there is either no change or the count of sporocarps is higher in the nitrogen-treated plots – H_0: $\mu_{Ctrl-N} \leq 0$. So, if we – for this

---

[5] If we do not water our control plots, then we could never dispel a possible reviewer's criticism that the observed effect might simply be a consequence of varying levels of water availability in the soil.

Example 5.2 One-sided t test of the effect of nitrogen addition on fructification of *Suillus variegatus*.

Here we start right away with the differences between the count of sporocarps in control plots and the count of sporocarps in corresponding N-treated plots: +5, +4, +3, −2, −5, +6, +1, +6, +9, +5.

$H_0: \mu_{\text{diff}} \le 0$ $\qquad\qquad$ $H_A: \mu_{\text{diff}} > 0$ $\qquad\qquad$ $\alpha = 0.05$

Estimated sample mean $\overline{X} = +3.2$

Estimated sample standard deviation $s_X = 4.158$

Standard error of the mean $s_{\bar{X}} = \frac{4.158}{\sqrt{10}} = 1.315$

Test statistic $t = \frac{\overline{X} - \mu}{s_{\bar{X}}} = \frac{+3.2 - 0}{1.315} = 2.434$ $\qquad\qquad$ $df = n - 1 = 10 - 1 = 9$

The significance level is $p = 0.0189$ and therefore we reject the H_0 at $\alpha = 0.05$.

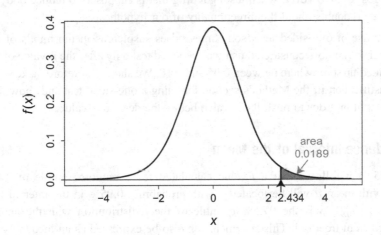

Figure 5.4 Density distribution curve for the t_9 distribution showing the position of the test statistic of our one-sided test from Example 5.2.

example – subtract the observed count of sporocarps in an N-treated plot from the count in a control plot in each plot pairing, only a large positive value of the t test statistic should lead to rejecting the null hypothesis, namely when the statistic is larger than the 95% quantile of the t_9 distribution. Please take careful note that we are using the 95% (and not the 97.5%) quantile for a one-sided test in order to make the correct decision at $\alpha = 0.05$. Because this new quantile has a lower value, we can deduce that a one-sided test has a higher power than a two-sided test. This is discussed further below.

The calculation of the one-sided paired t test on the N-treated plot data is illustrated in Example 5.2 below and in Fig. 5.4.

Our sporocarps example also nicely illustrates how we must always be careful to distinguish between effect significance and effect size. Although we showed that an average of approximately 3 sporocarps disappeared from the plots where nitrogen was added, this represents a very small change in terms of total observed counts. We can check this in the *Chap5* sheet within the example data Excel file, column *FB_Ctrl* – the average sporocarp count per control plot is 85.4, so the effect of nitrogen represents a decrease of 3.7%.

In our earlier example where we administered a drug that decreases body temperature and observed its effect, it should be noted that the experimental design was mostly incorrect. We can perhaps prove that the whole procedure of administering the drug leads to a temperature decrease in our patients by using this type of experiment. However, this approach cannot distinguish whether this was due to the chemicals present in the pills or simply due to some psychological effects of the administration. For a more correct design, we need to have another group of patients who are administered with a placebo drug. We must then compare their temperature change with the change in the original group (but this must be done with a two-sample *t* test, described in Chapter 6).

As we saw in the discussion above, one-sided tests have a higher power than the corresponding two-sided tests. It is therefore appropriate to use them on every occasion where our research question naturally leads to an asymmetrical hypothesis. In examples 1 and 2 in Section 5.1, we do not have any clear idea about a specific direction of change, so we should use a two-sided test. However, when testing a drug that is supposed to reduce body temperature, we have no doubts about the directionality of our hypothesis.

The use of one-sided tests sometimes raises suspicions in the minds of reviewers about whether the authors considered using a one-sided test only after the *p*-value of their two-sided test ended up somewhere between 0.05 and 0.10. We should therefore make sure that we provide a justification in the Methods section for using a one-sided test and show that we do not simply use it in order to push the *p*-value below the desired *α*-value.

5.5 Confidence Interval of the Mean

From Eq. (5.4) it follows that a *t*-value calculated for a random sample of a statistical population with mean μ will be located – with probability 0.95 – in the interval $(-t_{0.975,df}, t_{0.975,df})$, where $t_{0.975,df}$ is the 97.5% quantile of the *t* distribution with the appropriately selected degrees of freedom. This statement can also be expressed as an inequality

$$P\left(-t_{0.975,df} < \frac{\overline{X} - \mu}{s_{\overline{X}}} < t_{0.975,df}\right) = 0.95 \tag{5.5}$$

Eq. (5.5) can be modified (multiplying by $s_{\overline{X}}$, subtracting $\overline{X}$, multiplying by -1, with a consequent change of the inequality direction), yielding the following useful statement:

$$P(\overline{X} - t_{0.975,df}s_{\overline{X}} < \mu < \overline{X} + t_{0.975,df}s_{\overline{X}}) = 0.95 \tag{5.6}$$

The parentheses in Eq. (5.6) define an interval containing, with probability 0.95 (or 95%), the true mean value μ. This useful information is most often called the **95% confidence interval** (with its limits called *confidence limits*). We can also construct confidence intervals for confidence values other than 95%, with the most frequently used alternative being 99%.

> **When thinking about how we estimate means, it is good to remember that the true mean value of the sampled population is not a random variate, it is expected to be a fixed value: our estimates (whether a sample mean or confidence limits) are random variates, as shown in Fig. 5.5.**

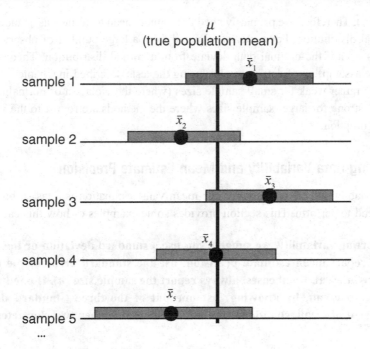

Figure 5.5 A hypothetical scenario in which we collect a large number of independent random samples from the same statistical population. For each sample, we get a different sample mean (black circles) and we compute different 95% confidence limits (the horizontal span of the grey rectangles). We can say that each confidence interval contains the fixed (but unknown) mean value (μ) for the statistical population with probability 0.95. So if our figure contained 20 random samples, we could expect that on average one of the confidence intervals (as a 1/20 fraction equals 5%) would miss the black vertical line representing the true μ-value and lie completely outside.

It can be shown that if a calculated confidence interval for a mean does not contain a particular value, then the mean is – at the α significance level – significantly different from that value. As an example, if the 95% confidence interval for the mean value of $\delta^{13}C$ in Example 5.1 does not contain the value −8, then we know that in a two-sided t test at 5% significance level we can reject the null hypothesis that $\delta^{13}C$ is equal to −8.[6]

5.6 Test Assumptions

When deriving the t statistic in Eq. (5.4) and its associated distribution, it is assumed that the X values are a random sample from a statistical population with a normal distribution. Therefore both the single-sample test, the paired t test and the estimation of confidence intervals assume the normality of data (while an estimate of the standard error of a mean does not have such an assumption). For all these methods, however, the larger the sample size (n), the more robust they are to violations of this assumption. This is because the formulas for these statistics do not use the original data values, but only the sample mean and its standard deviation

---

[6] In fact, given the p-value found in Example 5.1, we know that even a 99.9% confidence interval would not contain the value −8.

(standard error). Therefore, we primarily need the sample mean to come – as a random entity – from a normal distribution. For a mean estimated from a large number of observations, this usually holds even if the original data deviate from a normal distribution. Theoretically, we can verify the assumption of data normality using the tests described in Chapter 4. However, these tests are rather weak for small sample sizes (where the violation of normality matters), but are really strong for larger sample sizes where the methods are robust to the violation of normality assumption.

5.7 Reporting Data Variability and Mean Estimate Precision

Reporting variability or the precision of our mean value estimation is a task a biologist will frequently need to perform. This section provides some examples of how this can be done.

> **When reporting variability, we suggest you use a standard deviation or the range of values. To report mean estimate precision, use the standard error of the mean or a confidence interval. In all cases, always report the sample size (_n_). If one knows the sample size, one can, by knowing just one out of the three (standard deviation, standard error of mean, confidence limits), calculate the other two characteristics.**

The range of values (from minimum to maximum) is perhaps too dependent on the sample size to be a good description of data variability. The larger a sample, the larger the chance that extreme data values extend the range.

In text and tables, we often use the notation $\bar{X} \pm d$. Beware that this form can combine the mean estimate with a standard deviation, but also with a standard error of the mean, or with values implying limits of a confidence interval.[7] Unless we clearly state what the _d_-value means, everyone could interpret it differently. The arithmetic average is an appropriate measure of location for data with a symmetrical distribution, but for skewed distributions (which are quite common for biological data on a ratio scale) it is less informative. In such cases, you are better served by the median (see also Figs 5.7 and 5.8 and the related discussion). To indicate the spread of values, a median statistic is well supplemented by the lower and upper quartiles, but it does not make sense to combine a median with a standard deviation or a standard error of the mean. The median, together with the two quartiles (and possibly with other non-parametric estimates), forms the basis of the classical _box-and-whisker_ diagram, but we can also create a similar graph for parametric estimates (using e.g. the arithmetic average and standard deviation). In any case, an explanation of the statistics behind such graphs must be clearly provided.

Tables 5.1 and 5.2 represent just two of multiple possible ways of presenting summary statistics in research papers or reports. Similarly, Figs 5.6–5.8 show some of the possible graphical presentations for data summaries. Some variants of box-and-whisker plots (such as the notched box-and-whisker plot) allow you to show variability and estimation precision at the same time, albeit at the expense of increased graphical complexity. But most often we limit our presentations to simply plotting the mean using some symbol and – with the help of a bar – plotting one of the discussed characteristics: standard deviation (_SD_), standard

---

[7] In some research fields, this notation is also used for a single measured value combined with some _a priori_ known precision of the measuring instrument/device.

Table 5.1 *Number of observations and sample statistics for the concentration of nitrates in the soil of experimental plots: C = control plots, N = added nitrogen plots. Column n represents the number of observations, SD is the sample standard deviation and SE is the standard error of the mean*

Treatment	n	Average	Median	*SD*	*SE*
C	25	0.185	0.12	0.1642	0.0328
N	21	1.165	0.43	1.5593	0.3403

Table 5.2 *Summary of estimated soil chemistry parameters from an experiment (C = control plots, N = plots with added nitrogen). The arithmetic averages ± SE (standard error of the mean) are presented while the numbers in parentheses represent the observation count. Measurement scales were:* NO_3^- *mg* kg^{-1} *dry soil,* NH_4^+ ...

	Treatment	
Soil parameter	C	N
NO_3^-	0.185 ± 0.033 (25)	1.165 ± 0.340 (21)
NH_4^+	1.312 ± 0.636 (25)	3.863 ± 1.724 (20)
PO_4^-	14.278 ± 1.752 (25)	16.354 ± 1.925 (21)
Total nitrogen	15.21 ± 2.17 (25)	83.91 ± 5.31 (25)
Total phosphorus	2.372 ± 0.872 (25)	9.231 ± 1.382 (25)
pH	7.15 ± 0.22 (20)	7.04 ± 0.36 (20)

error (*SE*) or limits of a confidence interval (see Fig. 5.6). Whatever we plot, we must always describe precisely what it is.

Sometimes we plot the arithmetic average with ±2SD (or, using a higher precision, ±1.96SD). We do this to ensure that if the statistics being presented come from a statistical population with a normal distribution, then the interval constructed in this way would cover roughly 95% of all observations[8] (2.5% and 97.5% quantiles of a standardised normal distribution are −1.96 and +1.96).

Comparing the box-and-whisker plots in Fig. 5.7 with those in Fig. 5.8 nicely illustrates the inadequacy of parametric summaries for data with an asymmetrical distribution with substantial deviations from a normal distribution. The range of values in which 95% of observations should lie, as implied by the dashed bars in Fig. 5.7, suggests a frequent occurrence of negative values, but there are none: negative values make no sense for ion concentrations![9] On the contrary, Fig. 5.8 presents the real range of values as well as the asymmetry (skewness) of the distribution, which causes (among other things) much lower values for median estimates than those of the arithmetic averages (in Fig. 5.7).

This kind of data (which in addition to various concentration or density measurements also includes weights or dimensions) would have a more symmetrical distribution (and also a greater likeness to a normal distribution) after log-transforming the data (see Fig. 5.10 in Section 5.10.2). This transformation would also enable us to appropriately compare group means using parametric tests, which make the assumption that the variability within each

---

[8] Provided the *SD* is estimated from a large sample.

[9] In general, always check your graphs, and if your intervals suggest that the data should contain negative values for concentrations, sizes, counts or other data on ratio scale, check what is wrong.

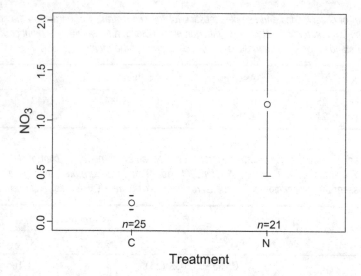

Figure 5.6 Graphical report showing the precision of mean estimates (see also Table 5.1). The graph contains averages (circles) and 95% confidence intervals for soil NO_3^- concentration in experimental plots of type C or N. The graph also contains information about the number of observations in each group, but perhaps this information would be better placed here in the caption.

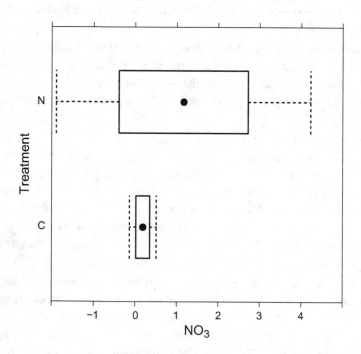

Figure 5.7 Graphical report on data variability (see also Fig. 5.8). The graph displays averages (black circles) with the range of $\pm 1SD$ from the averages (boxes) and the range of $\pm 1.96SD$ (dashed bars) for soil nitrate concentrations in experimental plots of types C and N. Number of observations was $n = 25$ for C plots and $n = 21$ for N plots.

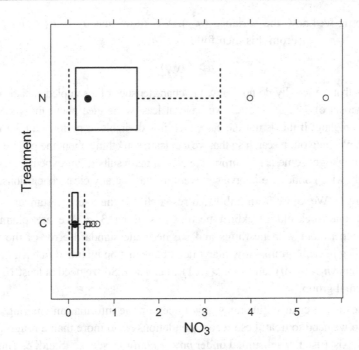

Figure 5.8 Graphical report on data variability (see also Fig. 5.7). The graph displays median values (black circles), the range from lower quartile (25% percentile) to upper quartile (75% percentile) as boxes, the range of so-called adjacent values (dashed bars) and the positions of outlying values (empty circles) for soil nitrate concentrations in experimental plots of types C and N. Number of observations was $n = 25$ for C plots and $n = 21$ for N plots.

group is similar (see Chapter 6). Displaying parametric estimates using log-transformed scales can be a viable alternative to presenting non-parametric statistics (as in Fig. 5.8).

Comparing Fig. 5.6 (reporting estimate precision) with the other two graphs (Figs 5.7 and 5.8) also demonstrates that a graphical report on precision would convince the reader that the two groups were different more so than the reports on variability.[10] Finally, the type of graph in Fig. 5.7 does not effectively use the plotting space that we have devoted to the graph (or which the editors allow us to devote to it). Even after using a relatively complex presentation, we have only managed to report about four values (two means and two standard deviations – if the reader sees the size of 1SD, she can certainly imagine the size of 2SD). It might be more effective to combine the information on variability with that of estimate precisions, or perhaps report in textual form, as illustrated in Tables 5.1 and 5.2.

5.8 How Large Should a Sample Size Be?

When we plan an experiment or an extensive observational study, it is useful to get at least an approximate idea of the size our random sample should be to achieve a sufficiently precise mean estimate (what 'sufficiently precise' actually means is for us to define and justify for the problem at hand). As a first approximation, we can reformulate this task in the following way: determine the size (n) of a random sample that leads to a standard error of the mean that is less

---

[10] Particularly for readers who do not sufficiently anticipate the differences between precision and data variability; all three graphs report on identical data values.

than q, assuming we know the variance (σ^2_X). We know that $\sigma_{\bar{X}} = \sigma_X/\sqrt{n}$. We therefore require that $\sigma_X/\sqrt{n} < q$. From this then follows

$$n > (\sigma_X/q)^2 \tag{5.7}$$

The problem is that we usually do not know the characteristics of a sampled statistical population (including its variance). But quite often we have at least some idea about the variability of the things we are sampling: if this is not the case, then it is desirable to perform a pilot study before starting or even planning our research so that we can learn something about the potential variability. Otherwise we might get some nasty surprises, such as the results of an expensive experiment in which extremely wide confidence intervals prevent us drawing any clear conclusions.

   Example: We know from published research that the average standard deviation of the weight of one-week-old blackbird nestlings is about 3 g. We are planning a field manipulative experiment with nestlings and we need the standard error of the mean to be no larger than 1 g in each group. How many nestlings must be included in each group? Using Eq. (5.7) we obtain $n > (\sigma_X/q)^2$ and so $n > (3/1)^2$, i.e. $n > 9$. So we need at least 10 nestlings in each experimental group.[11]

   This example clearly illustrates how uncertain the information entering our calculations can be, so we need to treat these recommendations as no more than a rough guide. More exact methods exist (usually subsumed under *power analysis*, see e.g. Steidl & Thomas, 2001) for sample sizes based on a pilot sample so that the confidence region is smaller than some desired value. Similarly, one can calculate the recommended sample size for a *t* test at a given α level and test power. This is useful information because we know that a non-significant result is either a consequence of a genuine lack of a difference or of a sample size that was simply too small. Carefully planning experiments using the methods outlined above can minimise the probability that H_0 will not be rejected on the basis of insufficient sample size alone. Figure 5.9 shows how the standard error of the mean decreases with increasing sample size.

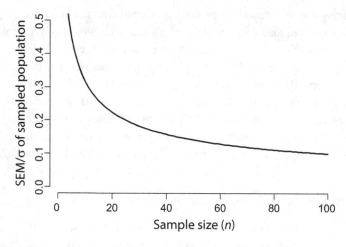

Figure 5.9 The dependence of the standard error of the sample mean (SEM) on sample size (n). The vertical axis shows the ratio of SEM to the standard deviation of the sampled statistical population.

---

[11] Here we simply ignore the fact that there are usually multiple nestlings in each nest, however measurement data from within a single nest is usually not independent.

5.9 Example Data

In order to illustrate the one-sample test we will use the example of ^{13}C concentrations in 10 plants (see Example 5.1). This data is stored in column *d13* in the *Chap5* sheet. For a classical paired *t* test we will use the data from Example 5.2, however this data is in the form recorded at the experimental site (column *FB_Ctrl* contains counts of fruiting bodies in the control plots while *FB_N* contains counts for the associated nitrogen-enhanced plots).

To illustrate the textual and graphical presentation of means, data variability and mean estimate precision, we will use the results of the experiment measuring nitrate ions (NO_3^-) in soil, with a specific focus on comparing the consequences of an experimental treatment (the variable *Treatment* with two levels – *C* for control plots and *N* for plots fertilised in the preceding year).

5.10 How to Proceed in R

Before carrying out the calculations, we first need to import the data into separate data frames – one for the first three columns (into the *chap5A* data frame) and another one for the following two columns (into the *chap5B* data frame), as they differ in observation counts.

5.10.1 Single Sample and Paired *t* Test

Both the single-sample and paired *t* tests (but also the two-sample *t* test which is handled in the following chapter) can be calculated using the *t.test* function. Of course, the way we enter data differs between the various types of *t* test. In the *t.test* function, we can also specify a one-sided hypothesis test, including the assumed direction of the deviation from the null hypothesis.

First we will calculate the single-sample *t* test to test a two-sided hypothesis:

```
with( chap5A, t.test( d13, mu=-8))

        One Sample t-test
data:  d13
t = -6.2868, df = 9, p-value = 0.0001432
alternative hypothesis: true mean is not equal to -8
95 percent confidence interval:
 -15.34306 -11.45694
sample estimates:
mean of x
    -13.4
```

We must specify the constant in the *t.test* function using the *mu* parameter. It is this constant that the mean of our variable is then compared with. If we were testing a one-sided hypothesis here, we would need to add the *alternative* parameter (see the following command for an example of how to do this). The main test results are in the output row starting with $t = -6.2868$.

We will perform a paired *t* test as follows:

```
with( chap5A,
      t.test( FB_Ctrl, FB_N, paired=T, alternative="greater"))
        Paired t-test
data:  FB_Ctrl and FB_N
t = 2.4337, df = 9, p-value = 0.01888
alternative hypothesis: true difference in means is greater than 0
95 percent confidence interval:
 0.7896908      Inf
sample estimates:
mean of the differences
                  3.2
```

If we are comparing two variables then we must specify *TRUE* for the *paired* parameter, so that the *t.test* function does not compute a two-sample *t* test. Moreover, our test is one-sided and this is specified by the *alternative* parameter. The value of this parameter implies that – in accordance with our alternative hypothesis – the values of the first variable (representing control plots) are expected to be larger than the values of the second variable (representing fertilised plots) in each plot pair.

5.10.2 Summarising Variability and Describing Mean Precision

The R software contains multiple versions of the classical box-and-whisker plot, with the *boxplot* function being the most easily accessible (implemented in the *graphics* package). You may use it in the following way:

```
boxplot( NO3~Treatment, data=chap5B)
```

The output for these two boxplots (separating the two experimental treatments) clearly indicates a strong positive skew in the distribution of nitrate concentrations. It might therefore be instructive to compare these box-and-whisker plots with those constructed for log-transformed concentrations:

```
boxplot( log(NO3)~Treatment, data=chap5B)
```

The two alternatives are shown side by side in Fig. 5.10 (see Chapter 10 for additional information about the use of log-transformations).

More advanced options are available with the *bwplot* function in the *lattice* library:

```
library( lattice)
bwplot( NO3~Treatment, data=chap5B, xlab="Treatment")
bwplot( Treatment~NO3, data=chap5B, ylab="Treatment")
```

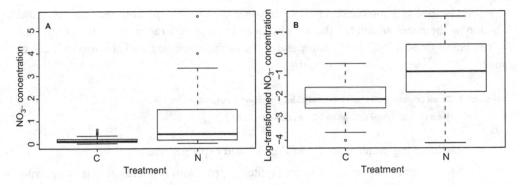

Figure 5.10 Classical box-and-whisker plots summarising the distribution of nitrate concentration in field plots of two treatments (control C vs. fertilised N). The left-hand plot A shows the original concentrations (mg g^{-1} of dry soil), while the right-hand plot B visualises the log-transformed data.

The alternative positioning of the two variables (*NO3* and *Treatment*) in the formula (the first parameter of the *bwplot* function) allows us to choose either a vertical or a horizontal direction for the summarised variable in the graph. The outcome of the second call to *bwplot* is shown in Fig. 5.8.

The R software is less willing, however, to produce a box-and-whisker plot displaying the arithmetic average and standard deviation. We must push a little more here. We first need to define a custom panel function used to draw the inner parts (located within the scale rectangle) of a *bwplot* graph. We can still leave most of the hard work to the default panel function (*panel.bwplot*); we just replace the plotted statistics by providing a new function called *my.stats* as the *stats* argument in the call to *panel.bwplot* (see the last line of the *my.bwplot.panel* function below).

```
my.bwplot.panel <- function( ...)
{
  my.stats <- function( x, ...)
  {
    x.mean <- mean( x)
    x.sd   <- sd( x)
    x.n    <- length( na.omit( x))
    x.t    <- qt( 0.975, x.n - 1)
    list( stats = c( x.mean - 1.96*x.sd, x.mean - x.sd, x.mean,
                     x.mean + x.sd, x.mean + 1.96*x.sd),
          n = x.n,
          conf = c( x.mean - x.t * x.sd / sqrt(x.n),
                    x.mean + x.t * x.sd / sqrt(x.n)),
          out=NULL)
  }
  panel.bwplot( ..., stats=my.stats)
}
```

The rest is simple, we just call the *bwplot* function, passing our custom panel function as the *panel* parameter. But we also need to adjust the range of the horizontal axis as it is based on observed *NO3* values and some of the computed statistics are well out of range:

```
bwplot( Treatment~NO3, data=chap5B, ylab="Treatment",
        panel=my.bwplot.panel, xlim=c(-2,5))
```

The resulting graph is shown in Fig. 5.7 and explained there.

More often, however, we are quite happy with simple graphs displaying summary statistics. For example, the following function *plotmeans* (in the *gplots* package) creates a diagram with means and 95% confidence intervals (see Fig. 5.6 earlier in this chapter):

```
library( gplots)
plotmeans( NO3~Treatment, data=chap5B,
           connect=F, barcol="black", ylim=c(0,2))
```

Giving the *connect* argument the value *FALSE* prevents the function from connecting two treatment means with a line segment, *barcol* makes the graph cheaply printable and *ylim* slightly adjusts the vertical axis range, so that the *n* = *25* label does not interact with the confidence interval plotted above it.

5.11 Reporting Analyses

5.11.1 Methods

Stable isotope $\delta^{13}C$ values of experimental plants were compared with the atmospheric isotope concentration using a one-sample *t* test.

A decrease in sporocarp counts of *Suillus variegatus* in plots with additional nitrogen was tested using the data from 20 paired plots using a one-sided paired *t* test.

Summary statistics such as arithmetic average, median, confidence intervals, etc. are considered as widely known, so their use is usually not even mentioned in the Methods section. For many journals, however, the same applies to t tests...

5.11.2 Results

The average $\delta^{13}C$ concentration in plants was -13.4, significantly lower than -8, the concentration in air ($t_9 = 6.287$, $p = 0.000143$).

The count of fungal sporocarps was significantly lower in fertilised plots when compared with nearby control plots ($t_9 = 2.434$, $p = 0.0189$), but the average effect size (decrease by 3.2 sporocarps per plot) was quite small.

Never ever forget to include information about degrees of freedom. They are usually presented as subscripts, but sometimes as a separate value (t = 6.287, df = 9, p = 0.000143).

5.12 Recommended Reading

Zar (2010), pp. 97–129 and pp. 179–182 (paired *t* test).

Quinn & Keough (2002), pp. 17–22 and pp. 35–37.

Sokal & Rohlf (2012), pp. 131–135, pp. 157–166 (confidence interval) and pp. 349–353 (paired *t* test).

R. J. Steidl & L. Thomas (2001) Power analysis and experimental design. In S. Scheiner & J. Gurevitch (eds), *Design and Analysis of Ecological Experiments*, 2nd edn. Oxford University Press, Oxford, pp. 14–36.

6 Comparing Two Samples

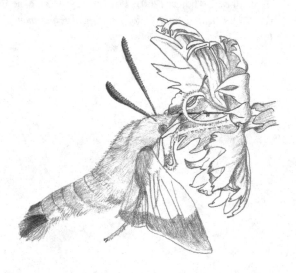

Let us assume that we want to compare two samples that come from target populations[1] characterised by a normal distribution. These populations may differ in their mean and/or variance (see Fig. 6.1) and we can test for both of these differences.

6.1 Use Case Examples

1. A plant population contains both diploid and tetraploid individuals. Anther length was measured for randomly selected individuals and their ploidy was then determined. Our task is to find out whether the diploids and tetraploids differ in their anther length.
2. Twenty plots were established in randomly chosen locations (preventing plot overlap) at a field site, and of these 20, 10 were randomly chosen and fertilised with a natrium phosphate solution. At the time of peak biomass in the following year, the aboveground parts of the plant community were harvested, dried to a constant mass and weighed. Does soil enrichment by P affect plant biomass, i.e. does the community's productivity differ in its average value between the two treatments, indicating it is limited by P availability?
3. A particular moth species was collected from light traps of two different designs. Ten traps of the first type and 10 traps of the second type were randomly spread across a site (in a non-segregated way). The moths in each individual trap were then counted after a whole-night exposure. Do the two trap types differ in their efficiency?

---

[1] Populations in a statistical sense, i.e. potentially infinitely large sets of plants that can be grown in pots, all moth individuals within a locality, all plots we can establish in the field in comparable conditions, etc.

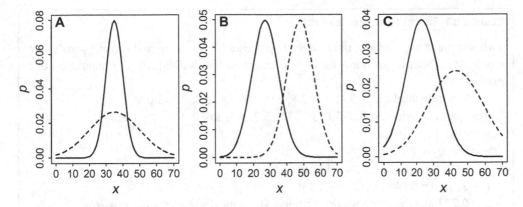

Figure 6.1 Probability density of two normal distributions, differing in variance (A), mean value (B) or both mean and variance (C). This last possibility will likely be the one we most frequently encounter.

6.2 Testing for Differences in Variance

We sample two populations and ask whether the variance differs between the two. Our null hypothesis is therefore H_0: $\sigma_1^2 = \sigma_2^2$ and our alternative hypothesis is H_A: $\sigma_1^2 \neq \sigma_2^2$. We perform the test in the following way: we calculate sample variances s_1^2 and s_2^2 and ask what is the probability that two random samples will differ in their variances as much or more than our two samples if they in fact come from populations with an identical variance (or from a single population) as the null hypothesis suggests. If this probability is small (usually less than 0.05 or 0.01, as in the tests described earlier), we reject the null hypothesis. If the probability is higher, we do not have sufficient evidence to reject the null hypothesis. We use the F test to test the hypothesis. The value of the F statistic is calculated as the ratio of the larger sample variance to the smaller one. So, if $s_1^2 > s_2^2$, we calculate the statistic as

$$F = \frac{s_1^2}{s_2^2} \tag{6.1}$$

The test statistic (F-value) comes – when the null hypothesis is true – from an **F distribution** (in reference to Sir R. A. Fisher, one of the fathers of statistical science). The properties of the F distribution depend (similar to the χ^2 distribution) on the number of degrees of freedom. But because the F statistic is calculated from two samples, we have to deal with two counts of degrees of freedom: the first for the sample with its variance estimate used as the numerator (**numerator df**) and the second for the sample with its variance estimate used as the denominator (**denominator df**). For each of the two samples, df is the sample size minus 1, i.e. $n - 1$.

The F statistic (as with any other test statistic) quantifies the deviation of our data from the expectation based on the null hypothesis. If the F statistic is larger than the critical value of the F distribution for appropriate degrees of freedom and for a given significance level α, we reject the null hypothesis at the chosen significance (probability) level. For a two-sided test (testing the null hypothesis $\sigma_1^2 = \sigma_2^2$) the critical value for a $100\alpha\%$ significance level (e.g. $\alpha = 0.05$) is the $(1 - \alpha/2)$ quantile (i.e. the 0.975 quantile for our example). Note that we divide α by two because we have arbitrarily decided that the larger variance estimate will become the numerator. Statistical software, however, supplements each calculated

---

Example 6.1 Two-sided test of variance ratio

Two-sample test of variance ratio for the hypotheses H_0: $\sigma_1^2 = \sigma_2^2$ and H_A: $\sigma_1^2 \neq \sigma_2^2$. Data represent anther lengths (mm) for diploid and tetraploid individuals in a population of a plant species.

Diploid individuals: 2.9, 3.1, 3.2, 2.8, 2.9, 3.3, 3.4, 2.8, 2.7, 3.0, 3.1

Tetraploid individuals: 3.5, 3.8, 3.7, 3.8, 3.7, 3.5, 3.6, 3.9

$n_1 = 11$, $df_1 = 10$

$n_2 = 8$, $df_2 = 7$

$s_1^2 = 0.0496$ mm^2, $s_2^2 = 0.0213$ mm^2

$F = s_1^2/s_2^2 = 0.0496/0.0213 = 2.336$

$p = 0.273$ and therefore we do not reject H_0 (critical value of $F_{10,7}$ is 4.76)

Because the variances do not differ, we can estimate the shared variance of both samples as

$s_p^2 = (0.496 + 0.1491)/(10 + 7) = 0.0379$ mm^2.

F statistic directly with the corresponding probability p (achieved significance level, usually called significance level or p-value). The calculations are illustrated in Example 6.1.

If we cannot reject the null hypothesis and decide to estimate the pooled variance of both samples (s_p^2), we can use the formula

$$s_p^2 = \frac{df_1 \cdot s_1^2 + df_2 \cdot s_2^2}{df_1 + df_2} = \frac{SS_1 + SS_2}{df_1 + df_2} \tag{6.2}$$

The test for a difference in variances is quite weak, particularly with small samples. If we compare two samples, each with a size of 10 (and in biology, often we do not have larger samples), the critical value for a two-sided F test at $\alpha = 0.05$ is 4.026. This means that one estimate of sample variance must be four times greater than the other to reject the null hypothesis stating the identity of population variances. We must therefore be very careful about a conclusion that two samples come from distributions with identical variance, as the probability of Type II error is high for this test.

The test description above refers to the two-sided version, but we can use a one-sided test as well: for example, we want to demonstrate that the variability of egg clutch size (characterised by variance) is larger in birds breeding under natural conditions than in captivity (our theory provides sufficient ground for expecting such a pattern, unlike the opposite, i.e. increasing variability in captivity). Our null hypothesis then states that the variance of clutch size under natural conditions is identical to or smaller than for clutches of birds kept in captivity. To test this at the significance level α, we use the $(1 - \alpha)$ quantile of an F distribution as its critical value. After our statistical software estimates the p-value for the two-sided test, we must check that the relative size of sample variances corresponds to our alternative hypothesis, and if so, we obtain the correct significance estimate for a one-sided test by dividing the p-value by two.

We can also estimate a confidence interval for the variance ratio. The value 1 is included within the $(1 - \alpha) \times 100\%$ confidence interval only when we cannot reject the null hypothesis about the equality of variances (in a two-sided test) at the significance level α. So if a 95% confidence interval for the variance ratio is (0.49, 9.23), as is the case in our example dataset (Example 6.1), this implies that we cannot reject the null hypothesis about variance equality at the 5% significance level. On the contrary, if a 99% confidence interval is (for a different dataset) estimated as (1.45, 6.54), we can reject the null hypothesis at the 1% significance level ($p < 0.01$).

6.3 Comparing Means

We can use a **two-sample t test** to compare the means of two samples. This must be the most frequently used statistical test throughout the history of statistics. It assumes that both samples come from populations where the observed variable has a normal distribution. In its standard form, the test further assumes that both samples come from populations with identical variance, but there are several ways to approach the problem where the populations being compared differ in their variance. With a two-sample t test, we test the null hypothesis $H_0: \mu_1 = \mu_2$ against the alternative hypothesis $H_A: \mu_1 \neq \mu_2$. In the typical version of the test, we use the following formula for the test statistic:

$$t = \frac{\overline{X}_1 - \overline{X}_2}{s_{\overline{X}1-\overline{X}2}} \tag{6.3}$$

Here, $s_{\overline{X}1-\overline{X}2}$ is the standard error of the difference between sample means. As we assume that the variance is identical for both sampled populations, we can estimate their pooled variance s_p^2 using Eq. (6.2) and then estimate the mean error of the mean difference as

$$s_{\overline{X}1-\overline{X}2} = \sqrt{\frac{s_p^2}{n_1} + \frac{s_p^2}{n_2}} \tag{6.4}$$

The formula in Eq. (6.3) can be rewritten as

$$t = \frac{\overline{X}_1 - \overline{X}_2}{\sqrt{\frac{s_p^2}{n_1} + \frac{s_p^2}{n_2}}} \tag{6.5}$$

The degrees of freedom for the t statistic equals the sum of the degrees of freedom for the two compared samples, i.e. $(n_1 - 1) + (n_2 - 1) = n_1 + n_2 - 2$. We reject the null hypothesis when the estimated significance (p-value) is smaller than the chosen α (i.e. when the calculated t statistic exceeds the critical value for our α). Example 6.2 illustrates the use of the two-sided t test. Here we compare the anther lengths of individuals with two ploidy levels (as in Example 6.1).

As in the one-sample t test, we can use (where appropriate for our research question) a one-sided version of the test instead of the two-sided method. In this case we test the null hypothesis $H_0: \mu_1 \leq \mu_2$ against the alternative hypothesis $H_A: \mu_1 > \mu_2$ (or vice versa).

Violation of the test assumptions. With this test we assume that both samples originate from populations with normal distributions and an identical variance. Luckily even a substantial distortion of these assumptions does not affect the test results too much (we say that the test is robust against such distortions), particularly if the size of the samples is

---

Example 6.2 Two-sample t test for a two-sided hypothesis.

Two-sample t test for a two-sided hypothesis $H_0: \mu_1 = \mu_2$ (and $H_A: \mu_1 \neq \mu_2$). The data again represent the lengths of anthers (mm) for diploid and tetraploid individuals in a population of a plant species.

Diploid individuals: 2.9, 3.1, 3.2, 2.8, 2.9, 3.3, 3.4, 2.8, 2.7, 3.0, 3.1

Tetraploid individuals: 3.5, 3.8, 3.7, 3.8, 3.7, 3.5, 3.6, 3.9

$n_1 = 11$, $df_1 = 10$

$n_2 = 8$, $df_2 = 7$

$\bar{X}_1 = 3.02$ mm, $SS_1 = 0.4964$ mm^2

$\bar{X}_2 = 3.69$ mm, $SS_2 = 0.1488$ mm^2

$$s_p^2 = \frac{SS_1 + SS_2}{df_1 + df_2} = \frac{0.4964 + 0.1488}{10 + 7} = 0.0379 \, \text{mm}^2$$

$$s_{\bar{X}_1 - \bar{X}_2} = \sqrt{\frac{s_p^2}{n_1} + \frac{s_p^2}{n_2}} = \sqrt{\frac{0.0379}{11} + \frac{0.0379}{8}} = 0.0905 \, \text{mm}$$

$$t = \frac{\bar{X}_1 - \bar{X}_2}{s_{\bar{X}_1 - \bar{X}_2}} = \frac{3.02 - 3.69}{0.0905} = -7.394$$

$p < 0.001$ and we therefore reject H_0 (critical value is $t_{0.05(2),17} = 2.11$).

---

sufficiently large and both samples are of approximately the same size. If there are large differences in sample variances (as in Fig. 6.1A), various 'approximate t' formulae are used, e.g. the *Welch approximate t*.

Warning: We should use a two-sample t test only when our aim is to compare just two samples. If we have multiple samples, we should use an analysis of variance with an additional multiple comparison procedure. In particular, we cannot compare all sample pairs using a series of t tests, because the Type I error probability is α in every such test and the individual comparisons are not mutually independent. Even if the null hypothesis is correct, the probability of finding a significant difference for at least one pair of samples is very high and grows with the number of tests performed.

6.4 Example Data

We will use the example comparing anther length between 11 diploid and 8 tetraploid individuals of a single species. This dataset is used to compare both the variances and the means – this is, in fact, the way we usually proceed (also in this order) when applying two-sample tests. This dataset is stored in the *Chap6* worksheet of the example data file. The variable *Ploidy* determines which group a particular specimen belongs to, while the variable *Anther* provides the anther length for each specimen.

6.5 How to Proceed in R

We recommend importing the data in the layout used in the *Chap6* sheet of the example data file. The resulting data frame can then be named, e.g. *chap6*.

6.5.1 *F* Test of Variance Equality

We can test the identity of variances using the *var.test* function as follows:

```
var.test( Anther~Ploidy, data=chap6)

        F test to compare two variances
data:  Anther by Ploidy
F = 2.3358, num df = 10, denom df = 7, p-value = 0.2726
alternative hypothesis: true ratio of variances is not equal to 1
95 percent confidence interval:
 0.4906053 9.2261131
sample estimates:
ratio of variances
          2.335829
```

If appropriate, we can also test a one-sided hypothesis by specifying a non-default value for the *alternative* argument ('*less*' or '*greater*'). When we need to compute the confidence interval with a coverage different from 95%, we must change the default value of the *conf.level* parameter (0.95) to the desired level (e.g. 0.99 for a 99% confidence interval).

6.5.2 Two-Sample *t* Test of the Equality of Means

The classical two-sample *t* test can be computed in the following way:

```
t.test( Anther~Ploidy, data=chap6, var.equal=T)

        Two Sample t-test
data:  Anther by Ploidy
t = -7.3944, df = 17, p-value = 1.048e-06
alternative hypothesis: true difference in means is not equal to 0
95 percent confidence interval:
 -0.8602919 -0.4783445
sample estimates:
mean in group 2n mean in group 4n
       3.018182          3.687500
```

This is a test of a two-sided (symmetrical) hypothesis; if we need to test a one-sided hypothesis, we must again choose a non-implicit value of the *alternative* parameter. If we cannot rely on the identity of variances in the two populations, we can compute the approximate Welch test:

```
t.test( Anther~Ploidy, data=chap6, var.equal=F)

        Welch Two Sample t-test
data:  Anther by Ploidy
t = -7.9052, df = 16.882, p-value = 4.5e-07
alternative hypothesis: true difference in means is not equal to 0
95 percent confidence interval:
```

```
 -0.8480473 -0.4905891
sample estimates:
mean in group 2n mean in group 4n
        3.018182        3.687500
```

We can use a confidence interval to show the difference between the means of two population samples. To obtain a confidence interval with a coverage other than 95%, we can again use the *conf.level* parameter.

Note that the same function is also used for a paired *t* test, but then the parameter *paired* must be explicitly set to *TRUE* (see Chapter 5).

We can then easily create a classified boxplot using the *plot* command in order to complement these statistical tests with a graphical presentation:

```
plot( Anther~Ploidy, data=chap6)
```

The resultant graph is shown in Fig. 6.2.

Note, however, that the individual boxplots do not display the sample statistics used in the *t* test or *F* test; the median represents the mean value (thick horizontal line within each box) and the lower and upper end of each box represents the lower and upper quartile, respectively. The following example demonstrates how to add arithmetic averages for each group to the plot, and how to improve the labelling of the groups and of the vertical axis (the label on the horizontal axis can be changed in a similar way by using the *xlab* parameter). This graph is shown in Fig. 6.3.

```
avg <- with( chap6, tapply( Anther, Ploidy, mean))
plot( Anther~Ploidy, names=c("diploids","tetraploids"),
     ylab="Anther length [mm]", data=chap6)
points( 1:2, avg, cex=2, pch=16)
```

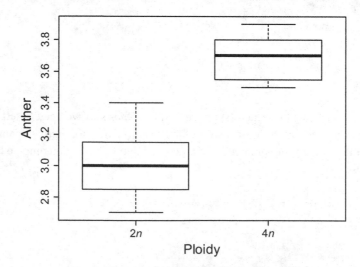

Figure 6.2 Graphical comparison of two samples using box-and-whisker plots.

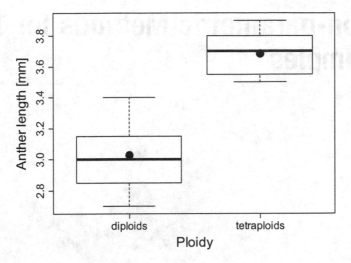

Figure 6.3 Graphical comparison of two samples using box-and-whisker plots, with customised descriptions of ploidy levels and additional solid circles representing sample arithmetic averages.

6.6 Reporting Analyses

6.6.1 Methods

We tested the homogeneity of variances between the groups of diploid and tetraploid individuals using an F-ratio test.

The difference in the mean length of anthers for diploid and tetraploid specimens was tested using a two-sample t test (with a Welch correction).

Most journals, however, consider the t test to be too trivial, so it is often sufficient to describe the results and assume that the reader will understand from the way the results are reported that a t test was performed.

6.6.2 Results

We found no differences in the variance of anther length between diploid and tetraploid plants ($F_{10,7} = 2.336$, n.s.).

Diploid individuals have significantly shorter anthers than tetraploids (means 3.0 and 3.7 mm, respectively, $t_{17} = -7.394$, $p < 0.001$).

6.7 Recommended Reading

Zar (2010), pp. 130–162.
Quinn & Keough (2002), pp. 37–42.
Sokal & Rohlf (2012), pp. 223–228 (t test) and pp. 182–190 (F test).

7 Non-parametric Methods for Two Samples

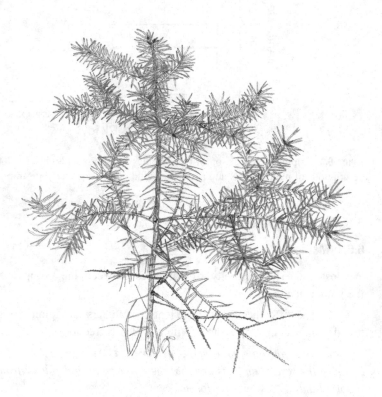

The one-sample (or paired) *t* test, two-sample *t* test, as well as the *F* test, all assume that the sampled statistical population has a normal distribution. In all these tests, we state and test hypotheses about **parameters** of this distribution. This is why we call them parametric tests. Luckily, all of them are quite robust, so that small deviations from their assumptions have a negligible effect. But what shall we do if the deviations are really large?

Essentially, we have three options for how to proceed:

1. We can use data transformations (e.g. a log-transformation) that could (under certain circumstances) change the distribution of data values so that they are sufficiently close to a normal distribution. We will handle data transformation in Chapter 10.
2. We can pick a distribution that is suitable for approximating the random variation in our data. A wide range of possibilities is available and this can be done e.g. by *generalised linear models* (GLM) that we introduce in Chapter 15.
3. Or we can use so-called non-parametric methods, discussed in this chapter, but also within parts of Chapters 8, 9 and 13.

Many of the parametric statistical methods have their non-parametric counterparts. Most of those non-parametric methods are based on the ranks (ordering) of sampled values. But another important group of non-parametric methods are those based on a permutation approach, which are also (mostly) independent of the data distribution. We will touch on permutation methods in this chapter as well.

7.1 Mann–Whitney Test

This test (sometimes with its statistic U included in the name, and sometimes also referred to as, somewhat confusingly, the Wilcoxon–Mann–Whitney test) is a non-parametric counterpart of a two-sample t test. With the Mann–Whitney test, we test a null hypothesis that both samples come from the same distribution (of whatever type). If we want to interpret the test result as a test of location[1] (which is something we usually want), we must assume that the two compared distributions have the same shape (of probability density curves). So the frequent claim that non-parametric tests have no assumptions is incorrect.[2]

To perform the test, we order the values from both samples into a single, shared ordering. From this we can then obtain ranks for all individual observations. The highest value might get a rank value of 1, while the lowest value gets the rank N ($N = n_1 + n_2$, i.e. the total number of observations within both samples). If there are groups of observations with an identical observed value (i.e. ties), we assign them the same rank value, which is the average rank in their arbitrary ordering. For example, we might follow counts of seedlings in plots with two treatments. These counts might be (the sample is too small, but it just illustrates the procedure): 17, 15, 12, 12, 12, 10. The ranks assigned to such observations will then be 1, 2, 4, 4, 4, 6, where rank 4 is an average of the implied ranks 3, 4, 5.[3] Subsequently, we use the ranks to calculate the test statistic U:

$$U = n_1 n_2 + \frac{n_1 (n_1 + 1)}{2} - R_1 \tag{7.1}$$

where R_1 is the sum of the ranks for observations in the first sample (but those ranks refer to the ordering of observations from both samples; see the description above). Analogously, we can calculate the statistic U' as

$$U' = n_1 n_2 + \frac{n_2 (n_2 + 1)}{2} - R_2 \tag{7.2}$$

where R_2 is the sum of the ranks for observations from the second sample. These two statistics are mutually related by

$$U + U' = n_1 n_2 \tag{7.3}$$

so that in practice we calculate just one of the statistics using Eq. (7.1) or Eq. (7.2) and find the other using Eq. (7.3). When performing a two-sided test (of a symmetrical hypothesis), we

---

[1] Typically, a test of median equality.

[2] On top of that, this test also assumes that the individual observations are mutually independent.

[3] As a matter of fact, rank-based methods like the Mann–Whitney test were originally developed with an assumption that all the values can be unequivocally ordered. The use of average rank is therefore just a quick fix for the problem with ties. Some rank-based methods have, however, a more precise correction for the presence of ties.

Example 7.1 Mann–Whitney test for testing a two-sided hypothesis regarding the difference in the health status of two tree cultivars.

The health status of spruce trees representing two cultivars (called here simply A and B) was subjectively assessed using a five-level scale ranging from 1 (fully healthy individual) to 5 (completely dead individual) for 20 trees, with 10 for each cultivar.
   Scores for individuals of cultivar A: 2, 2, 1, 2, 3, 4, 2, 3, 1, 5 $n_1 = 10$
   Scores for individuals of cultivar B: 4, 5, 3, 1, 4, 3, 5, 2, 1, 2 $n_2 = 10$
   H_0: The health of individuals does not differ between cultivars A and B
   H_A: The health of individuals differs between cultivars A and B
   After transforming the values into ranks (using average rank for tied values), we get

Cultivar A: 13.5, 13.5, 18.5, 13.5, 8.5, 5.0, 13.5, 8.5, 18.5, 2.0 $R_1 = 115.0$
Cultivar B: 5.0, 2.0, 8.5, 18.5, 5.0, 8.5, 2.0, 13.5, 18.5, 13.5 $R_2 = 95.0$

$$U = n_1 n_2 + n_1(n_1 + 1)/2 - R_1$$
$$= 10 \cdot 10 + 10 \cdot 11/2 - 115 = 100 + 55 - 115 = 40$$
$$U' = n_1 n_2 - U = 10 \cdot 10 - 40 = 60$$

$p = 0.481$ (exact estimate by a simulation, see above), so we cannot reject H_0.

---

select the smaller of the two statistics (U or U') and compare it with the distribution expected under the assumption that H_0 is correct. The Type I error (p) is determined in this way. In the event where we have a small sample size, we can estimate the distribution of the U statistic in an exact way by computer simulation: we can simulate all possible arrangements of the $n_1 + n_2$ values into two groups of size n_1 and n_2, respectively, and for each such arrangement we calculate the U statistic.

Example 7.1 illustrates how to compute the Mann–Whitney test for data on the health status of two spruce cultivars in a polluted city environment.

If the samples are sufficiently large (say more than 50 observations in either sample), we can assume[4] that the U statistic comes (if our H_0 is correct) from a normal distribution with mean value equal to

$$\mu_U = \frac{n_1 n_2}{2} \tag{7.4}$$

and with standard deviation equal to

$$\sigma_U = \sqrt{\frac{n_1 n_2 (N + 1)}{12}} \tag{7.5}$$

where $N = n_1 + n_2$. The value $Z = (U - \mu_U)/\sigma_U$ therefore has an approximate standardised normal distribution $N(0, 1)$. Sometimes the correction for continuity is added, and this is done by subtracting a constant value of 0.5 from the absolute value of the difference ($U - \mu_U$).

---

[4] We should recall that for large samples, the two-sample t test is quite robust to violations of the normal distribution assumption, so in many circumstances it is probably better to use the parametric test.

In contrast to a two-sample t test, we can also use the Mann–Whitney test for data on an ordinal scale, as illustrated in Example 7.1.

The Mann–Whitney test uses a null hypothesis about the identity of distributions from which the compared samples were taken. If we want to test a null hypothesis about the identity of position parameters (either median or arithmetic average), we must assume that the distributions do not differ in their shape.

Given this, you can often find a sentence, or one of its many variants, in scientific articles which states something like 'because we rejected homogeneity of variances, we opted for a non-parametric test' (in this context this would be the Mann–Whitney test). This statement is at the very least suspicious. If we find different variances, then we have no need to perform a further test of the null hypothesis that the distributions are identical (identical distributions cannot have different variances). Additionally, we should not interpret the test as a test for location because the shapes of the distributions are different. However, a non-parametric test would typically be less sensitive to differences in group variance, as it might happen that whereas the variances of the original data are very different, the rank variances of the two groups might be rather similar.

Finally, we should also be aware that the test statistics are based on ranks. So their values must be exactly the same, whether we use original data or whether we apply any monotonic transformation. Thus, the calculation of a Mann–Whitney test using log-transformed data does not do any harm, but neither does it help, because the results are exactly the same with or without the transformation.

Median test. This is a simple non-parametric method for comparing two samples by directly testing the hypothesis about the identity of the medians. We estimate the median from pooled groups and then compare the count of observations above and below this joint median estimate in each group using a χ^2 test on a 2×2 contingency table (see Section 3.1.5). This test is appropriately focused on median differences, but unfortunately it is very weak.

7.2 Wilcoxon Test for Paired Observations

While the Mann–Whitney test is a non-parametric alternative to a two-sample t test, the Wilcoxon test (often also called the Wilcoxon signed-rank test) is a non-parametric alternative to a paired t test. To perform the test, we first calculate the differences between the original (observed) paired values and eliminate the differences with a 0 value. The remaining differences are then sorted based on their <u>absolute</u> values from the smallest to the largest and replaced by their rank values in the subsequent computations (with tied ranks again replaced by an average rank value). We then calculate the sum of rank values for positive differences (T_+) and for negative differences (T_-). As the sum of a sequence of values from 1 to n is $n(n+1)/2$, we can easily calculate e.g. T_+ as $n(n+1)/2 - T_-$. The smaller value of the T_-, T_+ pair can either be compared with a known distribution of this statistic or (for larger samples) we can use an approximation by the standardised normal distribution, as we know the expected mean value

$$\mu_T = \frac{n(n+1)}{4} \tag{7.6}$$

and expected standard deviation

$$\sigma_T = \sqrt{\frac{n(n+1)(2n+1)}{24}} \tag{7.7}$$

and so we can again calculate the Z value (see above for the Mann–Whitney test procedure) and compare it with the $N(0, 1)$ normal distribution.[5]

It is important to realise that the first step of the Wilcoxon test is the calculation of differences using the original data and only then are the differences transformed into rank values. This means that when using this test, we assume that the original values can be subtracted one from another (this is why Example 7.2 uses allocated points). If we were using the Wilcoxon test of paired observations with data on an ordinal scale (e.g. the health status of spruces in Example 7.1), we would imply that there are constant differences among adjacent levels: e.g. that a difference between health status 1 and 2 (fully healthy tree vs. mostly healthy tree) is identical to the difference between e.g. health status 4 and 5 (critically ill tree vs. completely dead tree). In doing this we actually transform an ordinal scale into an interval scale. In fact, this is what we do when we calculate an average score of a pupil in school.

The use of the Wilcoxon test is illustrated in Example 7.2.

The Wilcoxon test for paired observations does not assume a normal distribution for the data under evaluation, but in contrast to the Mann–Whitney test it does assume that the

---

Example 7.2 Wilcoxon signed-rank test for data comparing the scoring of two expert groups.

Two expert groups were tasked with an evaluation of the success of agri-environmental measures on individual farms. Each group could allocate, based on a standardised protocol, 0 to 10 points to each farm. To standardise the scoring of the two groups, both were asked to independently score the same 10 farms in a pilot study. Our task is to find out whether there is a systematic difference between the two expert groups (one being more 'forgiving' than the other).

H_0: The valuation does not systematically differ between the two expert groups
H_A: The valuation systematically differs between the two expert groups
The results from 10 farms were as follows:

Expert group 1:	5, 4, 1, 8, 7, 3, 1, 0, 9, 2
Expert group 2:	7, 5, 1, 9, 6, 5, 4, 4, 10, 3
Differences:	$-2, -1, 0, -1, +1, -2, -3, -4, -1, -1$
Rank of absolute values:	6.5, 3.0, xxx (omitted), 3.0, 3.0, 6.5, 8.0, 9.0, 3.0, 3.0
Signed ranks:	$-6.5, -3.0, $ xxx$, -3.0, +3.0, -6.5, -8.0, -9.0, -3.0, -3.0$

$n=10$
$T_+ = 3.0$
$T_- = 6.5 + 3.0 + 3.0 + 6.5 + 8.0 + 9.0 + 3.0 + 3.0 = 42.0$
$p = 0.022$ so we reject H_0 and conclude that the valuation differs systematically between the two expert groups, the second group giving a systematically higher valuation.

---

[5] Again, we should consider whether a paired t test would provide a better solution.

distribution of the calculated differences is symmetrical around the median (but this assumption is often met). If this assumption is not fulfilled, one can use the **sign test** which compares the number of positive and negative differences. If the two samples do not differ, we expect the same count of positive as well as negative differences. The sign test is very weak (for our Example 7.2 we get the significance estimate $p = 0.0455$), but it comes in handy for cases when we cannot use either the paired t test or the Wilcoxon test.

7.3 Using Rank-Based Tests

There are quite different opinions among statisticians concerning the use of non-parametric tests. Some authors wish these tests were used more frequently when analysing biological data (Potvin & Roff, 1993), others (e.g. Johnson, 1995) warn against the frequently incorrect interpretation of their results (e.g. the Mann–Whitney test cannot generally be interpreted as a test of a difference between mean values) and also point to the incorrect interpretation of the assumptions of parametric tests (as an example, it is not really necessary that the analysed data have a normal distribution, this is important only for the estimated means).

Mann–Whitney and paired Wilcoxon tests are two of the most frequently used non-parametric tests, both of which have quite high power. If the assumptions of alternative parametric tests (t tests here) are fulfilled, their power is only slightly higher than that of the non-parametric tests. In contrast, if the assumptions are not met, the non-parametric tests are more reliable.

> Broadly, if you are sufficiently convinced that the assumptions of a parametric test are not violated, we recommend using the parametric test. However, the violation of those assumptions is more critical for small data samples.

7.4 Permutation Tests

The classical statistical tests (whether parametric or non-parametric) are based on an assumption that we know the distribution of the test statistic if a null hypothesis is correct, e.g. we know that a test statistic should have a t distribution with a particular number of degrees of freedom. In the case of the t test, however, it is then necessary to state certain assumptions about the distribution not only of the test statistic, but also of the unexplained variation in the data. The tests performed with so-called generalised linear models (see Chapter 15 for a brief introduction) allow us to generalise the assumptions about the distribution of unexplained variation from the normal distribution to additional distribution types, such as the Poisson or binomial distributions. But if we do not want to (or cannot) rely on the assumptions of a particular distribution, namely for the test statistic, we can simulate that distribution for a correct null hypothesis using **permutation tests**.

How can we perform a permutation test where we have to compare two samples? To demonstrate, we will use our example of anther lengths for 11 diploid and 8 tetraploid individuals (see Example 6.2). In total, we have 19 observations of anther length. We start by calculating the value of a classical t statistic based on the assignment of those 19 observations to the two groups. Next, we can imagine writing those 19 lengths onto small pieces of paper and throwing them all into a hat. Mixing them carefully, we draw 11 leaflets from the hat (ideally, we should be blindfolded) and consider them as representative of the group of diploid plants, with the remaining 8 leaflets providing values for tetraploid plants. We calculate the value of the t statistic based on this new assignment of observations into the two groups. Then we return the leaflets back to the hat, remix them and again choose 11 leaflets for the diploids (and take the remaining ones as tetraploid values), calculating the t statistic again. Now this starts to feel tiresome, although we did not yet suggest doing it another 997 times! Luckily, the random choice of values from a hat can be replaced with a computer algorithm based on generating random values, with much more reliable results.[6] If we perform the random splitting (permutation) of the 19 observed values into two groups (with 11 and 8 members) say 1000 times,[7] we will get a pretty good idea about the distribution of t statistic values in the event that the anther lengths do not differ between the two groups.

Now we have 1000 values of the t statistic (we will call them t^*_j), obtained from the randomly permuted data at hand. We should now focus primarily on estimating the percentage of cases where the absolute value of the test statistic coming from a particular permutation was equal to or larger than the absolute value of the t statistic calculated from the data with a real (correct) assignment of observations to two groups (i.e. where $|t^*_j| \geq |t|$). This percentage provides an estimate of the probability that we obtain the t statistic value (based on the true group memberships) if the null hypothesis is correct. So this is therefore the significance level of a permutation test. A more precise formula for estimating the significance level is $p = \frac{x+1}{n+1}$, where x is the number of random permutations that produced a t^*_j (absolute) value equal to or larger than the (absolute) value of the real t statistic and n is the number of random permutations performed. In our example, we suggested performing the random assignment of observed values into the two groups 1000 times, but looking at the formula (where a value of 1 is added to the number of permutations), it is hopefully obvious why some software recommends values like $n = 999$. As an example, if the value x were 14 and we had $n = 999$ random permutations, the estimate of p would be $(14 + 1)/(999 + 1) = 0.015$.

As we have worked with absolute values (ignoring the signs of the t statistics), we obtain a two-sided test (i.e. we were estimating the area of both 'tails' of the test statistic's distribution). A one-sided test would need a modification of the algorithm described above so that we do not use the absolute values and estimate the size of a single tail area, which is of interest in our alternative hypothesis. In the procedure above, we suggest an algorithm for comparing two independent samples. For each type of question, we must construct a different way of randomly permuting the data in order to address the specific null hypothesis we are testing.[8] In practice, we apply permutation tests to problems rather more complex than comparing the means of a single variable. But even in this simple example we should take care of our null hypothesis and the assumptions about our data, as we also do for rank-based tests: either we accept that we are testing the hypothesis about identical distributions for the two samples or – if we want to interpret the test results as speaking about the difference in

---

[6] To add some precision to our description, we should say that a classical computer is unable to generate truly random numbers, but it can generate so-called pseudo-random numbers which are not distinguishable from truly random numbers in the aspects that matter in our procedure.

[7] We can alternatively imagine there are 19 slots for the values, with the first 11 representing the diploid group and the remaining ones being tetraploids. Each random choice can then be seen as reordering (permuting) the collected values into a random order. This is where the label *permutation* test comes from.

[8] But, for example, to test the identity of variances we would modify our algorithm just slightly – calculating the F statistic (ratio of variances) instead of a t statistic.

positions – we must add an assumption that the distributions of the two populations represented by our two samples have the same shape.

7.5 Example Data

Data for this chapter are in the *Chap7* sheet. To illustrate the non-parametric two-sample test we will use data about the health status of two spruce cultivars (see Example 7.1). This dataset is presented in two columns, with one (*Health*) representing the health status of all individuals and the other (*Cultivar*) coding the assignment of individuals to a particular cultivar, using the labels *A* and *B*.

The non-parametric test for paired data will be demonstrated using the example comparing the judgements of two expert groups (Example 7.2). For this kind of paired data, we must specify the data in two columns, each representing a particular expert group, with the individual rows identifying the farms.

7.6 How to Proceed in R

You need to import the first two columns as one data frame (*chap7a*) and the remaining two columns as another one (*chap7b*). Somewhat confusingly, R uses the same function (named *wilcox.test*) to perform both the two-sample Mann–Whitney test and the paired-value Wilcoxon test. To differentiate these two test types, you must use the *paired = T* argument for the latter test.

7.6.1 Mann–Whitney Test

The most straightforward calculation of the Mann–Whitney test is as follows:

```
wilcox.test( Health~Cultivar, data=chap7a)
        Wilcoxon rank sum test with continuity correction
data:  Health by Cultivar
W = 40, p-value = 0.4619
alternative hypothesis: true location shift is not equal to 0
Warning message:
In wilcox.test.default(x = c(2L, 2L, 1L, 2L, 3L, 4L, 2L,
   3L, 1L,  :   cannot compute exact p-value with ties
```

The warning at the end is not a problem report (unless you consider the presence of tied values as a problem): the test is not able to calculate an exact significance level, but rather uses a Z value-based approximation. The p-value ($p = 0.4619$) provided is nevertheless similar to the one from Example 7.1, where it is reported as 0.481. Interestingly, R provides the cumulative probability function for the U statistic, so we can estimate the p-value for our two-sided test based on the reported U statistic (40) and the known size of both samples (10 and 10 observations):

```
pwilcox( 40, 10, 10) * 2
[1] 0.4812509
```

This is identical to the *p*-value reported in Example 7.1.

By default, the *wilcox.test* performs the correction for continuity when the significance value is estimated using the *Z* statistic approximation. If you do not wish to perform it, you can add the *correct = FALSE* parameter.

An interesting possibility is the calculation of a confidence interval (95% by default) for the median value of the differences between the compared samples:

```
wilcox.test( Health~Cultivar, data=chap7a, conf.int=T)
    Wilcoxon rank sum test with continuity correction
...
95 percent confidence interval:
 -2.0000486  0.9999876
sample estimates:
difference in location
          -0.03741339
```

It is not surprising that the confidence interval covers 0, as the null hypothesis about no difference is very plausible for this dataset.

7.6.2 Wilcoxon Paired Data Test

To perform this test, we must call the *wilcox.test* function with the addition of the *paired = TRUE* parameter and we must also specify the two paired samples as the first two parameters. However, when we do this, the *data* argument does not work, so we use a nested call using the *with* function:

```
with( chap7b, wilcox.test( ExpGrp1, ExpGrp2, paired=T))
    Wilcoxon signed rank test with continuity correction
data:  ExpGrp1 and ExpGrp2
V = 3, p-value = 0.02182
alternative hypothesis: true location shift is not equal to 0
Warning messages:
1: In wilcox.test.default(ExpGrp1, ExpGrp2, paired = T) :
   cannot compute exact p-value with ties
2: In wilcox.test.default(ExpGrp1, ExpGrp2, paired = T) :
   cannot compute exact p-value with zeroes
```

7.6.3 Permutation Tests

We will demonstrate the principles of constructing permutation tests in R using an example for a two-sided, two-sample test of the identity of medians. What follows is the definition of a function implementing the calculation of a test statistic (here just a plain difference of medians between the two samples) for the actual data and then repeating the same calculation under a null model, enforced on our data by randomly assigning observations into the two groups. The meaning of individual commands is hinted by the comments shown after # characters.

```
permtest.two.groups <- function( x, y, N=9999)
{
    xy      <- c( x, y)                     # pooled vector
    len1    <- length( x)                   # n1
    len2    <- length( y)                   # n2
    len12   <- len1 + len2                  # n1+n2
    # differences among group medians for each permutation
    diffs   <- numeric(N + 1)
    # observed value of the difference
    diffs[1] <- median( x) - median( y)
    for( i in 2:(N+1))
    {  # select subset corresponding to first group
       idx <- sample( 1:len12, size=len1, replace=F)
       xx  <- xy[idx]              # simulate first group
       yy  <- xy[-idx]             # simulate second group
       # median difference:
       diffs[i] <- median( xx) - median( yy)
    }
    # estimate p: how many differences greater than
    #     the observed one?
    mean( abs( diffs) >= abs( diffs[1]))
}
```

Note that we have calculated a standard difference of medians (with its sign retained), but when judging the Type I error probability, we work with absolute values of the differences (function *abs*). The last line is probably the most obscure piece of the whole implementation: the command works on the whole vector of median differences, and for each entry it determines whether its absolute value is larger than or equal to the absolute value of the first entry (which reflects the true, unpermuted arrangement). If it is, the logical comparison using the >= operator yields the value *TRUE*, which is transformed into a numerical value 1.0 by the enclosing function *mean*, while for the other entries the value *FALSE* is turned into 0.0. The function *mean* calculates the arithmetic average of those 1s and 0s, so you get the relative proportion of 1s, i.e. the relative proportion of the statistics from the permuted data larger than the real difference in medians. Because we also apply this comparison with the first entry to the first entry itself, this corresponds to the '+1' in the formula $p = (x + 1)/(n + 1)$ we have seen earlier. The random choice needed to generate a permutation is obtained with the function *sample*, which randomly selects indices of *len1* elements from the sequence from 1 to *len12*.

The above function can be used e.g. as follows:

```
with( chap7a,
      permtest.two.groups( Health[1:10], Health[11:20]))
[1]  0.6515
```

Note that we are performing a permutation test where we obtain just a random subset of, say, 9999 permutations out of all possible permutations. Therefore, when you perform this function on your computer, your *p*-value is bound to differ slightly. With a repeated call of this function, the authors were getting *p*-values like 0.6611, 0.6489, 0.6521, ...

You do not need to write your own functions in order to perform permutation tests as we have done above (although it is beneficial in order to achieve a fuller understanding of how they work). There is, for example, the package *lmPerm*, which offers permutation tests for linear methods and analysis of variance (ANOVA) models (handled in the following chapters). Here we can use the fact that a two-sample test comparing mean values is a special case of a one-way ANOVA (described in Chapter 8), where just two groups are compared. Note, however, that the following example uses permutations to test the hypothesis concerning arithmetic averages, not medians, so *health* is used as a variable on the interval scale. The two compared groups must come from distributions of similar shape and the arithmetic average must be a representative characteristic of location for both of them:

```
> library( lmPerm)
> summary( aovp( Health~Cultivar, data=chap7a, perm="Prob"))
[1] "Settings:  unique SS "
Component 1 :
              Df R Sum Sq R Mean Sq Iter Pr(Prob)
Cultivar       1    1.25    1.2500    51   0.6863
Residuals     18   34.50    1.9167
```

So there is no significant difference in health status among the two cultivars ($p = 0.6863$).

7.7 Reporting Analyses

7.7.1 Methods

To test the intensity of the health response of trees of two cultivars we used the Mann–Whitney *U* test, with the *p*-value estimated by normal approximation with a continuity correction.

Or, if we have an exact p estimate available

We used the Mann–Whitney *U* test with an exact Type I error calculation (based on enumerating all possible value assignments in the groups) to test the hypothesis ...

We used the Wilcoxon matched-pair test with the *p*-value estimated by a normal approximation in order to test for differences between the judgements of two expert groups.

7.7.2 Results

The distribution of health status values does not differ significantly between two compared cultivars ($Z = -0.7357$, n.s.).

We found a significant difference between two expert groups in their scoring of the success of agri-environmental measures ($Z = 2.311$, $p = 0.0218$).

7.8 Recommended Reading

Zar (2010), pp. 162–178 and pp. 183–188.

Quinn & Keough (2002), pp. 45–48.

Sokal & Rohlf (2012), pp. 446–452 and pp. 463–465.

D. H. Johnson (1995) Statistical sirens: the allure of nonparametrics. *Ecology*, **76**: 1998–2000.

C. Potvin & D. A. Roff (1993) Distribution-free and robust statistical methods: viable alternatives to parametric statistics? *Ecology*, **74**: 1617–1628.

8   One-Way Analysis of Variance (ANOVA) and Kruskal–Wallis Test

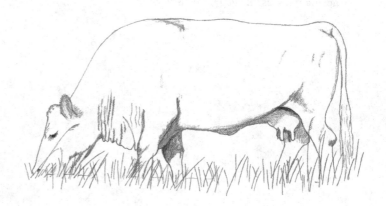

8.1 Use Case Examples

The following research tasks are representative of the problems solved with the one-way ANOVA method. We will introduce an example for the Kruskal–Wallis test in Example 8.2 (Section 8.10).

1. We want to explore the effect of substrate on the height of individuals of a certain plant species. Out of 15 pots in a greenhouse experiment: 5 were filled with sandy soil; 5 were filled with loamy soil; 5 were filled with a peat-based substrate. A single seedling was planted in each pot and grown for 8 weeks. Plant heights were then measured at the end of the experiment. We ask whether plant heights differ among the groups defined by the pot substrate.
2. We obtained red fescue seeds from five different populations. The plants germinated from these seeds were grown under comparable conditions (each individual in a separate pot). We then measured the number of tillers for each individual. Does the studied characteristic differ between groups of plants coming from different populations?
3. We need to compare the protein content of milk from three cattle breeds kept at the same farm. Milk from 10 individuals of each breed was collected on the same day and we determined the protein content. Does it differ between the three breeds?

8.2 ANOVA: A Method for Comparing More Than Two Means

As we have seen in Chapter 6, we can use a two-sample t test to compare the means of two groups. But when we compare more than two means, the t test (performed in a pairwise manner for all possible pairs) is not appropriate. This is because the Type I error probability has the value α in each pairwise comparison, and so the probability that we find at least one significant difference among the pairs is substantially higher than α, even when the null hypothesis is correct (and so there are no real differences among the means). For example, if we have four groups and carry out t tests for all of the six possible pairings using a nominal level $\alpha = 0.05$, the probability that we find at least one significant difference is 0.21, and this probability increases further with an increasing number of groups.

We must use an **analysis of variance** (usually called **ANOVA**) if we want to test a null hypothesis $H_0: \mu_1 = \mu_2 = \ldots = \mu_k$, where k is the number of observation groups being compared. The ANOVA model is actually much more general, so much so that it could even be considered an entire research field in its own right. As such, it is able to test much more complex hypotheses than the H_0 presented above: we use the **one-way ANOVA** or **single-factor ANOVA** for this simple type of hypothesis. The ANOVA model is part of an even wider group of statistical methods, most often called **general linear models** (see Section 14.4).

In our first example in Section 8.1, the individual observations (plants) are classified by type of substrate. In this context, we often refer to the substrate types as **factor levels**.[1] In this simple form of experimental design, each experimental group (in this case the five pots with an identical substrate type) is a random sample that is independent of other samples (groups). So we speak about a **completely randomised experimental design**.

We can judge differences among the groups only if we know the variability of the data within the groups. The principle of the (one-way) ANOVA method can be simply explained in the following way. We test the null hypothesis that there is no difference between group means. As the ANOVA test assumes the identity of group variances, we can imagine that if the null hypothesis is correct, the k groups of observations are in fact k random samples from the same statistical population. We can then estimate the variance of that population using the variance of the values within individual groups. Using this joint within-group variance estimate, we can predict the expected variation among the groups. This prediction can then be compared with the observed among-group variation. If the observed among-group variation is improbably large (we ascertain this using an F test), we must reject the null hypothesis about the equality of group means.

8.3 Test Assumptions

The primary assumption of the one-way ANOVA F test is that each group of observations represents a random sample of independent observations, chosen from a particular statistical population with a normal distribution and a constant variance that is unchanging across the groups. This is important as we expect our F test statistic to come from an F distribution. If the variances are different, the resulting F does not follow an F distribution, even when the null hypothesis is correct.

The requirement that individual groups come from statistical populations with an identical variance (σ^2) – referred to as the **homogeneity of variances** (or *homoscedasticity*) – is most frequently checked by **Bartlett's test**. This test uses the following test statistic:

---

[1] We can use a *factor* variable (often also called a *categorical* variable) to sort our observations into two or more groups (categories, such as substrate type, sampling location, breed of cow, etc.). Each group of observations has its own label (e.g. sandy soil, loamy soil, peaty soil for the substrate type factor) and we call those labels the *factor levels* in the context of statistical models such as ANOVA.

$$\chi^2 = \frac{(N-k)\ln\left(s_p^2\right) - \sum_{i=1}^{k}(n_i-1)\ln\left(s_i^2\right)}{1+\dfrac{1}{3(k-1)}\left(\sum_{i=1}^{k}\left(\dfrac{1}{n_i-1}\right)-\dfrac{1}{N-k}\right)} \tag{8.1}$$

where N is the total number of observations, n_i is the observation count in the i-th group, k is the number of compared groups, $s^2{}_i$ is the sample variance in the i-th group, $s^2{}_p$ is the pooled estimate of the within-group variance, calculated as $s_p^2 = \sum_{i=1}^{k}(n_i-1)s_i^2/(N-k)$ and ln is the natural log. The χ^2 statistic of Bartlett's test is compared with the χ^2_{k-1} distribution. This support test should be used with caution, however, as it is sensitive to departures from a normal distribution for our observations (if that happens, it is actually testing the normality).

8.4 Sum of Squares Decomposition and the *F* Statistic

We assume that our observations are split into k groups (sometimes called classes) so that for an observed variable X, its value for the j-th observation in group i (i ranging from 1 to k) is marked as X_{ij}. In example 1, $X_{2,4}$ is therefore the height of the fourth plant in the second experimental group (in pots with loamy soil). The number of observations in the i-th group is n_i, and the total number of observations in the dataset is $N = \sum_{i=1}^{k}n_i$. The average value in the i-th group is labelled as $\overline{X}_i$, the overall average value is $\overline{X}$. A core principle of the one-way ANOVA test is the comparison of variation within groups with the variation among groups. The variation within groups is characterised by the mean square of the deviation of observed values from a group's mean (*within-group mean square*), often also called the *residual mean square* or *error mean square* (MS_E). To calculate it, we first calculate the sum-of-squares deviation of observed values from the mean of the group to which the values belong – this is the *residual sum of squares* (RSS) or *error sum of squares* (SS_E):

$$SS_E = \sum_{i=1}^{k}\sum_{j=1}^{n_i}\left(X_{ij}-\overline{X}_i\right)^2 \tag{8.2}$$

The degrees of freedom corresponding to this sum (df_E) is the sum of the degrees of freedom within individual groups:

$$df_E = \sum_{i=1}^{k}(n_i-1) = N-k \tag{8.3}$$

The error mean square is then the sum of squares divided by the degrees of freedom:

$$MS_E = \frac{SS_E}{df_E} \tag{8.4}$$

and MS_E is an estimate of the variance σ^2 shared by all groups. It is useful to recall that we estimated the shared variance in the t test in a similar way, and also that our assumption of identical variance in the compared groups is similar to the assumption of a two-sample t test.

Variability <u>among</u> the groups is characterised by the mean square among the groups (MS_G) calculated from the among-group sum of squares (SS_G) with the aid of the among-group degrees of freedom (df_G). The following equations provide formulas for the calculation of these statistics:

$$SS_G = \sum_{i=1}^{k} n_i (\overline{X}_i - \overline{X})^2 \tag{8.5}$$

$$df_G = k - 1 \tag{8.6}$$

$$MS_G = \frac{SS_G}{df_G} \tag{8.7}$$

It is possible to demonstrate that if the null hypothesis (about the identity of group means) is correct, then MS_G is also an estimate of the shared variance σ^2. But if the null hypothesis is not correct, then the variation among the means (MS_G) is much larger than the variation within the groups (MS_E). We can use an **F test** to compare these two variance estimates.[2] So if the null hypothesis is correct, the test statistic $F = MS_G/MS_E$ comes from an F distribution with corresponding degrees of freedom df_G, df_E. As in the statistical tests introduced earlier, we can use the comparison of the F statistic with a given distribution in order to determine the probability that we can obtain such a large (or larger) F value if the null hypothesis is correct. This probability represents the achieved significance level p and as usual, if this p is smaller than an *a priori* chosen α (e.g. 0.05) then we reject the null hypothesis.

Often when the results of an ANOVA are displayed in statistical software there will also be another sum of squares shown. This is the *total sum of squares* (SS_{TOT}) together with the corresponding degrees of freedom (df_{TOT}):

$$SS_{TOT} = \sum_{i=1}^{k} \sum_{j=1}^{n_i} (X_{ij} - \overline{X})^2 \tag{8.8}$$

$$df_{TOT} = N - 1 \tag{8.9}$$

These two statistics can be combined together by a division (SS_{TOT}/df_{TOT}) and this is the usual variance estimate (s^2) for the whole dataset as if it were not split into distinct groups.

Although neither SS_{TOT} nor df_{TOT} are used when calculating the F statistic, they are usually shown in the ANOVA model summary and they were traditionally used for calculations due to their relation with the two components:

$$SS_{TOT} = SS_G + SS_E \tag{8.10}$$

$$df_{TOT} = df_G + df_E \tag{8.11}$$

We demonstrate how the one-way ANOVA test can be applied to our data in Example 8.1.

---

[2] We already used the F test to compare the variance estimates of two random samples (see Section 6.2).

Example 8.1 Calculating a one-way ANOVA test.

We use the data from example 1 of Section 8.1. The plant heights were (cm):

Sandy soil: 15, 16, 18, 15, 21
Loamy soil: 21, 20, 18, 25, 26
Peat: 22, 26, 27, 30, 29

We first calculate the averages:

$\overline{X}_1 = 17, \overline{X}_2 = 22, \overline{X}_3 = 26.8$, total average $\overline{X} = 21.9333$

The df value is 4 in each group:

$df_E = 4 + 4 + 4 = 12 (= 15 - 3)$

$df_G = 3 - 1 = 2$

$SS_E = (15 - 17)^2 + (16 - 17)^2 + (18 - 17)^2 + \ldots + (21 - 22)^2 + \ldots + (30 - 26.8)^2 + (29 - 26.8)^2 = 110.8$

$SS_G = 5 \times (17 - 21.9333)^2 + 5 \times (22 - 21.9333)^2 + 5 \times (26.8 - 21.9333)^2 = 240.13$

$MS_G = 240.13/2 = 120.07$

$MS_E = 110.8/12 = 9.23$

$F = MS_G/MS_E = 120.07/9.23 = 13.00$

The probability of obtaining an F value of 13.0 or larger from an $F_{2,12}$ distribution is equal to 0.00099. We therefore reject the null hypothesis about the identity of mean values in the three compared groups.

When we reject the null hypothesis of a one-way ANOVA, this only implies that at least one of the means differs, i.e. not *all* means are identical. However, the result of the *F* test does not identify which means differ. In order to get some idea about this, we must apply an additional statistical technique called *multiple comparisons*.

8.5 ANOVA for Two Groups and the Two-Sample *t* Test

We can also use the one-way ANOVA for two groups ($k = 2$), i.e. to compare two means. In this case the result (the *p*-value) is completely identical to the result of a two-sided two-sample *t* test. But when we use an ANOVA we cannot test a one-sided hypothesis and neither can we test a null hypothesis H$_0$: $\mu_1 - \mu_2 = c$ if *c* is different from zero (we can do this with a *t* test, however). The two-sample *t* test also offers a direct adjustment for the violation of the requirement of identical variances (see Section 6.3).[3]

8.6 Fixed and Random Effects

There are two basic models of ANOVA: the **fixed effect model** (also known as *model I*) and the **random effect model** (also known as *model II*). Examples 1 and 3 in Section 8.1 illustrate

[3] It is only fair to note that a modification of the *F* test for a one-way ANOVA, designed to account for unequal group variances, has also been described. This method is not so widely used however.

models with fixed effects. In example 1 we ask how the chosen substrate types affect plant height: we are only interested in the particular substrates defined in our experiment. Similarly, in example 3 we are only interested in comparing those three particular breeds of cattle.

However, in example 2 we ask whether the chosen morphological characteristic might differ among populations of that species. The five populations (locations) are just a random subset (sample) from many possible populations. Our task is not to find out whether the fescue plants from population B differ from those coming from population D, but to demonstrate that there might be a systematic difference among the various populations of the same species. The computations are identical for the two types of ANOVA model when our sampling design leads to a one-way ANOVA. But once we start to work with more complicated ANOVA models (see the following chapters), the calculations will differ.

Our decision on whether a factor represents a fixed or random effect depends on the context and the questions we are asking. The following rule of thumb can be used to come to this decision. If you carry out the same type of experiment again in order to answer the same question and you use identical factor levels, this factor should very probably be considered as a factor with a fixed effect (the same breeds of cow, the same soil types). On the contrary, if different levels of the factor may be chosen to answer the same question, the factor represents a random effect (you can use different populations of fescue to test the inter-population differences).

The twenty-first century saw an enormous expansion in the use of statistical models which include random effects. They represent not only the various models of analysis of variance, but also extend the family of general linear models (with the explanatory variables representing both categorical and quantitative data), as well as the generalised linear models. The models including both random and fixed effects are usually called **mixed effect models** (with two particular groups being the *linear mixed effect models*, *LMM* and the *generalised linear mixed effect models*, *GLMM*). Our example of an analysis of variance with just a single random effect and no fixed effect is the simplest form of a linear mixed effect model.[4]

Proponents of the mixed effect model methodology view the concept of degrees of freedom for random effects in a particular way. To illustrate this, we take a look at our example 2 (differences of a morphological parameter of red fescue among localities). In the eyes of a mixed effect model proponent, we would consider the random effect of locality as a model parameter specified by a single value, namely the estimate of variation of population means around the overall mean.[5]

8.7 *F* Test Power

As in the tests introduced earlier, we must realise that a non-significant outcome for an ANOVA *F* test suggests that either the mean values in the sampled populations are identical or that a Type II error occurred. While we know the probability of the Type I error (due to our *a priori* stated α level), we do not know the probability of the Type II error. But one can

---

[4] Strictly speaking, this model is too simple to be called a mixed effect model, as the 'mixing' part refers to a combination of fixed and random effects. But we often start our modelling with such a simple model type.

[5] We assume that those deviations come from a normal distribution $N(0, s^2_A)$ and so we use just a single degree of freedom for a random effect of population, whereas we would use $df = 4$ for a fixed effect.

estimate this probability under certain assumptions. Such an estimate is recommended when planning any extensive or complex experiment. The estimation procedure is quite complicated, but nicely described in the textbooks of Zar (2010, pp. 207–211) and Sokal & Rohlf (2012, pp. 390–395). For a one-way ANOVA model, R provides an easy-to-use function *power.anova.test*, which is described in Section 8.12.3.

For a start, it is good to remember that the test power increases with sample size and with the increasing differences among group means, but the power decreases with increasing variability within groups and with the number of groups. The test power also decreases when group sizes become increasingly unbalanced.

As an example of the use of test power analysis, let us imagine we want to increase the number of substrate types being compared in example 1 of Section 8.1. Limited resources imply we cannot afford more than 50 pots in our experiment. If we have an idea about the variability of height among the substrate types and about the height variability among plants grown on the same substrate types, we can calculate how many substrate types we can use to achieve the test power of at least 0.95 (i.e. 95%).

8.8 Violating ANOVA Assumptions

As we have seen in Section 8.3, an ANOVA test assumes data normality (within the groups) and homogeneity (identity) of variances (among the groups). We can test both assumptions – for normality we should test the normal distribution of model residuals, while for the homogeneity of variances we most often use the Bartlett test. Luckily, an ANOVA test is fairly robust against violations of either assumption. Perhaps more importantly, the desired outcome of the tests verifying these assumptions is that they are non-significant (i.e. when we cannot reject the null hypothesis about an agreement with a normal distribution or about the homogeneity of variances). When we are dealing with small data samples (when e.g. the Bartlett test is very weak), it might easily happen that a non-significant result will lure us into a false sense of assurance. In contrast, with a large number of observations even a minute violation of the assumption (for which the ANOVA test would be sufficiently robust) will lead to a significant test outcome, causing us to worry about how to handle the 'problem'. All in all, we recommend a visual inspection of the model residuals rather than performing formal tests of model assumptions. For data on a ratio scale (height, weight), the standard deviation is often dependent on the mean (which violates the homogeneity of variance assumption). It might be useful just to visually check whether standard deviations and means are independent across the groups.

A valid use of an ANOVA model does **not** require the same counts of observations across the groups. Nevertheless, when there are large differences between group sizes, ANOVA loses its robustness towards violating the requirement for the homogeneity of variances. In addition, we lose some test power. This is why we should strive to have all of our groups equally sized (at least when we compare all groups in a symmetrical manner, i.e. every group mean with all others, see Section 8.9.2) when planning our experiment or observation. If all groups in our data have the same size then we say that the design is balanced.

The larger the size of our groups, the more robust our test will be against violations of the assumption of normality within groups. If the normality assumption is extensively violated, we can employ data transformations (see Chapter 10), use a non-parametric alternative to ANOVA (Kruskal–Wallis test for one-way design, see Section 8.10) or use a generalised linear model. The last option would probably be appropriate for the data outlined in example 2: if the mean count of tillers was low, we could hardly consider it a continuous variable with a normal distribution and so it would be better to use a generalised linear model with an assumed Poisson distribution for the random variation.

8.9 Multiple Comparisons

A significant result (i.e. a rejection of the null hypothesis) in an ANOVA F test informs us that at least one of the compared means is different from the others. But there might be multiple significant differences among the group means. If our model uses a factor with a fixed effect,[6] then we will be interested in identifying where the means differ. To accomplish this we can use the **multiple comparisons** procedure.

The usual protocol starts with an ANOVA F test, after which we proceed with multiple comparisons only when we reject the null hypothesis. Because they are performed after the actual ANOVA test and are not based on any specific *a priori* hypothesis about which of the groups will differ, we call them *a posteriori comparisons* (or *post hoc tests*). In contrast, when we have intentions of performing a particular subset of comparisons even before we collect the data, corresponding to a more specific alternative hypothesis than just a statement like 'some mean(s) will differ', we perform *planned comparisons* (or *planned contrasts* or *a priori comparisons*) providing stronger statistical tests. We will not discuss them in this introductory text, but see for example Sokal & Rohlf (2012, pp. 228–237) or Quinn & Keough (2002, pp. 197–199).

When performing multiple comparisons, we are in fact dealing with a problem which is quite common in the practical application of statistical methods. The results obtained from a particular experiment or observation allow us to answer more than a single research question and so we are likely to perform more than one statistical test with our data. But if we set the acceptable probability of Type I error to the level α in each test, the probability that we commit at least one Type I error (i.e. we find a significant difference even though the null hypotheses are correct) while evaluating the whole experiment will be much higher. We must then decide whether we want to control the frequency (probability) of Type I errors in individual tests (*comparison-wise Type I error rate*) or whether we want to control it across the whole experiment (*experiment-wise Type I error rate*). The former approach will lead (at least for a larger number of tests) to the existence of many 'false positive' results.[7]

On the contrary, if we decide to control the Type I error across an experiment where many hypotheses are being tested, we need to be very demanding in individual tests and this will naturally lead to very weak tests, with our conclusions heavily affected by Type II errors (i.e. we miss many of the existing deviations from the null hypotheses). Therefore we usually control for the frequency of Type I errors within groups of logically related tests – e.g. when comparing all levels of one of the tested factors, as discussed in this section, or when selecting

---

[6] That is, if each group of observations is clearly defined and the groups do not represent a random sample from a much larger set of possible groups.

[7] Representing a situation sometimes jokingly labelled *statistical fishing*.

explanatory variables for a particular regression model (see Chapter 14). This approach is usually called *family-wise Type I error rate*.

There are several methods of multiple comparisons and this fact itself suggests that none of them is an ideal solution to the problem. Here we will demonstrate one that is generally accepted and available in most statistical programs – Tukey's HSD test (Section 8.9.1). From the others, we recommend the SNK (Student–Newman–Keuls) test and Scheffé's test. Both have the nice property of being constructed in such a way that the probability of Type I error in at least one of the partial tests is equal to the chosen significance level.

Aside from the multiple comparison procedures comparing all possible pairs of means, there is one alternative task: we compare all possible treatments with a control treatment only. This far more selective form of multiple comparisons is supported by Dunnett's test, described in Section 8.9.2.

Multiple comparisons assume that we work with an ANOVA model I, i.e. with a model containing fixed effects. If we compare three selected cattle breeds, we are naturally interested in where the differences, if any, lie. But if our task is to demonstrate that populations of a grass species collected from five randomly selected locations differ (i.e. a model II ANOVA), we do not test the differences among individual locations. If we get a significant result from a model II ANOVA, we sometimes estimate the relative effects on the variation (e.g. the relative size of the variability within locations and among locations), and these are known as *variance components*. Alternatively, these relative effects are expressed by an *intraclass correlation coefficient*.[8]

In everyday practice, sometimes it can be difficult to decide whether we are dealing with a situation that warrants a model I or a model II approach. Let us go back to the red fescue example. Under some circumstances, we can consider the five locations to be a random sample from a much larger set of locations; in this case we are not interested in specific differences, just in the extent of variability among and within the locations. But we often have additional information about the locations being compared and thus it might be interesting to state the locations that actually differ. In this circumstance, we would consider the location effect as fixed and if we find it to be significant, we would perform a multiple comparisons procedure on its levels.

When we compare populations of a particular species, readers of our report might be interested to find that populations from nearby locations do not differ, but a population from a more distant place does. However, let us now imagine we are carrying out a study comparing the offspring of eight randomly selected maternal plants that we know nothing about. If we specify in our paper that the offspring of individuals 1, 3 and 8 do not differ, but this group is different from the offspring of individuals 2, 4, 5, 6 and 7, this information is almost worthless to our readers: given the random choice of maternal individuals, those labeled 1, 3 and 8 could also simply be labeled 4, 5 and 7. But the fact that we get two well-separated groups (or, alternatively, that the offspring of individual parents have relatively constant values of the investigated parameter, but the means for individual parents cover the overall range of variation) can be communicated as useful information.

---

[8] For an intraclass correlation coefficient (ICC), the value 1.0 means that all observations are identical within the classes and only the classes differ, while the value 0.0 means that there are no differences among the classes – all variation happens within the classes (see Sokal & Rohlf, 2012, pp. 216–218).

Sometimes a class of observations is indicated by the results of multiple comparisons to belong to more than one group of mutually indistinguishable classes. In this event we might be tempted to interpret such overlaps. What we should recall, however, is that the overlaps between groups of factor levels are a consequence of committing a Type II error and this is the way to interpret them (see also the following Section 8.9.1).

8.9.1 Tukey's Test

We perform Tukey's test (also known as *Tukey's HSD*[9] *test*) analogously to a two-sample t test. The t statistic is replaced here by the q statistic, which can be calculated for any pair of means of groups i and j as

$$q = \frac{\overline{X}_i - \overline{X}_j}{SE} \tag{8.12}$$

where SE is the standard error of the estimated difference between the means of groups i and j, calculated as

$$SE = \sqrt{\frac{s^2}{2}\left(\frac{1}{n_i} + \frac{1}{n_j}\right)} \tag{8.13}$$

with s^2 being the estimate of shared variance – the residual (within-group) mean square MS_E from the analysis of variance (see Eq. (8.4)) and n_i, n_j are the observation counts in groups i, j. Please note that s^2 is computed using the variation within all groups, not just of the two currently being compared. Remember that we assume homogeneity of variances and that the recommendation that all groups should be of equal size is even more important for multiple comparisons than it is for the main ANOVA F test.

The q statistic comes (assuming the null hypothesis H_0: $\mu_i = \mu_j$ is correct) from its own specific distribution, parameterised by two values – the number of groups k and the residual degrees of freedom of the ANOVA model. R software offers specific functions to obtain cumulative probabilities (*ptukey*) or quantiles (*qtukey*) of this distribution.

The alternative *SNK test* is calculated similarly; in the SNK test, we order group means by their size and the critical value depends on the difference between these mean rankings, not on the total count of compared means. The SNK test is more powerful than Tukey's test, but it has a higher Type I error probability. It is said that the true Type I error probability is higher than the chosen α level for the SNK test and lower than the α for Tukey's test, but it is very difficult to state it more precisely.

We can present the results of multiple comparisons either as text or graphically in several ways. In the first case, we can display group means ordered by their value in a table and flag the absence of significant differences by using the same letter or by putting an asterisk or cross into a particular column.[10] Alternatively, we can create a square table comparing each factor level with all others,[11] or we can calculate and graph confidence intervals for the

---

[9] HSD stands for honestly significant difference.

[10] There will be as many columns of asterisks/crosses as there are number of separate groups of non-different levels. This count also matches the number of letters used for the alternative display method.

[11] But the information provided in such a table is mirrored across the main diagonal (difference between groups i and j is the same as between groups j and i), so typically the table space is not very efficiently used.

differences among group means. Any graph displaying individual group means (using symbols or bars) can also be supplemented by letters, where each letter labels the set of levels with non-different means. Some of the possibilities are illustrated alongside their corresponding commands in R in Section 8.12.2.

We encounter the following situation quite often when using multiple comparisons. We might be comparing, say, three groups of observations (representing three factor levels) and we find that group 1 differs from group 3, but group 2 does not differ from either group 1 or group 3. This is not logical and is very likely a consequence of committing a Type II error. The frequency of these errors increases with the number of compared means. We should realise that a report on multiple comparisons does not portray just the real difference, but also the degree of uncertainty about the truth caused by an insufficient sample size. Sometimes it also happens that although the main ANOVA F test is significant, the multiple comparisons do not identify even a single significant difference. This is also a consequence of the lower power of the multiple comparisons procedure compared with that of the F test itself. Under such circumstances we may expect that an experiment (or observation) with a larger number of observations would likely bring significant results, even for the multiple comparisons.

Also, as already noted, the power of the ANOVA F test decreases as the number of groups increases. This decrease in power is even more pronounced in Tukey's test (and other multiple comparison methods). This might lead to a paradoxical situation. Imagine that we are comparing, say, the amount of nuclear DNA in three species of buttercups (e.g. *Ranunculus acris*, *R. auricomus*, *R. nemorosus*), with each species represented by five populations from some selected area, using an ANOVA and a follow-up Tukey's test. After securing some additional funding, we decide to sample five populations of an additional species (say *R. bulbosus*) and re-analyse the data using all four species. If the differences were not very pronounced, but still significant in the original analysis, it might happen that some pairs of species that were significantly different in the original analysis will not be different any more, despite the fact that the data for them are exactly the same.

8.9.2 Dunnett's Test

If we want to compare a single reference level (*control level*) with multiple experimental treatments, we should use Dunnett's test. Let us take the example of a study of proposed changes in land management on farms, designed to encourage a higher abundance of song birds. The standard farm management will be taken as control and left running unaltered in a group of farms, while the new suggested measures (e.g. sown weed margins, stubble kept on grain fields until spring, planting of hedges) would be alternatives imposed on groups of other, randomly selected farms. If our task is to choose just a single, most effective one of the alternative measures then we will be interested in comparing them against the standard practice (control) rather than comparing them against the alternative measures.

Let us assume that we are comparing group i with the control group (*Ctrl*). The value of q for Dunnett's test is calculated the same way as it is for Tukey's test (Eq. (8.12)):

$$q = \frac{\overline{X}_i - \overline{X}_{Ctrl}}{SE} \tag{8.14}$$

where *SE* is the standard error of the difference between the means for groups *i* and *Ctrl*. We calculate it as

$$SE = \sqrt{\frac{s^2}{2}\left(\frac{1}{n_i} + \frac{1}{n_{Ctrl}}\right)} \tag{8.15}$$

The meaning of the symbols is analogous to Eqs (8.12) and (8.13). If we have an idea about the desired direction of change due to the type of treatment (we are striving to <u>increase</u> song bird abundance and/or their diversity in our example), it is advantageous to use a one-sided test. The power of Dunnett's test is higher than for multiple comparisons performed for each possible pair of groups, as we are performing a smaller number of comparisons. Because the control treatment enters the test multiple times (unlike the other levels), it is a good idea to estimate its mean more precisely. Therefore it is recommended that the number of observations in the control group should be roughly $\sqrt{k-1}$ times higher than in the other groups (*k* is the total count of groups, including the control) and that the other groups should not differ in their size.

8.10 Non-parametric ANOVA: Kruskal–Wallis Test

Data that can be appropriately analysed using a one-way ANOVA test (i.e. data from a completely randomised experimental design) can, alternatively, be tested using a non-parametric test based on ranks. This test is known as the **Kruskal–Wallis test** (sometimes also called *Kruskal–Wallis ANOVA* or *analysis of variance by ranks*). Like Mann–Whitney's test being a non-parametric counterpart of the two-sample *t* test, the Kruskal–Wallis test is a counterpart of the one-way ANOVA. But if we are comparing two groups only, the Mann–Whitney test is recommended instead.[12]

If the assumptions of the one-way ANOVA are met (data normality and homogeneity of variances), the power of the Kruskal–Wallis test is roughly 95% of the power of the parametric ANOVA. But the non-parametric test can be used, in some cases, when the ANOVA assumptions are violated. Additionally, we can use it for data on an ordinal scale.

The test is performed in the following way. First we rank all observations (irrespective of the group they belong to) based on their size. Then we calculate the *H* statistic as

$$H = (N - 1)\frac{\sum_{i=1}^{k} n_i(r_i - r)^2}{\sum_{i=1}^{k}\sum_{j=1}^{n_i}(r_{ij} - r)^2} \tag{8.16}$$

where n_i is the number of observations in group *i*, *N* is the total number of observations in our dataset, *k* is the number of groups, r_{ij} is the (global) rank of the *j*-th observation from the *i*-th group, r_i is the average rank for observations of group *i* and *r* is the total average rank in the data (equal to $(N+1)/2$). If the null hypothesis is correct, the *H* statistic has (approximately) the χ^2 distribution with $k-1$ degrees of freedom. The calculation of the Kruskall–Wallis test is illustrated in Example 8.2. We can also perform multiple comparisons after obtaining a significant result from the test, see Zar (2010, pp. 239–243).

---

[12] Although the one-way ANOVA with two groups gives identical results as a two-sample *t* test, the results for the Kruskal–Wallis test with two groups may differ from the results of the Mann–Whitney test.

Example 8.2 Kruskal–Wallis test (analysis of variance by ranks) for opinion poll data.

We need to evaluate the results of an opinion poll asking the residents of three settlement types about their attitude towards species extinctions on Earth. Possible answers had to be chosen from an ordinal scale: 0 for 'not a problem', 1 for 'a small issue without importance for humans', ..., 10 for 'a very serious problem endangering the existence of humans on Earth'. The respondents were randomly selected from three contrasting settlement types: large industrial towns, small towns without any extensive industry, villages (with up to 10,000 inhabitants). Does the attitude of respondents differ depending on the type of settlement they live in?

H_0: The attitude towards species extinctions does not differ among the three compared groups

H_A: The attitude towards species extinctions differs among the three compared groups

The collected data were as follows:

Industrial towns: 1, 0, 2, 1, 4
Small towns: 5, 7, 9, 5, 6, 4
Villages: 7, 9, 6, 8, 5, 5

When we replace the values with their global ranks (or rank averages for tied observations), we get

Industrial towns: 2.5, 1.0, 4.0, 2.5, 5.5
Small towns: 8.5, 13.5, 16.5, 8.5, 11.5, 5.5
Villages: 13.5, 16.5, 11.5, 15.0, 8.5, 8.5

$N = 5 + 6 + 6 = 17$
$H = 16(254.09/400.5) = 10.15098$
$p = 0.00625$ (comparing with χ^2_2).

So we reject the null hypothesis.

When interpreting the results of Example 8.2, we must be aware that it is risky to interpret the results as an effect of living environment on attitude. Perhaps the causality is directed in the opposite way, e.g. people respecting nature might try to avoid a life in industrial towns.

8.11 Example Data

To illustrate the classical one-way ANOVA, we will use example 1 from Section 8.1, which asks whether plant height is affected by substrate type (see also Example 8.1). You will find the data in the *Chap8* sheet of the example data file: the variable *Height* gives the plant height (cm), while the variable *Substrate* identifies the substrate in which each plant grew.

To illustrate how we can test a random effect, we will use the following data, which is somewhat similar to the second example of Section 8.1. In a project where genetically determined plant size variability was compared among different populations of red fescue (*Festuca rubra*), seeds from individual populations were germinated and individual plants were grown in comparable conditions. After two months the length of the longest tiller (cm) was determined. The lengths for individual plants are given in the *Till.Len* variable, while the *Population* variable identifies the population from which the plant originates.

The Kruskal–Wallis test will be illustrated with the data from Example 8.2. The settlement type is given by the *Settlement* factor, while the response is given by the *Importance* variable.

8.12 How to Proceed in R

Given the different number of observations, the last two columns of the *Chap8* sheet were imported into a separate data frame (*chap8b*), while the first four variables were imported into a data frame named *chap8a*.

8.12.1 One-Way ANOVA

We first illustrate how to check the homogeneity of variances using Bartlett's test:

```
bartlett.test( Height~Substrate, data=chap8a)

        Bartlett test of homogeneity of variances
data:  Height by Substrate
Bartlett's K-squared = 0.29587, df = 2, p-value = 0.8625
```

Based on these results, we cannot reject the null hypothesis that the three groups come from populations with identical variance, which is a conclusion allowing us to progress to fitting a one-way ANOVA model. Most of the variants of the classical ANOVA (including those handled in the following chapters) can be estimated with the *aov* function. The object returned from *aov* represents the fitted ANOVA model and can be passed to additional functions to obtain the traditional ANOVA table or to perform multiple comparisons:

```
aov.1 <- aov( Height~Substrate, data=chap8a)
summary( aov.1)

            Df Sum Sq Mean Sq F value   Pr(>F)
Substrate    2  240.1  120.07      13 0.000991 ***
Residuals   12  110.8    9.23
---
Signif. codes:  0 '***' 0.001 '**' 0.01 '*' 0.05 '.' 0.1 ' ' 1
```

The *p*-value suggests that the mean plant height from at least one substrate differs from the mean height in other substrate type(s). Now we can find which differences are involved in the deviation of our data from the null hypothesis with the aid of a multiple comparisons procedure.

8.12.2 Multiple Comparisons

Tukey's HSD method is available in an accessible form in the *TukeyHSD* function:

```
TukeyHSD( aov.1, which="Substrate")
   Tukey multiple comparisons of means
     95% family-wise confidence level
Fit: aov(formula = Height ~ Substrate, data = chap8a)
$`Substrate`
            diff        lwr        upr      p adj
sand-peat -9.8 -14.9271129 -4.6728871 0.0007081
soil-peat -4.8  -9.9271129  0.3271129 0.0672929
soil-sand  5.0  -0.1271129 10.1271129 0.0561479
```

We have specified the *which* parameter to identify the factor to use for multiple comparisons. This is of course redundant for a one-way ANOVA, but its use illustrates how to proceed e.g. with a two-way factorial ANOVA introduced in the next chapter.

Apparently, only the difference between *sand* and *peat* is strong enough to be statistically significant (the plant height in pots with peat is, on average, 9.8 cm larger when compared with the plants from pots with sand, $p = 0.0007081$). The other differences are close to a conventional α level ($p = 0.0673$ when comparing soil with peat and $p = 0.0561$ when comparing soil with sand), but the test is not sufficiently powerful to demonstrate those differences clearly (we would need more than five replicates for each treatment).

A small but handy improvement for reading and interpreting the differences among the means is if we order the groups according to their mean estimates before the comparison. This results in all of the average differences being presented as positive values:

```
TukeyHSD( aov.1, which="Substrate", ordered=T)
   Tukey multiple comparisons of means
     95% family-wise confidence level
     factor levels have been ordered
Fit: aov(formula = Height ~ Substrate, data = chap8a)
$`Substrate`
            diff        lwr        upr     p adj
soil-sand  5.0 -0.1271129 10.127113 0.0561479
peat-sand  9.8  4.6728871 14.927113 0.0007081
peat-soil  4.8 -0.3271129  9.927113 0.0672929
```

You can see that the *p*-values are identical to those calculated earlier, as are the other values, except for some sign changes and a reversal of order for the confidence intervals.

The results of the *TukeyHSD* function can also be visually summarised in a graph, using the function *plot* applied to the *TukeyHSD* return value. To work more extensively with multiple comparisons, we need to move to the more specialised *multcomp* package (Bretz et al., 2010). We start by illustrating how to perform the same Tukey's comparisons as above using *multcomp* functions:

```
library( multcomp)
glht.subst <- glht( aov.1, linfct=mcp(Substrate="Tukey"))
summary( glht.subst)
```

```
        Simultaneous Tests for General Linear Hypotheses
Multiple Comparisons of Means: Tukey Contrasts
Fit: aov(formula = Height ~ Substrate, data = chap8a)
Linear Hypotheses:
                Estimate Std. Error t value Pr(>|t|)
sand - peat == 0   -9.800      1.922  -5.099   <0.001 ***
soil - peat == 0   -4.800      1.922  -2.498   0.0675 .
soil - sand == 0    5.000      1.922   2.602   0.0560 .
---
Signif. codes:  0 '***' 0.001 '**' 0.01 '*' 0.05 '.' 0.1 ' ' 1
(Adjusted p values reported -- single-step method)
```

The *glht* function (its name is an acronym of 'general linear hypothesis test') defines the hypothesis we will be testing using multiple comparisons. The simplest use of the *glht* function is with Tukey's method. Here the identity of the pairs being tested is specified using a call to the *mcp* function, inserting the name of the factor we are testing (*Substrate*) in combination with the name of the 'Tukey' method. The value that is returned from *glht* can be used in multiple ways, as illustrated above with the *summary* function and also with the code below.

We discussed in Section 8.9.1 that we can present the conclusions of multiple pairwise comparisons in a compact way with letters labelling groups of mutually indistinguishable means. When we have to compare multiple means, devising the letters correctly is sometimes tricky (due to the overlaps discussed earlier), but the *multcomp* package comes to our aid with the *cld* function:

```
cld( glht.subst)
```

```
peat sand soil
 "b"  "a"  "ab"
```

The chosen letters nicely summarise our finding that while *peat* and *sand* produce plants with significantly different average heights, neither of these two groups can be distinguished from plants grown in *soil*. If we plot the value returned by the *cld* function, we get one of the most frequently used graphical presentations of one-way ANOVA results (see Fig. 8.1):

```
plot( cld( glht.subst))
```

Please note that while our ANOVA model tests hypotheses about means estimated as arithmetic averages, there are no such averages plotted in Fig. 8.1. A classical box-and-whisker plot which displays medians and quartiles is most often used. Therefore the fitted ANOVA model is reflected only in the letters near the upper edge of the graphing area. To plot the averages, we can e.g. create a graph with bars or symbols and supplement them with confidence intervals. The confidence intervals (for group means, rather than for the differences

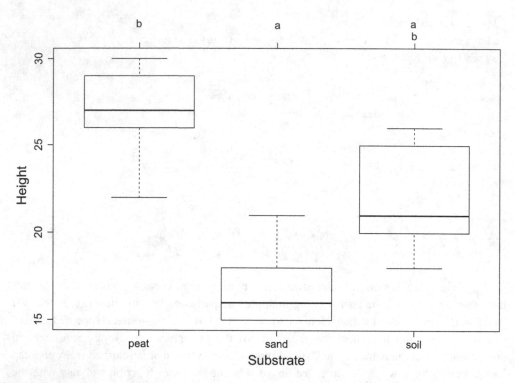

Figure 8.1 Data summary of plant heights with a box-and-whisker plot, classified by substrate type. The results of multiple comparisons for a one-way ANOVA model are indicated by the letters above the graph. The *Substrate* types which are not indicated as significantly different by Tukey's multiple comparisons share the same letter.

among group means, which are plotted in Fig. 8.2) can be obtained for this simple model in the following way (note that the range of confidence intervals is again family-wise adjusted for multiple comparisons):

```
confint( glht( aov( Height~Substrate-1, data=chap8a)))
        Simultaneous Confidence Intervals
Fit: aov(formula = Height ~ Substrate - 1, data = chap8a)
Quantile = 2.7459
95% family-wise confidence level
Linear Hypotheses:
                  Estimate lwr      upr
Substratepeat == 0 26.8000  23.0685 30.5315
Substratesand == 0 17.0000  13.2685 20.7315
Substratesoil == 0 22.0000  18.2685 25.7315
```

Here we have employed a 'trick' with the *aov* formula (inserting −1) that leads to a different parameterisation: normally, one of the levels (the first, 'reference' level) has its mean value estimated in a parameter called 'intercept' (see Chapter 12 for more details), while the other levels are presented as differences against the reference level. By adding the −1 term

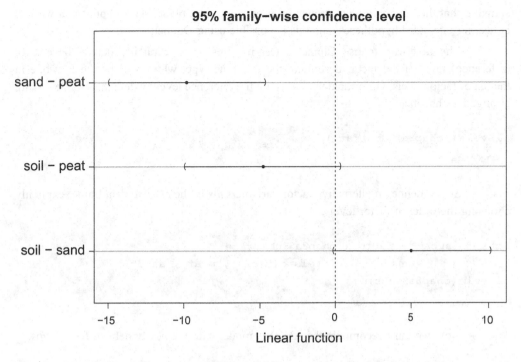

Figure 8.2 Plot of 95% confidence intervals for the differences among mean heights of plants grown in three different substrate types.

into the model formula, we remove the intercept from the estimated model (implicitly setting it to 0), so every factor level is then represented by its true average. However, we do not recommend this form of ANOVA model formula for any other use, particularly not for testing.

We can plot the confidence intervals for the estimated differences among group means in the following way:

```
par.def <- par( mar=c(5,6,4,2)+0.1)
plot( glht.subst)
par( par.def)
```

We increased the size of the area reserved for the labels of the vertical axis using the *mar* argument in a call to the *par* function (and restored the original settings after plotting the graph), otherwise the three long labels would not fit. The resulting graph is illustrated in Fig. 8.2.

Note that the overlap between the two pairs of treatments is again reflected in the graph by the two confidence intervals spanning the zero value (dashed vertical line in the graph).

Now we will demonstrate the use of Dunnett's test in two ways, illustrating additional aspects of the use of multiple comparisons for factor levels. Please note that our example dataset is not exactly suited for the type of hypothesis the Dunnett test addresses. But you can hopefully still imagine the scenario mentioned earlier where we are considering using two substrates as an alternative to traditional soil, namely peat and sand, with the aim of showing that they improve plant growth by producing taller plants. This implies that we will be testing one-sided hypotheses, and this is possible using Dunnett's test.

The first way to use Dunnett's test requires us to explicitly define the control (reference) level of the factor describing the substrate type, which will be the first one in the list of factor levels. Unfortunately, *soil* is not the reference level by default as the levels are arranged alphabetically:

```
levels( chap8a$Substrate)
```
```
[1] "peat" "sand" "soil"
```

So we define an alternative factor variable *subs* in the *chap8a* data frame, explicitly choosing the order of factor levels:

```
chap8a$subs <- factor( chap8a$Substrate,
                       levels=c("soil","peat","sand"))
levels(chap8a$subs)
```
```
[1] "soil" "peat" "sand"
```

Now we must recompute the ANOVA model with the newly defined factor *subs*:

```
aov.2 <- aov( Height~subs, data=chap8a)
```

And finally, we can compute Dunnett's multiple comparisons, also specifying the one-sided alternative hypothesis (implying that plant height should be <u>greater</u> for the levels being compared to the reference level, i.e. to the *soil* level):

```
glht.subs.dunnett <- glht( aov.2, linfct=mcp( subs="Dunnett"),
                           alternative=c("greater"))
summary( glht.subs.dunnett)
          Simultaneous Tests for General Linear Hypotheses
Multiple Comparisons of Means: Dunnett Contrasts
Fit: aov(formula = Height ~ subs, data = chap8a)
Linear Hypotheses:
                 Estimate Std. Error t value Pr(>t)
peat - soil <= 0    4.800      1.922   2.498 0.0252 *
sand - soil <= 0   -5.000      1.922  -2.602 0.9978
```

Given that we are now dealing with a one-sided hypothesis, the corresponding test has more power and thus rejects the null hypothesis for the *peat/soil* comparison seen above ($p = 0.0252$). In contrast, the direction of the difference in plant height between the pots with sand and those with soil conflicts with our alternative hypothesis (because the plants grew smaller in sand compared with the plants grown in soil) and the difference cannot therefore be significant.

Now we will illustrate an alternative way to specify Dunnett's test, using the original factor *Substrate* and the *aov.1* model of the one-way ANOVA. Let us first recall the order in which the levels of *Substrate* are presented:

```
levels( chap8a$Substrate)
```

```
[1] "peat" "sand" "soil"
```

So, to compare *peat* and *sand* pairwise with *soil*, we must subtract the mean for the third factor level from that of the second level or the first level. This is encoded in a matrix created by the following command (function *rbind* combines passed vectors as rows of a matrix):

```
CompSoil <- rbind( "sand vs. soil" = c( 0, +1, -1),
                   "peat vs. soil" = c(+1,  0, -1))
CompSoil
```

```
              [,1] [,2] [,3]
sand vs. soil    0    1   -1
peat vs. soil    1    0   -1
```

The second command just verified the resulting *CompSoil* matrix by displaying it for us. Each row of the matrix represents a single comparison, with the −1 value in the third column ensuring that the mean of the *soil* level is always subtracted from the mean of another level, indicated by the 1 value. We can also test the planned (*a priori*) contrasts in the same way as discussed earlier in this chapter (at the beginning of Section 8.9):

```
summary( glht( aov.1, linfct=mcp(Substrate=CompSoil),
alternative=c("greater")))
```

```
        Simultaneous Tests for General Linear Hypotheses
Multiple Comparisons of Means: User-defined Contrasts
Fit: aov(formula = Height ~ Substrate, data = chap8a)
Linear Hypotheses:
                    Estimate Std. Error t value Pr(>t)
sand vs. soil <= 0    -5.000      1.922  -2.602 0.9978
peat vs. soil <= 0     4.800      1.922   2.498 0.0252 *
---
Signif. codes:  0 '***' 0.001 '**' 0.01 '*' 0.05 '.' 0.1 ' ' 1
(Adjusted p values reported -- single-step method)
```

As we can see, the estimated *p*-values are identical to those provided by Dunnett's procedure implemented in the *mcp* function, albeit presented in a different order.

8.12.3 Power Analysis

There are specialised packages in R for solving important questions about test power for many types of models (e.g. the *pwr* package). Their flexibility is also reflected in their higher complexity. But for a basic one-way ANOVA model with equally sized groups, R offers a simple function called *power.anova.test*. This function has six parameters, and you can pass five of them in any combination while the sixth is computed.

In our substrate type example (see Example 8.1), we can check how many replicates we need per substrate type if we want the power of the test to be 0.95

(i.e. to have no more than 5% Type II error chance) and we consider the mean difference as significant at $p < 0.05$:

```
power.anova.test( groups=3, between.var=120, within.var=9.2,
sig.level=0.05, power=0.95)
     Balanced one-way analysis of variance power calculation
          groups = 3
               n = 2.02144
     between.var = 120
      within.var = 9.2
       sig.level = 0.05
           power = 0.95
NOTE: n is number in each group
```

The calculated n (two pots per group) suggests that with five replicates, we have even higher power than is needed.[13] This outcome is due to the high ratio of between-group and within-group variation: the values were taken as the mean squares (MS_G and MS_E, respectively) from the ANOVA table.

8.12.4 Testing a Random Effect

Although we will be using the classical ANOVA model just a little in this section, the check for homogeneity of variances across our groups is important even when working with models where the groups are represented by a factor with a random effect:

```
bartlett.test( Till.Len~Population, data=chap8a)
          Bartlett test of homogeneity of variances
data:  Till.Len by Population
Bartlett's K-squared = 12.072, df = 4, p-value = 0.01682
```

We can see that the variability of tiller lengths differs among the populations. The log-transformation often comes in handy if we want to stabilise the variance (and also make the distribution curve more symmetrical) for measurements of dimensions, concentrations or weights (such as biomass data) – you can find more about this topic in Chapter 10. So let us check how the log-transformation of tiller lengths affects the outcome of Bartlett's test:

```
bartlett.test( log(Till.Len)~Population, data=chap8a)
          Bartlett test of homogeneity of variances
data:  log(Till.Len) by Population
Bartlett's K-squared = 5.9544, df = 4, p-value = 0.2026
```

---

[13] Although the power analysis suggests that two replicates per group provides sufficient power, there are other reasons why comparing three groups using two replicates in each is not a good idea. One of the reasons is that such a small dataset (with six observations) would have an extremely low robustness to assumption violations and given the number of replications, there is no way of reliably checking for such violations.

The significant heterogeneity of variances is no longer present, so we will use the log-transformed tiller lengths in our subsequent analyses. We will test the random effect using the *nlme* package (Pinheiro & Bates, 2008), which allows us to estimate (fit) both linear and non-linear models with and without the random effects:

```
library( nlme)
lm.0  <- lm( log(Till.Len)~1, data=chap8a)
lme.1 <- lme( log(Till.Len)~1, random=~1|Population,
            data=chap8a)
```

In the above commands, we first fitted a simple linear regression model (see Chapter 12 for its introduction) *lm.0* with no explanatory variable (essentially stating that the length of tillers is only subject to homogeneous random variation) and then an alternative model *lme.1* with a single random effect of *Population*. The *lme.1* model implies that the length of tillers is subject to random variation, but that the variation is composed of random variation among the populations and random variation within the populations. Next, we compare (using the **likelihood ratio test**) the quality of these two models in terms of their ability to describe our data:

```
anova( lme.1, lm.0)
        Model df     AIC      BIC     logLik   Test  L.Ratio p-value
lme.1     1   3 25.09871 27.01588  -9.549356
lm.0      2   2 27.55328 28.83139 -11.776639 1 vs 2 4.454568  0.0348
```

The probability that we obtain the value of the *L.Ratio* statistic (4.45), or an even larger value, from a χ^2_1 distribution is quite low ($p = 0.0348$). We therefore reject the null hypothesis that the two models are of the same quality (predictive power) and pick the model with the larger likelihood (and a higher parsimony measured by the Akaike information criterion, AIC – inversely related to parsimony, see Chapter 15), i.e. the *lme.1* model containing the random effect. So the significance level ($p = 0.0348$) can be presented as an outcome of a test of the random effect of population.[14] As the *L.Ratio* statistic (with a χ^2 distribution assumed under H_0) compares two models implied by the two table rows, we must deduce its corresponding degrees of freedom as a difference between the two *df* values (i.e. here $3 - 2 = 1$).

We can even check the relative size of the among-population and within-population variabilities. This is provided by the summary of the mixed effect model:

```
summary( lme.1)
Linear mixed-effects model fit by REML
...
Random effects:
 Formula: ~1 | Population
         (Intercept)  Residual
StdDev:   0.4066099 0.3432269
...
```

---

[14] Classical one-way ANOVA model testing the fixed effect of population (using *aov(log(Till.Len)~Population, data = chap8a*) yields $p = 0.0157$, leading to an identical conclusion.

The among-population variability is given by the column (*Intercept*) as a standard deviation of the (plant) population means around the global mean, while the value in the *Residual* column represents the within-population variation, measured as the standard deviation of measured lengths from the mean of the population to which a plant belongs (i.e. as a square root of the error mean square).

The standard deviations for random effects are one of the simplest ways to quantify the *variance components* of an ANOVA model with random effect(s). We can see that the variation among the populations is slightly larger, but likely does not differ significantly – as evidenced by the confidence intervals of those estimates computed using the *intervals* function:

```
intervals( lme.1)

Approximate 95% confidence intervals
 Fixed effects:
               lower      est.      upper
(Intercept) 2.136281 2.587004 3.037727
...
 Random Effects:
  Level: Population
                  lower       est.      upper
sd((Intercept)) 0.1713998 0.4066099 0.9645963

Within-group standard error:
    lower      est.      upper
0.2214352 0.3432269 0.5320052
```

We note that the first confidence interval displayed in the function output (for (*Intercept*)) represents the confidence interval for the total average of tiller lengths (on the log-transformed scale). The confidence intervals for the two standard deviations, i.e. (0.1714, 0.9646) for among-population variability and (0.2214, 0.5320) for within-population variability, overlap extensively.

8.12.5 Kruskal–Wallis Test

We can compute the Kruskal–Wallis rank-based test with the *kruskal.test* function:

```
kruskal.test( Importance~Settlement, data=chap8b)
        Kruskal-Wallis rank sum test
data:  Importance by Settlement
Kruskal-Wallis chi-squared = 10.151, df = 2, p-value = 0.006248
```

There is a significant difference among the three settlement types, so we can identify which settlement types are responsible using multiple comparisons implemented for this non-parametric test in the *pgirmess* package (Giraudoux 2018):

```
library( pgirmess)
kruskalmc( Importance~Settlement, data=chap8b, p=0.05)
Multiple comparison test after Kruskal-Wallis
p.value: 0.05
Comparisons
                         obs.dif critical.dif difference
industrial-town          7.566667     7.320256        TRUE
industrial-village 9.150000     7.320256        TRUE
town-village             1.583333     6.979591       FALSE
```

Here we have to choose the α level of significance (using the p parameter in the function call) and then see which pairwise comparisons lead to a rejection of the null hypothesis. People from villages do not differ in their opinion from small-town people, but the opinion of those living in industrial cities differs from the other two groups.

8.13 Reporting Analyses

8.13.1 Methods

The homogeneity of variances was checked using Bartlett's test. Differences in plant height among the three substrate types were tested with a one-way ANOVA followed by *post-hoc* comparisons using Tukey's HSD method.

The results of the Bartlett test are not usually described in the Results section, but if it identifies a significant departure from homogeneity of variances and a log-transformation would fix that issue, we could add the following to the Methods section: 'Tiller length values were log-transformed to achieve homogeneity of variances required for the F test in the one-way ANOVA.' *But even if the chosen transformation does not fix the problem completely (paradoxically, this often happens with a large number of observations), we would still give a similar statement to the one above, just replacing the words* 'to achieve' *with* 'to improve'.

We tested the differences in the attitude of people towards species extinctions among the three social groups using a Kruskal–Wallis test with subsequent non-parametric *post-hoc* comparisons.

Based on the pilot study results (group means and data variation estimates), we performed a power analysis of the single-factor design to determine the number of replicates needed in each group in order to achieve the target test power 0.95 with $\alpha = 0.05$.

The random effect of population on longest tiller lengths was tested using a likelihood ratio test in the *nlme* package of the R program *[R citation here]*.

8.13.2 Results

Plant heights differed significantly among the substrate types ($F_{2,12} = 13.0$, $p = 0.001$) and follow-up tests demonstrated a significant difference between the plants grown in sand and in peat ($p < 0.001$). The difference between plants grown in soil and in other substrates was nearly significant ($p = 0.056$ for sand/soil difference and $p = 0.067$ for peat/soil difference) and the lack of stronger evidence is likely due to the limited size of our sample. The average values, together with the group confidence intervals and highlighted significance differences, are shown in Fig. X.[15]

Under standard circumstances, the text would probably be much shorter, as the differences between pairs of groups can be (roughly) read from the graph.

There were significant differences in the attitude towards species extinctions among the respondents from different types of residential areas ($H = 10.15$, $p = 0.006$). *Post-hoc* tests revealed that this is due to a strong difference between the respondents from industrial centres on the one hand, and those from small towns or villages on the other hand. There was, however, no difference between the respondents from small towns and those from villages.

We found significant variation in tiller length among the five sampled populations ($\chi^2_1 = 4.45$, $p = 0.035$).

8.14 Recommended Reading

Zar (2010), pp. 189–248.
Quinn & Keough (2002), pp. 173–207.
Sokal & Rohlf (2012), pp. 177–276 (ANOVA), pp. 440–446 (Kruskal–Wallis test).
F. Bretz, T. Hothorn & P. Westfall (2010) *Multiple Comparisons Using R*, CRC Press, Boca Raton, FL.
P. Giraudoux (2018) *pgirmess*: spatial analysis and data mining for field ecologists. R package version 1.69. https://cran.r-project.org/package=pgirmess
J. Pinheiro & D. Bates (2008) *Mixed-Effects Models in S and S-PLUS*, 3rd printing 2002 edn. Springer, New York, 548 pp.

---

[15] Figure not shown here, but it would look similar to Fig. 8.1 in this chapter.

9 Two-Way Analysis of Variance

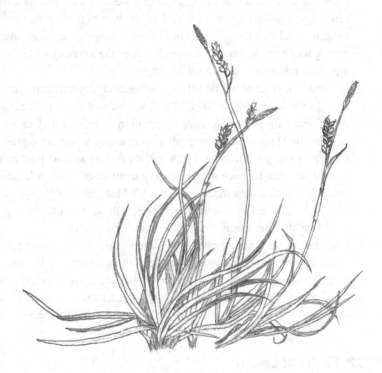

9.1 Use Case Examples

The following examples illustrate research questions that can be addressed with the help of two-way ANOVA models with or without interactions, their extensions with more than two factors, or the non-parametric Friedman test.

1. We studied the response of a wetland sedge (*Carex panicea*) to eutrophication by a nitrogen fertiliser and its interaction with reduced water availability. In a garden experiment, sedge individuals were grown for two seasons under manipulated conditions with either high or low water availability and high or low nitrogen supply. The response was measured by the dry weight of aboveground biomass at the end of the experiment. Is the biomass affected by water availability? Is the biomass affected by the availability of nitrogen? Does the response of sedges to high nitrogen supply differ depending on water availability?
2. We studied the effect of fertilisation on the length of tillers of red fescue (*Festuca rubra*). We used two treatment levels: unfertilised and fertilised, with individual tussocks being our experimental units. The experiment was conducted at three localities as we expected that the response to fertilisation might be different in different localities due to natural conditions. There were several tussocks (replicates) in each group in each locality. The response variable was the length of the longest tiller of each tussock.

3. We were quantifying the response of plant seedling emergence to a manipulation of vegetation cover in a grassland community (Špačková et al., 1998). Besides the control (non-modified) plots, some plots had the dominant grass species (*Nardus stricta*) removed, other plots had the plant litter removed, and another group of plots had both the plant litter removed and mosses at the soil surface weeded out. The experiment was established in four experimental blocks, with each of the blocks containing four plots – one plot for each experimental treatment. The number of emerging seedlings was recorded in each plot throughout a single vegetation season. Does the intensity of seedling emergence depend on the manipulations imposed on the vegetation?

4. In a study investigating the effect of arbuscular mycorrhizal symbiosis on a plant community (Šmilauer & Šmilauerová, 2000), we wanted to check the effect of fungicide addition combined with phosphate supplementation (resulting in four experimental treatments in combination) upon the aboveground biomass of a dominant grass species, *Poa angustifolia*. The plots were arranged in a grid of four rows and four columns, so that there was always one plot for each of the existing treatments in any column or any row (Latin square design). Are there any detectable effects of fungicide or phosphate addition on the biomass of *Poa*? Is there any interaction between these two effects (e.g. the effect of fungicide might be stronger when phosphate is added as well)?

5. The allergic response of people to pollen grains of three allergenic species was studied in the following manner. A small sample of three allergens (*Artemisia*, *Ambrosia*, *Betula*) was injected subcutaneously into each of 10 persons, and the allergic response at the three skin patches was recorded after two days using a subjective ordinal scale ranging from 0 (no response) to 4 (strongest response). Does sensitivity differ among the three pollen sources?

9.2 Factorial Design

The two-way ANOVA method is also sometimes called the *two-factor ANOVA*, as the observations on the response variable are sorted based on the values of two classification criteria (two factor variables). In this chapter we extend the topic by presenting an example involving more than two factors, i.e. example 4 above.

If we investigate the effects of more than a single factor, then our experimental design usually represents a so-called **factorial design**. This means that we are investigating the effects of all possible combinations of the levels of the factors of interest. If we, for example, follow the effect of two factors each with two levels (water availability high vs. low and nitrogen (N) supply high vs. low), there are four ways we can combine them (low water with low N, low water with high N, high water with low N, high water with high N). It is also best if each combination is represented by the same number of replicates.[1]

Our factorial design can of course include more than two factors or (some of) our factors may have more than two levels. The factorial design is one of the most effective experimental arrangements. It makes efficient use of time and money (compared with studying the effects of each factor in a separate experiment) and it also allows us to study the interactions between individual factors. In biological research, it is quite rare to find successful experiments with more than three or four factors. For example, if we have five factors, each with just two levels, there are 32 experimental groups to study. Each of these

---

[1] Replicates are independent sampling units sharing identical experimental treatments.

groups need a number of replicates, thus requiring a high number of individual experimental units (which might be difficult to manage in field experiments).

But factors can also be combined in a way which differs from the factorial design, namely in a **hierarchical design**. This type of arrangement is primarily characterised by the fact that not all of the levels of one factor are combined with every level of another factor. We can illustrate this with a hypothetical extension of example 2 from Section 8.1, where we collect red fescue seeds from five populations, but at each population we also collect multiple seeds from each of five different mother plants. We can then investigate the differences not only among populations, but also among different mother plants within each population. Plant identity is one of the factors (with a random effect) and it is plain to see that its particular level (particular mother plant) cannot be combined factorially with all the populations – it can only come from a single population. This kind of data can be processed by a *hierarchical ANOVA* (or *nested design ANOVA*), which is described in more detail in Chapter 11.

Returning to a factorial two-way ANOVA, we note that in terms of computing the test statistics, there is a large difference between a balanced and an unbalanced design. The **balanced design** has the same number of replicates for each factor combination. This allows simpler computations but also – more importantly from the user's perspective – the highest power in subsequent tests. If for some reason we cannot retain a balanced design (e.g. due to the availability of experimental units), we should strive to achieve at least a **proportional design**. If we imagine presenting the combinations of factor levels for a two-way ANOVA in a two-dimensional table with its rows representing levels of one factor and its columns representing levels of the other factor, the individual combinations of rows and columns can be called *cells*, addressed by the identity of the two factor levels as i, j. For a proportional design, the number of observations in a cell i, j must be

$$n_{ij} = \frac{R_i C_j}{N} \tag{9.1}$$

where R_i is the total number of observations with level i of the first factor, C_j is the total number of observations with level j of the second factor and N is the total number of observations in the data. If you recall the contingency tables of Chapter 3, you will find that a contingency table with the observation counts of an experiment with a proportional design is a table completely matching the null hypothesis of the χ^2 test, i.e. with test statistic $\chi^2 = 0$. This implies that the two experimental factors will be mutually independent. If there is a dependency between the factors then it is more difficult to separate their individual effects. In this case, we must pay particular attention to the chosen type of decomposition of the total sum of squares. In R, *summary* and *anova* functions for objects produced by *aov* or *lm* decompose the effects of multiple predictors in a sequential manner, which can be a risky approach (see Section 10.7).

Under certain circumstances, a two-way ANOVA is even able to test data where each combination of factors is represented just by a single replicate.

The model of a <u>one-way</u> ANOVA (introduced in the preceding chapter) can be represented by the following equation:[2]

$$\text{observation} = \text{total mean} + \text{factor effect} + \text{random variation} \tag{9.2}$$

---

[2] Honestly, we should rather call it a symbolic statement as it is not sufficiently precise to be an equation.

		factor A	
		a1	a2
factor B	b1	15	25
	b2	18	28

		factor A			
		a1	a2	a3	a4
factor B	b1	21	29	14	25
	b2	18	26	11	22

Figure 9.1 Possible values of cell means for data from a factorial experiment, if the effects of factors A and B are purely additive, with no interaction, and we ignore the random variation. In the example on the left, both factors have just two levels, while in the example on the right, factor A has four levels and factor B has two levels. For each level of factor A, we can say that its mean value differs between the two levels of factor B by 3 units (so this is the size of the main effect of factor B). A similar statement can also be made for factor B.

and we test the null hypothesis H_0: factor effect = 0 across all groups (levels). We can describe the two-way factorial ANOVA model in a similar way, labelling the two factors as A and B:

$$\text{observation} = \text{total mean} + \text{effect of } A + \text{effect of } B + \text{interaction } A \times B + \text{random variation} \quad (9.3)$$

Consequently, we can test three null hypotheses here: (1) the effect of factor A is 0 across all its levels; (2) the effect of factor B is 0 across all its levels; (3) the effect of the interaction $A \times B$ is 0 for all factor-level combinations.

> **What does it mean that an interaction effect is zero (we also speak about 'zero interaction' or 'no interaction between the factors')? Zero interaction means that the effect of factors is purely additive. This means that the differences among the means of groups defined by factor A levels are constant, they do not change depending on the levels of factor B.**

If we label the average of all observations with the i-th level of the first factor as $\overline{X}_{i\bullet}$, the average of all observations with the j-th level of the second factor as $\overline{X}_{\bullet j}$ and the overall mean (calculated from all observations) as $\overline{X}$, then if there is no interaction and we ignore the random variation, we can describe the average value of a cell with the i-th level of the first factor and the j-th level of the second factor as

$$\overline{X}_{ij} = \overline{X}_{i\bullet} + \overline{X}_{\bullet j} - \overline{X} \quad (9.4)$$

A hypothetical example of cell means when there is complete additivity of factor effects (ignoring the ever-present random variation) is shown in Fig. 9.1. The same pattern can be shown in a graph using an *interaction plot* (see Section 9.10.1 for guidelines to its construction).

9.3 Sum of Squares Decomposition and Test Statistics

Here we will demonstrate just one part of the total sum of squares decomposition in a balanced two-way ANOVA model. Let us denote the number of levels of factor A as a, the number of levels of factor B as b and, because we assume a balanced design, we can specify the number of replicates for each combination of factor levels by a single value n. We can then write

$$SS_{TOT} = SS_A + SS_B + SS_{AB} + SS_E \tag{9.5}$$

where SS_{TOT} is the total sum of squares, i.e. a sum of squared differences of all observations from the overall mean, with the corresponding $df_{TOT} = N - 1$, where N is the total number of observations, so that $N = abn$. The SS_{TOT} value is a measure of the total variability in the response variable. SS_A is the sum of squared differences of the means of groups defined by factor A from the total mean, multiplied for each group by the corresponding number of observations (i.e. by nb). So SS_A is computed as the SS_G in a one-way ANOVA, and like there, it is a measure of the variability in the response variable explained by the factor A. The corresponding number of degrees of freedom is $df_A = a - 1$. In an analogous way, we can calculate SS_B and df_B for the B factor. The residual sum of squares (SS_E) is the sum of squared differences of the values in cells from the corresponding cell means; the corresponding degrees of freedom are $df_E = ab(n - 1)$. The interaction sum of squares (SS_{AB}, i.e. a measure of the variability explained by the non-additivity of effects) is the sum of squared differences of the cell means from their means expected according to Eq. (9.4), multiplied by the number of observations in the cell. The corresponding degrees of freedom are then

$$df_{AB} = (a - 1)(b - 1) \tag{9.6}$$

If we divide a particular SS statistic by its corresponding degrees of freedom (df), then we obtain the mean square value (MS).

As in the one-way ANOVA, the residual sum of squares (i.e. within-cell variation) is an estimate of the variance σ^2, common to statistical populations represented by ab samples in the cells. It can be shown that if the effect of factor A is absent (equal to zero), even MS_A is an estimate of the common variance, as is also the case for the factor B with MS_B being an estimate of the common variance. If the interaction effect is zero, then MS_{AB} is an estimate of common variance. If we handle each cell (i.e. each combination of levels for factors A and B) as a separate group in a one-way ANOVA, we obtain (as SS_G of that ANOVA model) the sum of squares among the cells with value $SS_{cell} = SS_A + SS_B + SS_{AB}$. If none of the factors has any effect on the values of the response variable then the corresponding mean square is also an estimate of the common variance σ^2. This hypothesised identity of the variance estimates is then used when testing corresponding null hypotheses about the individual effects in an ANOVA model.

The tests of hypotheses in a two-way ANOVA depend on whether the factors represent fixed effects (model I ANOVA) or random effects (model II ANOVA). We can also have a model III ANOVA (with one factor having a fixed effect, while the other has a random effect). In the case of a two-way ANOVA with two fixed effect factors (probably the most frequent pattern), we always compare the MS of the tested term with the residual mean square (MS_E). So the value of the test statistic for a particular factor (or factor interaction) is then

$$F = \frac{MS_{factor}}{MS_E} \tag{9.7}$$

Most statistical programs have the model I tests as their default choice, but some allow us to choose the denominator of the F statistic.

The computation procedure is quite complex, so we will not demonstrate it here but suggest that the reader checks the results obtained in Section 9.10.1 for example 1 (of Section 9.1). There we see that the F tests for both main effects, as well as for the interaction term, yield highly significant results. The significance of the interaction implies (at least for our data!) that the joint effect of both factors is larger than the sum of their independent effects (synergy of their effects). This is probably because in drier conditions, the plants are not able to use the increased availability of nitrogen.

When the model of two-way ANOVA includes one random effect, we must calculate the F statistic for the fixed effect with the value of the denominator set to MS_{AB} instead of MS_E. The reasons why the calculations of the F statistic must differ depending on the effect type can be illustrated by example 2 of Section 9.1, for which we can treat the locality either as a fixed or a random effect factor. We performed this experiment at three locations, in each of which we have randomly chosen 5 plants to be fertilised and 5 control plants (in reality, we should use a considerably better-replicated setup). So we have a factorial design with two factors – fertilisation and location. *Fertil* is clearly a fixed effect factor, but we can deal with *Locality* either as a fixed effect factor (we are interested in comparing the three particular locations and the average effect of fertilisation seen just on those three locations) or as a random effect factor. In the latter case, we ask whether various locations differ in the growth parameters of the grass (with our three locations being just a random sample from existing locations) and, mainly, we want to test whether there is an effect of fertilisation if we generalise across all possible locations of the sampled geographical region.

In the first case (*Locality* as a fixed effect factor), we will use the residual mean square for the F statistic testing the effect of *Fertil*, but in the second case (*Locality* as a random effect factor), we will use the interaction mean square in the F statistic denominator. We will almost certainly get a more powerful test in the first case. But this is alright: if we considered *Locality* to be a factor with fixed effect, it means that we only generalise our results to all plants at the three examined locations. But if we consider *Locality* to have a random effect, we intend to generalise our results to the populations of all plants over the whole set of locations in the region, of which our three locations are just a random sample (and we suspect that the effect of fertilisation is not the same in all the localities). This is why the observed effect is contrasted with the variation of the tiller length's response to fertilisation among individual localities, i.e. the interaction mean square. This suggests one important conclusion concerning the power of our test: if we have factor A as a fixed effect in our model and factor B as a random effect, then the power of the test for A increases with the number of levels of factor B. For our example this means that if we want to generalise across all possible locations, then the test will be stronger with an increasing number of locations included in our study.

9.4 Two-Way ANOVA with and without Interactions

For the two-way ANOVA model, we have so far considered that the effects of two factors are not purely additive – we have considered their possible interaction. However in some cases, we can decide *a priori* that we reject the possibility of an interaction (or rather, we consider it as a part of the random variation). We are therefore only testing the main effects, in a model often called a **main effects ANOVA**. In this case, we compare the mean squares of individual factors (A or B) with a mean square calculated (from the perspective of a full two-way

ANOVA model) as $(SS_E + SS_{AB})/(df_E + df_{AB})$. Any observed deviations from additivity then become a part of the random (unexplained) variation. Zar (2010) uses the term *remainder SS* for the sum $SS_E + SS_{AB}$. Most statistical programs allow us to specify whether we want to calculate the ANOVA with or without interactions.[3]

As seen in this and the preceding section, there are multiple decisions we can make in a two-way ANOVA that allow us to adjust our analysis to the nature of the issues we want to address. These decisions reflect which variation should be explained by the model and which variation should be considered as random. With more than two factors, the ANOVA model becomes even more flexible. There are interactions between all possible factor pairs, but also interactions of higher order – among more than two factors. The choice of the model we will use should be based on our *a priori* knowledge of the problem at hand. Alternatively, there are methods to select a model best describing our data.

9.5 Two-Way ANOVA with No Replicates

We can also use the two-way ANOVA to evaluate an experiment with two factors, but with just a single replicate for each combination of factor levels. In this situation we must use the two-way ANOVA without an interaction: we cannot test the interaction term as there is no variation within cells, and to estimate the residual variation we can only use the deviations from additivity.

9.6 Experimental Design

In this section we will briefly discuss some general principles of experimental design, particularly the distribution of experimental units such as plots. In our description, we will use examples of experimental plots spatially located in a field experiment, but the same principles can also be applied to lab experiments and the spatial separation can be replaced by temporal separation in other types of studies. We will not discuss problem-specific aspects of experimental design related to the nature of the particular subject here, such as issues related to the influence of margins in experimental plots or the effect of plot surroundings.

When designing our experiments, we must follow certain rules in order to be able to statistically evaluate the resulting data (see e.g. Mead, 1988). Most of the influential biotic and abiotic characteristics vary continually – nearby plots tend to be more similar to each other than distant plots. Field experiments have a great tradition in agricultural research where standard procedures for their design were developed. One of the main tasks of such designs is to eliminate the effects of environmental heterogeneity as much as possible without breaking the requirements of statistical methods (namely the independency of individual observations). As shown by Hurlbert (1984), such rules are not sufficiently followed in field ecology. This leads to limited trust in the results and often also to wrong conclusions being drawn. Although the conclusions of Hurlbert are based on an analysis of ecological research papers, an insufficient respect for design rules and subsequent unreliability of results is obviously a more general pattern in biological research.

---

[3] In R, we specify it directly with the model formula, see Sections 9.10.1 and 9.10.3.

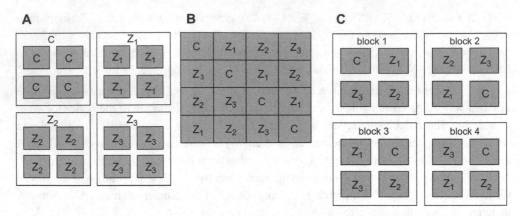

Figure 9.2 Some of the possible patterns of experimental design: A is not too rare, but an entirely wrong design; B is the Latin square design; C is the (complete) randomised blocks design.

So what is an appropriate spatial design for a field experiment? Let us assume we have a single type of control treatment level (C) and three alternative treatments (Z_1, Z_2, Z_3). The possible arrangements for an experiment with four replicates (16 experimental plots in total) are shown in Fig. 9.2. It is grossly inappropriate to keep each treatment type in a single contiguous area, from which we then collect separate 'samples' (replicates) (see Fig. 9.2A). Such replicates are not independent, and statistical analysis based on such a design might lead to totally incorrect conclusions. Hurlbert (1984) uses the term *pseudoreplication* for this kind of replicate. An experimental design similar to Fig. 9.2A is a frequent reason for rejecting manuscripts submitted to research journals.

The most frequently used (and correct) arrangements are illustrated by parts B and C. Part B represents a **Latin square design**, with each row and each column containing exactly one replicate of each treatment type. Figure 9.2 does not, however, show a **completely random design**. For this we would start with a set of randomly placed experimental plots, assigning a treatment type to each plot by some random process (e.g. using a random number generator), so that each plot has an identical probability of becoming a plot with any of the possible treatment types. Another possibility is to vary the treatment types in a systematic way so that we prevent aggregation of plots with the same treatment type.

The **complete randomised blocks** design (similar to Fig. 9.2C) has some advantages, especially if the total area in which the plots are located is large. We choose the number of blocks to correspond to the required number of replicates. The blocks are positioned to maximise the homogeneity within each block, but to ensure that the differences among the blocks cover as much variability as possible in the (environmental) conditions over which we want to generalise our conclusions. Within each block, there will be as many plots as there are different treatment types (levels) and for each plot we assign its treatment by a random process. This arrangement allows us to effectively separate the spatial variation of the studied phenomenon from the effects of the experimental treatments. In contrast, if we impose such a design in a homogeneous area (where the differences among the blocks are negligible) then the power of the test is decreased (in comparison with a completely random arrangement), particularly for a small number of replicates.

Analysis of variance and linear models can also be used to evaluate data collected through other types of design, such as the incomplete randomised blocks. The overall tendency is to adjust the experimental design to the properties of the biological subjects under investigation. As an example, an appropriate experimental block of observations for experiments with young mammals is juveniles from the same litter. We need to compare five treatment levels, but typically the number of young in each litter is three. Under these circumstances it might be necessary to use the incomplete randomised block design. There are more possibilities for how to define block design under various constraints, and there are rules for how to maximise power using the resources available. The calculations for such non-balanced models are then more complicated. We also want to stress again that some designs (such as that of Fig. 9.2A) cannot be evaluated with <u>any</u> statistical method. If you feel you need to use a non-standard design, we advise you to first seek the advice of a statistician. A detailed description of these issues can be found in Mead (1988).

9.6.1 Evaluating Data from Randomised Blocks and Latin Squares

The design of complete randomised blocks is in fact a generalisation of a pairwise design. The ANOVA of randomised blocks evaluates experiments in a manner similar to a paired t test, but we compare more than two groups. This ANOVA actually represents a mixed effect model without replicates. The factor with a fixed effect is the factor representing experimental treatments, while the factor with a random effect represents the blocks. We cannot quantify the interaction between these two factors as there are no replicates (of a particular treatment) within the blocks.

A similar ANOVA model is also used when we perform repeated measurements on each examined object. As an example, we can offer three different types of food (e.g. different grass species) in a defined amount to 10 snails sequentially and we can measure how much food they eat per hour. We will let the snails become hungry before each feeding. Our research question concerns a possible preference for a particular food type. Each snail individual is a single 'block' (level of a factor with a random effect), food type is a factor with a fixed effect. We cannot use this experimental design if there is a danger that one treatment could in some way influence the response to a later treatment. But we can at least mitigate such a problem by increasing the count of snail individuals, combined with randomising the order in which the food types are offered for each snail.

Data coming from a Latin square experiment can be evaluated by a specific three-way ANOVA model where the three explanatory factors are the identity of the row, the identity of the column and the type of treatment. We again cannot quantify the interactions in this case.[4]

9.7 Multiple Comparisons

When we find that a factor with a fixed effect and more than two levels has a significant effect, then we can use any of the approaches discussed in Chapter 8 for performing multiple comparisons (we recommend Tukey's test or – when comparing treatment levels just with

---

[4] More precisely, for our model, we cannot include the interactions between row and column factors and the experimental factors. But see Section 9.10.3 for an example ANOVA model with an interaction between the experimental treatment factors.

the control treatment – Dunnett's test). Instead of k (number of groups), we will use a or b in the equations, i.e. the number of levels of that particular factor, and we use the number of observations for the given factor level as n. For a model I ANOVA, we use MS_E for s^2 (i.e. the within-cell mean square) with the corresponding number of degrees of freedom. If we perform an ANOVA without replications (e.g. for complete randomised blocks), we must use the *remainder mean square* as s^2 with the corresponding DF (i.e. the DF value belonging to the denominator of the F statistic).

In some cases (particularly when we examine a significant interaction effect), we are not so much interested in comparing the levels of a particular factor, but instead we want to compare the means of individual cells, i.e. to compare the combinations of levels of the factors entering the interaction. We proceed here as in a one-way ANOVA, i.e. as if each cell was one of k mutually independent groups (where k is the total number of cells, therefore equal to $a.b$ for the simplest case of an A and B factor interaction). In contrast, with a significant interaction term, we do not usually perform multiple comparisons for each of the factors separately: if their effects are not additive, then the results comparing levels of one factor depend on the actual level of the other factor.

9.8 Non-parametric Methods

The ANOVA model and its F tests are quite robust to violations of its assumptions. But if the discrepancy is too large, one way of getting around it is to use non-parametric methods. The Kruskal–Wallis test is a non-parametric counterpart of the one-way ANOVA, however reliable generalisations of this test for two explanatory factors do not exist (Zar, 2010, p. 249). Sometimes we use the *rank transformation* approach, where we replace the original data values with their rank orders and then analyse the new values in a standard ANOVA model. Such an approach can only be used, however, for an ANOVA model with main effects, not for models with interaction terms.

For a non-parametric analysis of data from randomised block design experiments, we can use the **Friedman test**. It is based on using ranks of values **within blocks**. For example, if we have four types of treatments, we can assign a value from 1 to 4 to each value in a block, depending on the value's order within the block. We can then calculate a test statistic

$$\chi_r^2 = \frac{12}{b\,a\,(a+1)} \sum_{i=1}^{a} R_i^2 - 3b(a+1) \tag{9.8}$$

where a is the number of levels of the factor representing the treatment, b is the number of blocks and R_i is the sum of rank orders for the i-th level of the tested factor. As an example, if we have five blocks and for the first factor level, the value was smallest in four out of the five blocks, and second smallest in the last block, then $R_1 = 6$ (i.e. $4 \times 1 + 1 \times 2$). If the null hypothesis is true, this test statistic comes from a distribution close to a χ^2 distribution with $a - 1$ degrees of freedom. The larger the values of a and b, the better the agreement with that distribution. We can continue with multiple comparisons when we get a significant result. There are methods to compare each level with all others (a modification of Tukey's method), as well as to compare the control with other treatment levels (a modification of Dunnett's test), see Zar (2010, pp. 280–281). Unfortunately, those multiple comparison methods are not available in R.

9.9 Example Data

To illustrate a classical two-way ANOVA (with both factors having a fixed effect), we use the data described in the first example of Section 9.1. The experimental treatments are described by two factor variables: *Nitrogen* and *Water*, the resulting aboveground biomass of the sedge plants is in the *Weight* variable.

We will use example 2 of Section 9.1 to illustrate the effect of considering a factor as having either a fixed or a random effect. The fertilisation experimental treatment is in the variable *Fertil*, and the location is in the *Locality* variable. The response variable is *TillerLen* – the length of the longest tiller in a tussock (mm). We are primarily interested in the effect of fertilisation, but we are also interested in how general the effect is, i.e. whether the effect is the same in all three localities. This will provide a hint about whether we can generalise our findings past the three experimental localities. We will also test the locality effect, although the fact that the sizes of individuals are not identical in various localities is rather trivial.

To illustrate the analysis of data coming from a complete randomised blocks design, we will use the results of the experiment described in example 3 of Section 9.1. The treatments manipulating the vegetation are stored in the *Treatment* variable, the four experimental blocks are coded by the factor variable *Block* and the response (count of seedlings) is in the *SeedlSum* variable. In our example analyses, the response variable was used without any transformation, but it would actually be better to transform it (either log-transform or square-root transform), and even better would be to use a GLM with an assumed Poisson distribution (see Chapter 15).

To illustrate how to analyse data collected from a Latin square-arranged experiment, we use the data described in example 4 of Section 9.1. The use of fungicide is coded by the *Bav* factor, the addition of phosphates is coded by the *P* factor, while the biomass of *Poa* is stored in the numerical variable *PoaAngus*. Additionally, the position of each experimental plot within the Latin square is encoded by two factors: *Row* and *Column* (each with four levels).

The final set of example data is used to illustrate the Friedman test and represents example 5 of Section 9.1, evaluating allergies to three different types of pollen grains. Individual treatments (pollen types) are coded by separate variables (*R.Artemisia*, *R.Ambrosia*, *R.Betula*), while all three observations for a particular person are located in the same data row.

9.10 How to Proceed in R

In our example code below, we assume that the data from the *Chap9* sheet was imported into multiple data frames that differ in the number of cases (rows): *chap9a* contains data for a factorial analysis of variance, *chap9b* contains data on tiller lengths from three localities, *chap9c* contains data for the completely randomised blocks and Latin square examples, and finally *chap9d* contains data illustrating the Friedman test.

9.10.1 Factorial ANOVA with Two Factors

We start by checking the assumption of homogeneity of variances. Because we consider creating a factorial two-way ANOVA model including an interaction among the two factor variables (*Nitrogen* and *Water*), it is probably best to perform Bartlett's test on the four cells representing the combinations of the two levels of each of the two factors. The utility function *interaction* provides an easy way to create a new factor out of two or more existing factor variables, using the factorial combinations of the levels of the original factors as its new levels:

```
bartlett.test( Weight ~ interaction( Nitrogen, Water),
               data=chap9a)

        Bartlett test of homogeneity of variances
data:  Weight by interaction(Nitrogen, Water)
Bartlett's K-squared = 2.4762, df = 3, p-value = 0.4796
```

Bartlett's test suggests that there is no important difference in the variation among the four compared groups. We will now fit the complete two-way model of ANOVA using the *aov* function. The result of this fitting is then passed to the function *summary*, which will display the traditional ANOVA table:

```
summary( aov( Weight ~ Nitrogen * Water, data=chap9a))
                Df Sum Sq Mean Sq F value   Pr(>F)
Nitrogen         1 1140.0  1140.0   288.6 1.17e-11 ***
Water            1 2101.3  2101.3   532.0 1.05e-13 ***
Nitrogen:Water   1  414.0   414.0   104.8 1.98e-08 ***
Residuals       16   63.2     3.9
```

We have now described the explanatory variables in the *aov* model formula using a *Nitrogen * Water* expression. This notation represents both two main effects of *Nitrogen* and *Water*, as well as their interaction. It is a shorthand notation equivalent to writing *Nitrogen + Water + Nitrogen:Water*. This longer version separates the two main effects from the interaction term *Nitrogen:Water*.

The ANOVA table itself is often shown in this or similar forms in research papers, as it nicely summarises the findings about individual model terms. The first two rows describe the main (independent) effects of the two factors, the third row presents the last part of the explained variation in *Weight* values and the final row describes the unexplained variation, represented by SS_E and MS_E values. For each row, we can see the corresponding degrees of freedom in the *Df* column, followed by the values of an appropriate sum of squares in the *Sum Sq* column (SS_A, SS_B, SS_{AB}, SS_E using the notation of Section 9.3). Dividing the *Sum Sq* values by the *Df* values yields the values in the third column (*Mean Sq*), representing mean squares. When the mean square statistics of the first three rows are divided by the error mean square of the fourth row, we obtain the *F* values seen in the *F value* column. Finally the *Pr(>F)* column represents the achieved significance level of the test for a particular model term, followed by a commonly used notation where significances $p < 0.001$ are labelled with three asterisks, *p*-values larger than 0.001 but smaller than 0.01 are labelled with two asterisks and those *p*-values above 0.01 but smaller than 0.05 with a single asterisk. Please also note that with this arrangement of the ANOVA table, you must collect the degrees-of-freedom parameters applicable to the reference *F* distribution from two rows – that of the tested term and that of the error mean square. So, for example, the test statistic of the interaction term would be reported for our example as $F_{1,16} = 104.8$.

All of the model terms reported here are highly significant. For the main effect of *Nitrogen*, this implies that the mean weights of aboveground biomass differ significantly between fertilised and control plants, and similarly for the *Water* factor – the biomass means differ significantly between plants with high and low water availability. The significant interaction term tells us that the extent of the difference between fertilised and control plants depends on water availability. But an interaction between factors is symmetrical in its meaning, so we can also describe it by saying that the extent of weight differences between plants with higher and lower water availability depends on nitrogen addition. But note that a significant interaction can actually represent multiple alternative patterns depending on your actual data: possibly (but not likely), the fertilised plants may be heavier than the control plants under higher moisture, but with a lower biomass than the non-fertilised ones at lower moisture level. The best way to determine the nature of an interaction is to plot it with an interaction plot. This is done in the following command (see also Fig. 9.3):

```
with( chap9a,
        interaction.plot( Water, Nitrogen, Weight, lwd=2))
```

The resulting graph clearly shows that the effect of nitrogen addition (the distance between the dashed and solid lines) is larger for plants with high water availability (at the left end of the lines). If the interaction has a different nature than illustrated by our data (e.g. if the order of levels switches, depending on the level of the other factor), we sometimes encounter a strange situation where one or even both main effects of factors are non-significant, but the interaction effect is strong and significant.

The *interaction.plot* function provides only a limited set of possible adjustments (such as line colours, legend attributes and the decision on which factor is presented by different lines and which factor is presented by different positions along the horizontal axis).

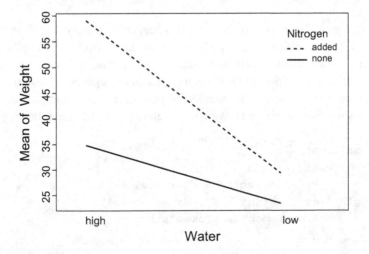

Figure 9.3 Interaction diagram illustrating the size and direction of an interaction term for a two-way ANOVA model with crossed effects of nitrogen and water availability.

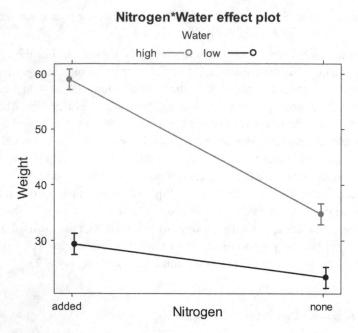

Figure 9.4 An interaction plot (created with the *effects* package) explaining the nature of an interaction term for the same two-way ANOVA model as used in Fig. 9.3.

For a more advanced presentation, you can use the *effects* package (Fox & Weisberg, 2018), which also works nicely for more complex models than that of our two-way ANOVA. Here is an example of plotting an interaction plot with confidence intervals for individual groups (see also Fig. 9.4):

```
library( effects)
plot( allEffects( aov.1), multiline=T,
      confint=list(style="auto"))
```

While the confidence intervals in Fig. 9.4 suggest that every combination of the two factors' levels differs significantly from others, it is better to check with a multiple comparisons procedure. Let us recall that for our model with a significant interaction term, it is not appropriate to perform multiple comparisons for each factor separately (nevertheless, as each of the factors has just two levels, we would not perform multiple comparisons even if the interaction term was non-significant). We will therefore proceed in the following way:

```
library( multcomp)
chap9a$NW <- with( chap9a,
                   interaction( Nitrogen, Water))
summary( glht( aov( Weight ~ NW, data=chap9a),
               linfct=mcp(NW="Tukey")))

        Simultaneous Tests for General Linear Hypotheses
Multiple Comparisons of Means: Tukey Contrasts

Fit: aov(formula = Weight ~ NW, data = chap9a)
```

```
Linear Hypotheses:
                             Estimate Std.Error t value Pr(>|t|)
none.high - added.high == 0  -24.200    1.257  -19.252  < 0.001 ***
added.low - added.high == 0  -29.600    1.257  -23.548  < 0.001 ***
none.low - added.high == 0   -35.600    1.257  -28.322  < 0.001 ***
added.low - none.high == 0    -5.400    1.257   -4.296  0.00277 **
none.low - none.high == 0    -11.400    1.257   -9.069  < 0.001 ***
none.low - added.low == 0     -6.000    1.257   -4.773  0.00112 **
--
```

All the pairwise differences among group means are significantly different from zero at $p < 0.01$, but most differences are much stronger.

We should also mention here that the current attitude towards presenting statistical models puts less emphasis on presenting the significance of effects, but rather places the focus on the actual **effect size**, allowing us to better grasp the existence or absence of the biological importance of the patterns revealed by our models. Although multiple sophisticated measures of effect sizes have been suggested, a simple yet still quite good measure is the value of the F statistic, comparing the explained and unexplained variation. If we compare the F statistics in the ANOVA table presented earlier, we can say that the aboveground biomass is affected more by the changes in water availability than by nitrogen addition, and the changes in weight against a hypothetical additive effect of *Water* and *Nitrogen* were the smallest.

9.10.2 Using a Fixed vs. Random Effect for a Factor

In this example (with data in the *chap9b* data frame), we focus on the response of tiller lengths (*TillerLen*) to fertiliser addition (*Fertil*). Aside from this factor, which clearly has a fixed effect, we also use another factor representing the experimental location (*Locality*). If we consider the locality to have a fixed effect, then computation is straightforward using the two-way factorial ANOVA model:

```
summary( aov( TillerLen ~ Fertil * Locality,
data=chap9b))
                 Df Sum Sq Mean Sq F value   Pr(>F)
Fertil            1  35707   35707  148.52 9.07e-12 ***
Locality          2 163940   81970  340.95  < 2e-16 ***
Fertil:Locality   2  27420   13710   57.03 7.62e-10 ***
Residuals        24   5770     240
```

Model results show that the tiller length is affected by fertilisation, tiller lengths differ among localities and – importantly – there is a strong interaction between the two factors.

When we plot the group averages using an interaction plot, we can see that the fertilisation increases tiller length in two localities, but not in the third (Fig. 9.5).

```
with( chap9b,
      interaction.plot( Fertil, Locality, TillerLen))
```

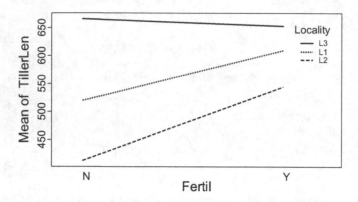

Figure 9.5 Interaction plot for *Locality* and *Fertil* factors, using the length of red fescue tillers as a response variable.

Nevertheless, on average the tiller length is positively affected by fertilisation **in the three studied localities.** Because we have chosen to use *Locality* as a factor with a fixed effect, we do not consider any other localities in which this species might grow.

But if we take the *Locality* factor as having a random effect and additionally we expect that the *Fertil* effect might vary across localities (see Fig. 9.5), we must test the effect of fertilisation against the interaction term of both factors:

```
summary( aov( TillerLen~Fertil+Error(Locality/Fertil),
         data=chap9b))

Error: Locality
          Df Sum Sq Mean Sq F value Pr(>F)
Residuals  2 163940   81970

Error: Locality:Fertil
          Df Sum Sq Mean Sq F value Pr(>F)
Fertil     1  35708   35708   2.604  0.248
Residuals  2  27420   13710

Error: Within
          Df Sum Sq Mean Sq F value Pr(>F)
Residuals 24   5770   240.4
```

When you locate the mean square (*Mean Sq*) terms, you will see that they agree with those computed in the earlier two-way ANOVA model. The only difference is how the *F* statistic is computed for the *Fertil* effect: the interaction term mean square (13,710) is used in the denominator, yielding a substantially smaller (and non-significant) *F* statistic estimate. But this makes perfect sense, because by declaring *Locality* as a random effect factor, we specify that our three localities are just a random selection from all possible localities of a given type and that we want to generalise our conclusions across all such localities. Consequently, if fertilisation increases tiller lengths in just two localities and has no substantial effect in the third, we can hardly say something specific about this response across all localities in the region.

If we consider *Locality* as the only error term[5] in our model (as is routinely done with this kind of random effect), then the results will be very different, showing a highly significant effect of fertilisation:

```
summary( aov( TillerLen~Fertil+Error(Locality),
             data=chap9b))
Error: Locality
          Df Sum Sq Mean Sq F value Pr(>F)
Residuals  2 163940   81970

Error: Within
          Df Sum Sq Mean Sq F value    Pr(>F)
Fertil     1  35707   35707   27.97 1.57e-05 ***
Residuals 26  33190    1277
```

But we apparently made an assumption about a constant effect of fertilisation across all locations which is too simplistic, because it does not fit with the content of Fig. 9.5 or with the significant interaction term we found in the two-way ANOVA model.

9.10.3 Analysing Randomised Blocks and Latin Squares

In our simplest possible example of data from a randomised block design, we can use a standard ANOVA model without an interaction, with the *Block* presented as a factor with a fixed effect:

```
aov.2 <- aov( SeedlSum ~ Block + Treatment, data=chap9c)
summary( aov.2)
          Df Sum Sq Mean Sq F value Pr(>F)
Block      3    647     216   0.202 0.8926
Treatment  3  13540    4513   4.223 0.0403 *
Residuals  9   9620    1069
```

We can see that there is no significant difference among block averages, but there is a stronger (and significant, $p = 0.040$) difference among the treatments. To get an ecologically interpretable view of our results, we must perform multiple comparisons here:

```
library( multcomp)
summary( glht( aov.2, linfct=mcp( Treatment="Tukey")))
         Simultaneous Tests for General Linear Hypotheses
Multiple Comparisons of Means: Tukey Contrasts
Fit: aov(formula = SeedlSum ~ Block + Treatment, data = chap9c)
```

---

[5] See the following Section 9.10.3 for a brief explanation of the *Error* term in the *aov* formula.

```
Linear Hypotheses:
                       Estimate Std. Error t value Pr(>|t|)
rem_litt - ctrl == 0      -1.00     23.12   -0.043   1.0000
rem_litt_moss - ctrl == 0 54.75     23.12    2.368   0.1533
rem_NS - ctrl == 0       -24.50     23.12   -1.060   0.7207
rem_litt_moss - rem_litt == 0 55.75 23.12    2.412   0.1438
rem_NS - rem_litt == 0   -23.50     23.12   -1.017   0.7444
rem_NS - rem_litt_moss == 0 -79.25  23.12   -3.428   0.0316 *
```

We obtained just a single significant difference,[6] with significantly higher seedling density in plots where plant litter and the moss layer was removed when compared with plots where *Nardus* grass was weeded out.

If our model becomes more complicated (particularly with multiple random effects), we can use the *aov* function with an *Error* term in the formula. We demonstrate this approach with the same data: the results are identical to those above, except now the differences among blocks are not tested:

```
summary( aov( SeedlSum ~ Treatment + Error( Block),
              data=chap9c))
Error: Block
          Df Sum Sq Mean Sq F value Pr(>F)
Residuals  3  646.7   215.6
Error: Within
          Df Sum Sq Mean Sq F value Pr(>F)
Treatment  3  13540    4513   4.223 0.0403 *
Residuals  9   9620    1069
```

An analysis of variance with an *Error* term splits the variation in the seedling counts into two parts (layers). The layer labelled in the above output as *Error: Block* represents the variation among blocks. There is no factor changing at the among-block level (except the *Block* factor, but this is used to define the layer here), so all among-block variation is presented as random in its *Residuals* row. On the contrary, the other layer (*Error: Within*) is the within-block variation and the *Treatment* factor explains part of the variation among values in blocks – so its mean square is compared against the error mean square within the blocks using the same *F* statistic as in our earlier main effect ANOVA example. If we had a factor with a fixed effect, changing its value on the block level (of course, we would need more than four blocks!), then our ANOVA design would represent a *split-plot ANOVA* design, which we will discuss in Section 11.2.

We can fit an ANOVA model for our Latin square design example with the following command. Note that the model formula provides separate effects of row and column identity (without any interaction), followed by an expression describing two main effects of phosphate addition (factor *P*) and fungicide application (factor *Bav*) and an interaction between them:

---

[6] Multiple comparisons tend to have a lower power than the ANOVA *F* test, which is a consequence of our asking more specific questions.

```
summary( aov( PoaAngus ~ Row + Column + P * Bav,
             data=chap9c))
```

	Df	Sum Sq	Mean Sq	F value	Pr(>F)	
Row	3	64.41	21.47	4.865	0.04779	*
Column	3	107.91	35.97	8.150	0.01544	*
P	1	127.41	127.41	28.868	0.00171	**
Bav	1	127.07	127.07	28.792	0.00172	**
P:Bav	1	43.53	43.53	9.863	0.02006	*
Residuals	6	26.48	4.41			

From the resulting ANOVA table, we can see strong and significant effects of phosphate and fungicide applications (judging from the F statistic values they appear to be similarly sized effects), as well as a significant interaction term. To interpret the meaning of the interaction in this model, we can either present it graphically (e.g. as an interaction diagram, see Fig. 9.4 for an example) or we can interpret it using the estimates of the ANOVA model parameters. This is because any ANOVA model can be considered to be a special case of linear regression models, in which the effects of individual variables are described numerically by the regression coefficients (see Chapter 14 for more details). We can extract the regression coefficients for our ANOVA model with the *coef* function:

```
coef( aov( PoaAngus ~ Row + Column + P * Bav,
          data=chap9c))
```

(Intercept)	Rowr2	Rowr3	Rowr4	Columnc2
4.23625	2.76000	-0.75250	-2.84500	-3.09500
Columnc3	Columnc4	Pyes	Bavyes	Pyes:Bavyes
0.58000	4.21750	2.34500	2.33750	6.59750

The values of regression coefficients show us (we will ignore the differences among rows and columns) that the plots with added phosphate (whether the fungicide was applied or not) have on average a biomass which is 2.345 g greater (*Pyes* coefficient). Similarly, the plots with added fungicide (averaging across plots with and without phosphates) had on average a biomass 2.3375 g greater when compared with plots without phosphate or fungicide addition. Because the interaction term is significant, the effect of *P* and *Bav* is not additive and so the plots where both the phosphates and the fungicide were applied do not see biomass increases (compared to the no phosphates/no fungicide plots) equivalent to (2.345 + 2.3375) g, but rather (2.345 + 2.3375 + 6.5975) g – see the coefficient *Pyes:Bavyes*.

9.10.4 Friedman Test

We have the response data arranged into three separate variables, one for each type of pollen (allergen). Therefore the easiest way to submit these data to a function for the Friedman test is in the form of a matrix with three columns:

```
with( chap9d, friedman.test(
            cbind( R.Artemisia, R.Ambrosia, R.Betula)))
        Friedman rank sum test
data:  cbind(R.Artemisia, R.Ambrosia, R.Betula)
Friedman chi-squared = 15.765, df = 2, p-value = 0.0003773
```

Alternatively, we can use data arranged the same as that of the main effect ANOVA with completely randomised blocks, i.e. with all response values in a single numerical variable and with two factors coding the type of allergen and the identity of the person. This is illustrated below:

```
Resp <- with( chap9d,
            c(R.Artemisia,R.Ambrosia,R.Betula))
Person <- as.factor( rep(1:10,3))
Allergen <- as.factor( rep(c("Artem","Ambros","Betula"),
                        rep(10,3)))
friedman.test( Resp ~ Allergen | Person)
        Friedman rank sum test
data:  Resp and Allergen and Person;
Friedman chi-squared = 15.765, df = 2, p-value = 0.0003773
```

We can see a significant difference among allergen types. To better understand the nature of these differences, we could simply use a classified box-and-whisker plot (see Fig. 9.6):

```
plot( Resp ~ Allergen)
```

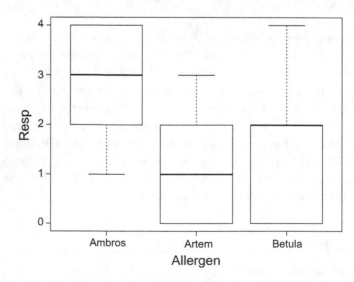

Figure 9.6 Differences in allergic response (measured on 10 persons) between three types of allergens (pollen types).

The strongest allergic response was observed with the pollen grains of *Ambrosia*, followed by *Betula*.

9.11 Reporting Analyses

9.11.1 Methods

The effects of nitrogen addition and manipulated water availability on aboveground biomass were studied in a factorial experiment (with five replicates at each combination of treatment levels), with a completely randomised arrangement of individual plants. Data were analysed with a two-way ANOVA model, using a *post-hoc* test of differences among the four combinations of experimental treatments by Tukey's HSD method.

The effects of plant cover manipulation on the establishment of plant seedlings throughout the season were evaluated using an ANOVA with added effect of block.

Or alternatively ... using a GLM with the main effects of manipulation and block identity.

The differences in the reaction of skin to three allergens were tested using a Friedman (ANOVA) test.

9.11.2 Results

The positive effect of higher water availability on plant biomass was more pronounced than the effect of nitrogen addition (with both effects being significant, see Table X, Fig. Y); moreover, the joint addition of both had a synergistic positive effect (significant interaction, see Table X).

We do not show Fig. Y here, but it would probably be a bar plot with the four combinations of watering and fertilisation treatments, displaying the mean aboveground biomass value for each group on the vertical axis (probably with ranges added indicating standard errors of mean estimates). The same diagram can also contain letters (above the bars) indicating significant differences found in multiple comparisons (see Chapter 8 for an example). But in our case (rather than having the a, b, c, d letters above the individual bars), it might be easier to state in the figure caption that all the combinations differed from all others at p < 0.01.

Another possibility would be to display an interaction plot (such as that in Fig. 9.4). It would then be necessary to mention in the caption that the intervals represent 95% confidence intervals of group means and probably also to stress that the lines connecting

Table X *Results of a two-way ANOVA showing the effects of nitrogen and water availability upon aboveground biomass. The F column represents values of the test statistic (with df = 1, 16) for each model term, p represents the significance of the tests*

	F	p
Nitrogen	288.6	<0.001
Water	532.0	<0.001
Nitrogen:Water	104.8	<0.001

the means do not represent an interpolation, but rather they visualise the strength of the interaction between the two factors.

We found significant differences among the soil cover treatments ($F_{3,9}$ = 4.22, p = 0.040). Multiple comparisons suggest that the only significant contrast was between the removal of both the plant litter and the moss layer and the removal of the dominant grass (p = 0.032), with highest seedling density in plots with imposed litter and moss removal.

The results of an ANOVA for the Latin square data are summarised in Table W (*we do not give Table W here, but it would be a simplification of the ANOVA table produced by the R software, similar to Table X above*). Both phosphate and fungicide applications significantly increased the aboveground biomass of *Poa*. We also demonstrate their synergistic effect, with biomass almost four times higher in plots which were subject to joint application of phosphate and fungicide compared to control plots – see Fig. Z (*again, we omit Fig. Z here*).

Skin response differed significantly among the three allergen types (χ^2_2 = 15.76, p = 0.0004), with the strongest response observed for *Ambrosia* pollen.

9.12 Recommended Reading

Zar (2010), pp. 249–281.

Quinn & Keough (2002), pp. 221–259 (factorial design) and pp. 262–300 (randomised blocks and simple repeated measurements).

Sokal & Rohlf (2012), pp. 319–378.

J. Fox & S. Weisberg (2018) Visualizing fit and lack of fit in complex regression models with predictor effect plots and partial residuals. *Journal of Statistical Software*, **87**(9). DOI: 10.18637/jss.v087.i09.

S. H. Hurlbert (1984) Pseudoreplication and the design of ecological field experiments. *Ecological Monographs*, **54**: 187–211.

R. Mead (1988) *The Design of Experiments. Statistical Principles for Practical Applications*. Cambridge University Press, Cambridge.

P. Šmilauer & M. Šmilauerová (2000) Effect of AM symbiosis exclusion on grassland community composition. *Folia Geobotanica*, **35**: 13–25.

I. Špačková, I. Kotorová & J. Lepš (1998) Sensitivity of seedling recruitment to moss, litter and dominant removal in an oligotrophic wet meadow. *Folia Geobotanica*, **33**: 17–30.

10 Data Transformations for Analysis of Variance

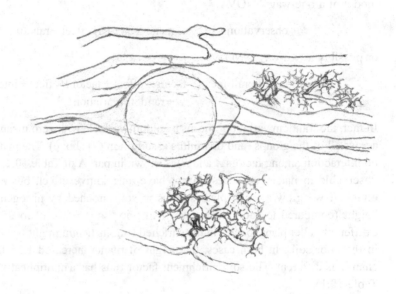

10.1 Assumptions of ANOVA and their Possible Violations

We make specific assumptions about the data being analysed in both the Student's t test and analysis of variance. One of the essential assumptions is the independence of observations. If our data do not meet this assumption (e.g. the individuals deemed to be 'typical' were selected or we used an inappropriate experimental design, see Fig. 9.2A in the preceding chapter), the trust in our statistical analysis is seriously broken and no statistical procedure can fix this problem.

Three additional assumptions concern: (1) *the normality*, each case (observation) comes from a statistical population with a normal distribution;[1] (2) *the homogeneity of variances* (homoscedasticity), statistical populations compared by their means do not differ in their variances; and (3) *the additivity* among the effects of individual factors and also in the random variation.

---

[1] *Beware:* if you want to test this assumption (and we do not recommend you doing so – see Section 4.4), you must realise that our cases may not come from a single statistical distribution. If, for example, in a one-way ANOVA model with a factor having three levels the null hypothesis is incorrect, the data for the three groups should originate from three normal distributions differing by their means and so we cannot compare all the data with a single test against a particular normal distribution: we must check the distribution for each group separately. But in doing this we diminish the test power even further for small data. Alternatively (and more appropriately), we should test model residuals (differences of the response variable values from group means), comparing them with a normal distribution with zero average.

We have already discussed assumptions (1) and (2) and we know that an ANOVA (as well as a t test) is fairly robust to their violation, as long as it is not too large. For a two-sample t test, we even have an approximate method for performing it without the assumption of homoscedasticity. But what does the assumption of additivity mean? It refers to the correctness of summing up the effects of individual predictors (here the factor variables) – any deviances from such a sum are considered to represent an interaction. We can start from the model of a one-way ANOVA:

$$\text{observation} = \text{overall mean} + \text{factor } A \text{ effect} + \text{random variation} \quad (10.1)$$

or possibly a two-way ANOVA:

$$\text{observation} = \text{overall mean} + \text{factor } A \text{ effect} + \text{factor } B \text{ effect} + \text{interaction of } A \text{ and } B + \text{random variation} \quad (10.2)$$

In fact, the 'random variation' means a random variable with zero mean and constant variance across all of the groups (and this fulfils assumption (2) above). The pattern of additivity (with no interaction among factors A and B) is shown in part A of Table 10.1. But many phenomena observable in natural sciences do not have an additive effect, but rather a **multiplicative effect**. If we grow a small plant species in soil enriched by nitrogen, it might increase its height (compared to individuals grown in poor soil) from 20 to 25 cm. But if we grow a different, taller plant species in the enriched soil, its height might be 50 cm (instead of 40 cm in the poor soil). In both cases, the height of plants increased 1.25 times, but the additive change is different. The soil enrichment factor thus has a multiplicative effect (see part B of Table 10.1).

An appropriate model for a multiplicative effect in a one-way ANOVA is

$$\text{observation} = \text{overall mean} \times \text{factor } A \text{ effect} \times \text{random variation} \quad (10.3)$$

Here, the random variation means a random variable, the logarithm of which has a normal distribution with zero mean (and so our random variables have a log-normal distribution). In this model, both the mean and the random variation are multiplied by the effect of factor A. This means that we can expect a linear dependency of the variation (at the scale of the standard deviation) on the mean. If we log-transform Eq. (10.3), we get:

$$\log(\text{observation}) = \log(\text{overall mean}) + \log(\text{factor } A \text{ effect}) + \log(\text{random variation}) \quad (10.4)$$

Table 10.1 *Additive and multiplicative effects in a two-way ANOVA for an experiment where daisies and sunflowers were grown in containers under four levels of nutrient addition (level 0, no added nutrients; level 1, 10 g of N; level 2, 15 g of N; level 3, 20 g of N) and their height was measured as a response variable*

Part A: Hypothetical values of mean height in cells of a two-way ANOVA for additive factor effects

Species	Nutrients			
	Level 0	Level 1	Level 2	Level 3
daisy	10	15	18	20
sunflower	100	105	108	110

Table 10.1 *(cont.)*

Part B: Hypothetical values of mean height in cells of a two-way ANOVA for multiplicative factor effects

Species	Nutrients			
	Level 0	Level 1	Level 2	Level 3
daisy	10	15	18	20
sunflower	100	150	180	200

Part C: Hypothetical values obtained by log-transforming the mean heights from Part B above, demonstrating the restoration of additivity by log-transformation.

Species	Nutrients			
	Level 0	Level 1	Level 2	Level 3
daisy	1.000	1.176	1.255	1.301
sunflower	2.000	2.176	2.255	2.301

This means that if a factor has a multiplicative effect on a response variable, it has an additive effect on log-transformed values of the response. This is illustrated in part C of Table 10.1. If factor A has no influence, this means that in a multiplicative relation its value is 1.0 for all its levels, and so it is equal to log(1), i.e. 0, for an additive model obtained by log-transforming the response variable. Multiplicative effects are probably quite common in the data we collect – actually, if a biologist says that nutrient addition has the same effect on daisies (*Bellis perennis*) as it does on sunflowers (*Helianthus annuus*), she usually means the situation described in part B below, i.e. a multiplicative effect.

If some or all of the assumptions of the ANOVA model are not sufficiently fulfilled, we have several options for how to proceed: we can use some alternative non-parametric statistical model, or we can consider using GLMs (see Chapter 15), or we can perform some **data transformation**. By data transformation, we mean a mathematical operation that changes a numerical variable X into another one (let us call it X'). In some instances, a single transformation can change our data so that they meet all of the three assumptions discussed above (normality, homogeneity of variances, additivity of effects). The most frequently used transformation is the log-transformation, but for specific data types it might be more appropriate to use arcsine transformation (for relative fractions) or square-root transformation (for counts of cases). All of these three transformation types are discussed in the following sections.

10.2 Log-transformation

This transformation is recommended for numerical data on a rational scale which are often affected by factors (or numerical predictors also) in a multiplicative way while their standard deviation size is linearly related to the mean value.[2] From the perspective of distribution shape

---

[2] As we have already discussed with reference to Eq. (10.3), both patterns often occur together.

or the change from a multiplicative relationship into additivity, it does not matter which base we choose for the log function.[3] The simple log-transformation looks as follows:

$$X' = \log(X) \tag{10.5}$$

If our data contain zeros (we assume there are no negative values), we use

$$X' = \log(X + c) \tag{10.6}$$

where c is a constant value, most often set to 1.[4] Both transformations have a similar effect. As demonstrated in Table 10.1, the log-transformation is able to turn multiplicative effects into additive ones, but for the $\log(X + c)$ transformation this holds only in an approximate way. So, if our data do not contain zeros, Eq. (10.5) should be used.

The use of log-transformation is quite common, and for field-based observations of abundance or biomass of organisms, zeros are also common.[5] Thus, biologists use the $\log(X + c)$ transformation quite frequently. Because it is nice to retain zero values for absent organisms even after such transformation, we often opt for $c = 1$, therefore using a $\log(X + 1)$ transformation. This usually works well for counts, but might fail to do an adequate job (i.e. to decrease the skewness and stabilise the variance of our data) if the values are mostly smaller than one.

Although for most types of statistical models negative values for the response variable do not represent a problem, graphs look better if zero on the transformed scale corresponds to zero on the original scale (e.g. the absence of some studied species). Consequently, instead of $\log(X + c)$ which will yield negative values for $c < 1$, we often use a $\log(aX + 1)$ transformation, which has similar effects on the distributional properties of transformed values. Actually, if $a = 1/c$, the effect is exactly the same, just the values are shifted so that zero in the original data yields zero in the transformed data.[6]

We will illustrate the effects of a $\log(aX + 1)$ transformation using the example of a set of dry weight values of *Prunella vulgaris* biomass collected from experimental plots (0.5 × 0.5 m). This plant species is relatively rare, and sometimes missing (implying the presence of zero values in our data), and most values are between 0 and 0.2 g. If we apply a $\log(aX + 1)$ transformation, its effect changes with the value of a (see Fig. 10.1). For example, if we use $a = 1000$, we are in fact first transforming weight values from grams to milligrams before adding 1. Consequently, whenever you use the $\log(X + 1)$ transformation, you should be aware that the results depend on the units in which the x variable is measured. On the contrary, when using a $\log(X)$ transformation, the results are not affected by the choice of units for X.

Also, when using a $\log(X + 1)$ transformation, the change from multiplicativity (on the original scale) to additivity (on the transformed scale) is only approximate. The range of values being transformed must not be too close to zero, otherwise we must use the $\log(aX + 1)$ transformation.

---

[3] We generally recommend the natural log (with base e) for data transformation; in this book we use ln where the natural log is required and log elsewhere.

[4] More generally, c is set to a value roughly matching the smallest positive value in the data.

[5] Zero abundance or biomass implies that the studied species is absent from the corresponding site. Zeros can also be present in concentrations (and other variables with data on the ratio scale) when the given ion or element is missing or at a concentration below the detection limit of the measuring device.

[6] Because in this case $\log(ax + 1) = \log(x + c) + \log(1/c)$.

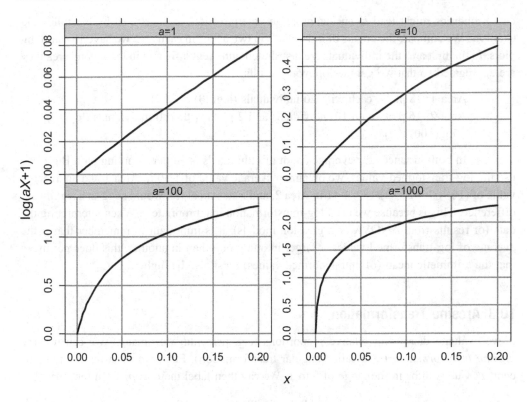

Figure 10.1 The effects of changing the multiplicative coefficient a in the generalised $\log(aX + 1)$ transformation.

Further, if our response variable has the property that the size of the standard deviation changes (e.g. across the groups in ANOVA models) linearly with the mean value (i.e. if the coefficient of variation is constant), then the log-transformed values have their variance estimates approximately constant.

The log-transformation also changes the type of distribution: for example, with data on a ratio scale, it can change a positively skewed distribution (e.g. of the weights of individuals) into a more symmetrical distribution. If the $\log(X)$ values have an (approximate) normal distribution, then the distribution of the original X values is often called the *log-normal distribution* (or Galton distribution).

The log-transformation is useful, in the majority of cases, for measures representing weights or dimensions or concentrations of ions, but also for counts of individuals, particularly if those individuals are distributed across space in an aggregate manner.[7]

But we should warn the reader about some additional dangers of log-transforming their data. If we undo the log-transformation of a mean calculated (as an arithmetic average) from log-transformed values, we do not obtain the arithmetic average, but rather the geometric mean of the original values, which is always lower than the arithmetic average. Mindless use of log-transformation (as well as any other statistical approach) without understanding the

---

[7] Although for such count data the so-called contagious distributions (such as the negative binomial distribution) are more appropriate, the log-normal distribution also matches the data reasonably well.

data properties might lead to an inappropriate interpretation, as illustrated by the following example. We compare the counts of individuals in two areas, in each area we have 18 sampling plots. In the first area the individuals are distributed quite regularly and in the second area they are aggregated so that we get the following results:

Area 1: 18 plots, each with 20 individuals (log(20) = 1.30)
Area 2: 16 plots with 10 individuals and 2 plots with 100 individuals (log(10) = 1, log(100) = 2)

In both instances the average count of individuals is 20 per sampling plot. But if we use the log-transformed values, we obtain an average value of 1.30 in Area 1 and an average value of $(16 \times 1 + 2 \times 2)/18 = 1.11$ in Area 2, and a statistical test would suggest a significant difference. This is because we used log-transformation inappropriately. When interpreting the data (or results from ANOVA or regression models), it is important to remember that if the average of log-transformed values is larger in one group than in another, this does not mean that the arithmetic mean (of untransformed values) must also be higher.

10.3 Arcsine Transformation

If we evaluate data using relative proportions (e.g. percentage estimates), we can use the *arcsine transformation* (also called angular transformation). First, we must rescale the percentage values to be in the range of 0 to 1. We can then label them as p. Then the variable

$$p' = \arcsin \sqrt{p} \qquad (10.7)$$

has an approximately normal distribution (or at least, the distribution is approximately symmetrical). This transformation is recommended if the data contain values either <0.3 or >0.7. If all the p-values are between 0.3 and 0.7, their distribution would be sufficiently close to a normal distribution and there is no need to transform. If we use this transformation in a factorial ANOVA model, we should be aware that for the test of the interaction, the null hypothesis is about the additivity on the transformed scale, which is quite difficult to interpret on the scale of the original values.

We should note that the use of this transformation, particularly for situations where the proportion is estimated as a count of success events from total events (e.g. each experimental pot will be characterised by a proportion of surviving seedlings out of the 10 planted), might be considered obsolete, being succeeded by the use of GLMs with a binomial distribution (see Chapter 15).

10.4 Square-Root and Box–Cox Transformation

If the data is sampled from a population characterised by a Poisson distribution, we can use the square-root transformation.[8] We will address the Poisson distribution in greater detail later in this book (Chapter 18), but we should mention here that one of its important properties is that its variance is equal to its mean. A typical example of data with a Poisson distribution is

---

[8] But a log-transformation would also be a good choice in this case.

the counts of individuals in sampling units, if the individuals have a random (and independent) spatial distribution (for sampling units like plots) or if they find their way into the unit fully independently (for sampling units like soil traps).

For the square-root transformation we either use a direct application of the square root, or better yet

$$X' = \sqrt{X + 0.5} \tag{10.8}$$

which is recommended particularly if the variable X also contains zero values. The resulting variable X' has a distribution closer to the normal distribution and also the variance is less dependent on the mean value. However, even here, a more appropriate approach would be to use GLMs (see Chapter 15).

Sometimes so-called Box–Cox transformation is recommended (see Sokal & Rohlf, 2012, pp. 435–438 for details), which has a varying parameter λ. The value of λ is determined using the data to be transformed (X values) so that the effect of transformation on the data normality (and sometimes also the homogeneity of variances) is maximised. The formula of this general transformation with the parameter λ is as follows (if λ is not zero):

$$X' = \frac{X^\lambda - 1}{\lambda} \tag{10.9}$$

or (if λ is zero)

$$X' = \ln(X) \tag{10.10}$$

where ln is a natural logarithm. The above equations apply for positive values only, but formulas also exist for computing with negative X values.

10.5 Concluding Remarks

All data transformations can also be employed when computing the mean and its confidence interval. To do so, we first compute the mean and confidence interval for transformed values and then we back-transform the resulting estimates. As a consequence, however, the mean estimate will be somewhat biased (see Section 10.2 above) and the confidence interval will not be symmetrical around the mean (which makes sense, as the original distribution of non-transformed data was also not symmetrical). It is not, however, sensible to provide back-transformed values of the standard error of the mean. The estimates of the mean and confidence intervals based on back-transformation are very robust towards extreme values that might be present, particularly in positively skewed distributions.

The use of data transformations is sometimes treated as a controversial issue and some authors warn against their use. But as a matter of fact, we use them routinely in multiple circumstances without even knowing it. As an example, if we measure the acidity of soil or water using pH values, we employ the log-transformation of the concentration of hydrogen ions. The values of this concentration usually have a log-normal distribution, so their variability depends on the mean and one can also expect that the effect of various factors – as well as the random variation – will be multiplicative for such concentration data. No one argues, however, that the log-transformation is inappropriate and that one should work with the original concentrations. Another way to address this supposed controversy is to point out that even leaving the data on the scale coming directly from our instruments is a (rather arbitrary) transformation. Very often the measurement scale is given by the physical or chemical method being employed, and we have no guarantee that it represents a scale optimal for describing processes taking place in nature. This is the case for the example of nutrient concentrations in soil or water, not just the example of hydrogen ion concentrations.

For simple statistical models like ANOVA or linear regression, the use of GLMs is usually a more appropriate solution than directly transforming the data. The GLMs also include the implicit transformation of the scale of the response variable (see Chapter 15). But even for GLMs and similar types of more advanced models (GAM, GLMM, etc.), the issue of an appropriate scale for explanatory (independent) quantitative variables still remains. Further, for more complex statistical methods (including multivariate ordination methods, see Chapter 22), the generalisations similar to a change from linear models to GLMs are not readily available and so data transformation is a vital tool.

10.6 Example Data

We return to data from a previous chapter for our first example, describing the relation of grassland plant seedling frequency (*SeedlSum*) to the manipulation of experimental plots (*Treatment* variable). This experiment has a complete randomised blocks design, with the identity of blocks described by the *Block* factor. If we were examining the homogeneity of variances in our analyses in the preceding chapter (but we cunningly avoided the check of this assumption ☺), we would find a significant departure from this assumption, and so now we will verify that a log-transformation solves the issue.

The second example (starting from column *D*) represents the data describing the percentage frequency of arbuscular mycorrhizal (AM) fungi in the roots of the grass species *Holcus lanatus*, collected from grassland plots differing in their management (factor variable *Mown* with values *yes* or *no* for, respectively, mown or unmown plots) and in the supply of phosphates (factor variable *P* with values *yes* or *no*). The frequency of AM fungi (*PercArb*) represents the count of how many out of 100 intersections of stained roots (observed under the microscope with a grid raster) had root parts with a developed AM fungal colony. Each observation (each root sample) comes from a separate experimental plot.

The third example (starting from column *G*) examines the effects of low vs. high water availability (*water*) and of nitrogen addition (*nitrogen*) on the dry weight of plant aboveground biomass, based on the results of a greenhouse experiment. The values of the response variable are provided either in grams (variable *biomass.g*) or in kilograms (*biomass.kg*).

10.7 How to Proceed in R

The variables for our three examples must be imported separately into data frames *chap10a*, *chap10b* and *chap10c*.

Let us first check the homogeneity of variances in the non-transformed seedling counts between the four treatment groups:

```
bartlett.test( SeedlSum ~ Treatment, data=chap10a)
```

```
        Bartlett test of homogeneity of variances
data:  SeedlSum by Treatment
Bartlett's K-squared = 9.0096, df = 3, p-value = 0.02916
```

So here we must reject the null hypothesis about the homoscedasticity; the data do not seem to fulfil this assumption sufficiently well. What about log-transformed values?

```
bartlett.test( log( SeedlSum) ~ Treatment, data=chap10a)
```

```
        Bartlett test of homogeneity of variances
data:  log(SeedlSum) by Treatment
Bartlett's K-squared = 4.3472, df = 3, p-value = 0.2263
```

This is much better, so we settle on log-transformed counts and perform the analysis:

```
summary( aov( log( SeedlSum) ~ Block + Treatment,
        data=chap10a))
```

	Df	Sum Sq	Mean Sq	F value	Pr(>F)
Block	3	0.1324	0.0441	0.413	0.7479
Treatment	3	1.4204	0.4735	4.427	0.0358 *
Residuals	9	0.9626	0.1070		

Luckily, the conclusions based on the model using the transformed data are identical, perhaps even better, with a slightly lower Type I error probability.

Now we proceed to the example with relative proportions of arbuscular mycorrhizal fungi in grass roots. The appropriate transformation is arcsine on square-root-transformed proportions:

```
summary( aov( asin( sqrt( PercArb/100)) ~ Mown * P,
        data=chap10b))
```

	Df	Sum Sq	Mean Sq	F value	Pr(>F)
Mown	1	0.0569	0.0569	4.851	0.0449 *
P	1	0.3842	0.3842	32.773	5.25e-05 ***
Mown:P	1	0.0322	0.0322	2.745	0.1198
Residuals	14	0.1641	0.0117		

Both main effects are significant, although barely so for mowing ($F_{1,14} = 4.851$, $p = 0.045$). It might be interesting to see what happens if we swap the order of the two factor variables in the ANOVA formula. This should not change anything, right?

```
summary( aov( asin( sqrt( PercArb/100)) ~ P * Mown,
        data=chap10b))
```

	Df	Sum Sq	Mean Sq	F value	Pr(>F)
P	1	0.4104	0.4104	35.003	3.76e-05 ***
Mown	1	0.0307	0.0307	2.621	0.128

```
P:Mown        1 0.0322  0.0322   2.745    0.120
Residuals    14 0.1641  0.0117
```

Wrong! The effect of mowing is no longer significant and the F statistics for both main effects have changed. In contrast, the results for the interaction term or in the *Residuals* row (representing the variance not explained by the ANOVA model) remain unchanged. What is going on? Our first clue comes from looking at the count of observations in the two-way ANOVA cells:

```
with( chap10b, summary( interaction( P, Mown)))
```
```
no.no  yes.no  no.yes yes.yes
  4       4       4       6
```

The experimental design is not balanced, and neither is it even proportional (see Section 9.2)! The number of observations is four for all combinations, except the fertilised and mown plots. It is possible that the experimenters felt this combination is more important, or perhaps the individuals of the grass species under study were found in just four plots of the other three treatment combinations. Anyway, this results in the effects of the P and *Mown* factors being correlated: they share a part of their explanatory ability.

The function *summary* for the *aov* models (but also the function *anova* for the linear models, fitted with the *lm* function – see Chapters 12 and 14) use so-called *sequential decomposition* of the model sum of squares into the contributions of individual model terms. This decomposition always starts with accounting for all the main effects, and only after their contributions are calculated does the algorithm quantify the interactions. This is why we get the same values for the interaction term in both ANOVA tables. But the main effects of the factors are evaluated in the order given by the formula. In our example we see that the main effect of *Mown* has the estimate of *SS* equal to 0.0569 in the first instance and 0.026 lower in the second instance, when it is considered after the effect of P (the values of *SS* for P change in a complementary way). So the difference 0.026 represents the explained variation shared between the two model terms.

When you have an imbalanced design and use the Type I sum of squares (the default in R, but not necessarily in other statistical software), you should always think carefully about the order in which you enter individual explanatory variables (this also applies to the quantitative variables that will be discussed in subsequent chapters) and take the implications of their ordering into account when interpreting the results.

This sequential decomposition of the model sum of squares (also called *Type I Sums of Squares*) is not particularly good for unbalanced designs. Alternative decomposition methods exist; choosing one depends on the type of hypotheses being tested, but for our example with a non-significant interaction term, the so-called *Type II Sums of Squares* is probably the best choice. To perform it in R, we recommend using the *Anova* function in the *car* package (Fox & Weisberg, 2018):

```
library( car)
Anova( aov( asin( sqrt( PercArb/100)) ~ Mown * P,
           data=chap10b), type=2)
Anova Table (Type II tests)
Response: asin(sqrt(PercArb/100))
            Sum Sq Df F value    Pr(>F)
Mown       0.03073  1  2.6212    0.1277
P          0.38423  1 32.7730 5.252e-05 ***
Mown:P     0.03218  1  2.7451    0.1198
Residuals 0.16414 14
```

With this *SS* decomposition, we cannot reject the null hypothesis that there is no effect of mowing on the frequency of mycorrhizal fungi in the roots of the grass ($p = 0.128$). We can cross-check that the order of factors specified in the model formula does not matter for this type of decomposition:

```
Anova( aov( asin( sqrt( PercArb/100)) ~ P * Mown,
           data=chap10b), type=2)
Anova Table (Type II tests)
Response: asin(sqrt(PercArb/100))
            Sum Sq Df F value    Pr(>F)
P          0.38423  1 32.7730 5.252e-05 ***
Mown       0.03073  1  2.6212    0.1277
P:Mown     0.03218  1  2.7451    0.1198
Residuals 0.16414 14
```

Finally, let us remind the reader that the choice of decomposition type for the model sum of squares in linear models is not really important if their data come from a balanced (or at least a proportional) design.

The issues identified above demonstrate that even for relatively straightforward statistical methods (as the two-way ANOVA is), we can obtain different results depending on the software we are using and/or the options we choose. This implies that even for these methods, we should identify the software we used for calculations. In general it is useful to know what options the software uses as its defaults.

Finally, using our third example, we examine the effects that a particular choice of log-transformation procedure might have on the results of a two-way ANOVA. The response variable values are presented on two scales – in grams and in kilograms. When we apply a log ($aX + 1$) transformation, use of the *biomass.g* response with *a* set to 1 implies exactly the same results as using *bomass.kg* with *a* set to 1000.

When our response variable does not contain any zero, it is preferable to use a $\log(X)$ transformation, i.e. not to add 1 to the values we transform. In doing so, we can choose either the response scaled in grams:

```
aovlog.g <- aov( log10( biomass.g) ~ water * nitrogen,
                 data=chap10c)
summary( aovlog.g)
               Df Sum Sq Mean Sq F value   Pr(>F)
water           1 0.4505  0.4505 373.829 1.61e-12 ***
nitrogen        1 0.4266  0.4266 354.004 2.45e-12 ***
water:nitrogen  1 0.0000  0.0000   0.003    0.956
Residuals      16 0.0193  0.0012
```

or in kilograms:

```
aovlog.kg <- aov( log10( biomass.kg) ~ water * nitrogen,
                  data=chap10c)
summary( aovlog.kg)
               Df Sum Sq Mean Sq F value   Pr(>F)
water           1 0.4505  0.4505 373.829 1.61e-12 ***
nitrogen        1 0.4266  0.4266 354.004 2.45e-12 ***
water:nitrogen  1 0.0000  0.0000   0.003    0.956
Residuals      16 0.0193  0.0012
```

with exactly the same results, confirming no deviation from multiplicativity.[9] The conclusions might change, however, when we decide to use a $\log(X + 1)$ transformation.[10] When we analyse the response variable scaled in grams, our results are quite similar to those we obtained earlier:

```
aovlog.g1 <- aov( log10( biomass.g+1) ~ water * nitrogen,
                  data=chap10c)summary( aovlog.g1)
               Df Sum Sq Mean Sq F value   Pr(>F)
water           1 0.4408  0.4408   373.8 1.61e-12 ***
nitrogen        1 0.4174  0.4174   354.0 2.45e-12 ***
water:nitrogen  1 0.0000  0.0000     0.0    0.991
Residuals      16 0.0189  0.0012
```

But when we use biomass values measured in kilograms, we get a striking difference in the results of the analysis. Now there is a highly significant interaction:

```
aovlog.kg1 <- aov( log10(biomass.kg+1) ~ water*nitrogen,
                   data=chap10c)
summary( aovlog.kg1)
```

---

[9] In fact, the results seem to be 'too good to be true', as we have invented the data to get a close match to the model of multiplicativity.

[10] As the response variable contains no zeros, it is pointless to add 1 before log-transforming (see Section 10.2). But we might often have zero values (e.g. if the effects of water and nitrogen availability were studied under field conditions and we focused on a particular species that might be missing from a locality) and our example dataset allows us to compare pure $\log(X)$ transformation with $\log(X + 1)$ transformation.

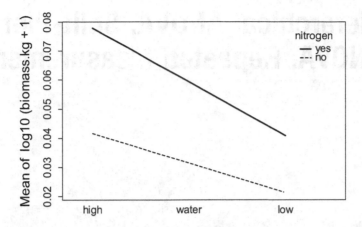

Figure 10.2 Interaction plot for water and nitrogen availability predictors in a two-way ANOVA model with the response data log-transformed after the addition of an inappropriately large constant value.

```
                Df   Sum Sq   Mean Sq  F value   Pr(>F)
water            1  0.004102  0.004102  282.00  1.39e-11 ***
nitrogen         1  0.003901  0.003901  268.15  2.04e-11 ***
water:nitrogen   1  0.000350  0.000350   24.08  0.000158 ***
Residuals       16  0.000233  0.000015
```

Also the interaction plot (Fig. 10.2) suggests that the effect of nitrogen addition is more pronounced at a high water level.

```
with( chap10c, interaction.plot( water, nitrogen,
                    log10(biomass.kg+1)))
```

10.8 Reporting Analyses

10.8.1 Methods

Seedling counts were log-transformed (frequency of mycorrhizal symbionts in roots was arcsine-transformed) to meet the assumptions of ANOVA (*or alternatively*, to achieve homogeneity of variances).

10.8.2 Results

We are not usually concerned with the transformations that have been applied when describing the results.

10.9 Recommended Reading

Zar (2010), pp. 286–295.
Quinn & Keough (2002), pp. 64–67.
Sokal & Rohlf (2012), pp. 426–440.
J. Fox & S. Weisberg (2018) *An R Companion to Applied Regression*, 3rd edn. Sage, Los Angeles, CA, 608 pp.

11 Hierarchical ANOVA, Split-Plot ANOVA, Repeated Measurements

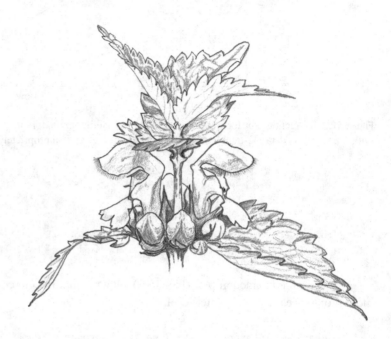

In this textbook we will use the term *hiearchical analysis of variance* or *nested analysis of variance* for any ANOVA model with multiple, hierarchically arranged sources of random variation, but with the fixed effect predictors either totally absent or present just at a single hierarchical level. We call models containing fixed effects at two or more hierarchical levels of variability *split-plot ANOVA* models. We will describe these later in the chapter, alongside ANOVA models for repeated measurements.

11.1 Hierarchical ANOVA

11.1.1 Use Case Examples

Here are two example studies in which the hierarchical ANOVA would be a suitable model choice.

1. We compare the effects of three fertiliser types (represented by a factor with three levels) on the nitrogen content of plant leaves. In each experimental group, we have five plants of the test species and from each plant we collect four leaf samples in a random manner and analyse their nitrogen content. We ask whether nitrogen concentration differs among the leaves from plants treated with different fertiliser types. To properly account for our experimental design, we should use another factor – aside from the fertiliser type – which

identifies the plant from which each leaf sample was collected (a factor with 15 levels representing 3×5 experimental plants).

These two factors (*fertiliser* and *plant*) do not have a factorial (crossed) arrangement, as each plant can only be combined with a single fertiliser type. The factors have a hierarchical arrangement, with the factor *plant* being nested within the *fertiliser* factor. Alternatively, we can describe this experimental design as having two sources of random variation (in contrast to an alternative design where just one leaf sample would be taken from each plant): the differences among the plants grown with the same type of fertiliser, and the differences among leaf samples taken from the same plant. The individual plants (rather than individual leaf samples) are our independent replicates[1] when testing for differences due to fertiliser type.

In a hierarchical ANOVA, the highest hierarchical level can be either a factor with a fixed effect (we would primarily be interested in that effect, as in our example 1) with lower levels then represented by factors with random effects, or all factors represent random effects. We may have more than two hierarchical levels in the sampling/experimental design, as is the case in the following example study where all levels represent random effects.

2. We performed a study in which we measured the length of the corona tube in flowers of a deadnettle species (*Lamium* sp.). We selected three geographical regions of interest. In each region we randomly selected five locations, at each location we randomly selected four plants, and on each plant we measured seven randomly chosen flowers. We are interested in the differences among the regions, among the locations within their region, and also among the plants within the same location (from the same population). We are most likely interested in comparing the size of variation across groups at different hierarchical levels.

Figure 11.1 shows a simplified version of the sampling arrangement in example 2. Here we compare three locations, with three plants chosen at each, and with five flowers measured on each plant. For this example, we will label the highest hierarchical level *location* with a (=3) levels, the factor nested within each location is *plant* with b (=3) levels, and n is the number of replicates at the lowest hierarchical level (five flowers

Factor

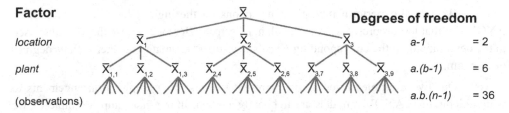

Degrees of freedom

location	$a-1$	$= 2$
plant	$a.(b-1)$	$= 6$
(observations)	$a.b.(n-1)$	$= 36$

Figure 11.1 A simplified schematic view of the sampling design for example 2 illustrating a dataset appropriate for the hierarchical ANOVA. The graphical part depicts the objects at the three levels of random variation (among locations, among plants and among flower samples), as well as the mean estimates for each recognised group of observations. Formulas are shown on the right for calculating the degrees of freedom matching the random factor for a particular hierarchical level.

---

[1] Assuming the plants are properly treated as far as their position in the greenhouse is concerned – typically mixed thoroughly in a random manner.

measured on each plant). For each hierarchical level, Fig. 11.1 shows the calculation of the degrees of freedom.

11.1.2 Decomposing Variation in a Hierarchical ANOVA Model

Generally, we express the variation at a particular hierarchical level as a sum of squared differences of the means estimated at that hierarchical level (see Fig. 11.1) from the corresponding mean at the next higher level, multiplied (weighted) by the count of observations in the particular group. For example, the sum of squares for the factor *plant* is

$$(\overline{X}_{1,1} - \overline{X}_1)^2 + (\overline{X}_{1,2} - \overline{X}_1)^2 + (\overline{X}_{1,3} - \overline{X}_1)^2 + (\overline{X}_{2,4} - \overline{X}_2)^2 + (\overline{X}_{2,5} - \overline{X}_2)^2 +$$
$$(\overline{X}_{2,6} - \overline{X}_2)^2 + (\overline{X}_{3,7} - \overline{X}_3)^2 + (\overline{X}_{3,8} - \overline{X}_3)^2 + (\overline{X}_{3,9} - \overline{X}_3)^2$$

with the result of the above expression then further multiplied by 5. The corresponding mean square (*MS*) statistic is calculated by dividing the sum of squares by the appropriate degrees of freedom (see Fig. 11.1 again).

To test the null hypothesis that there is no difference among the levels of a factor representing a particular hierarchical level, we calculate the *F* statistic by dividing the *MS* of the hierarchical level under consideration by the *MS* of the closest lower hierarchical level.

We often want to estimate the extent to which individual hierarchical levels contribute to the total variation in our data. One way to calculate such estimates, called *variance components*, is to subtract the *MS* estimate of the closest lower level from the *MS* estimate of the hierarchical level of interest, and divide the result by the count of observations in the groups defined at that level, i.e. by 5 for the *plant* factor (number of flowers measured per plant) and by 15 (3 plants × 5 flowers) for the *location* factor in our example in Fig. 11.1. The variance component for the lowest level is then represented by its *MS* value. If the *MS* value for our hierarchical level of interest is smaller than the *MS* of the level we should subtract from it, then we consider the contribution of the target level to be zero. The contributions of individual hierarchical levels are often presented on a percentage scale.

We can also perform multiple comparisons on the highest level in a hierarchical ANOVA, if that level represents a factor with fixed effects. Here we choose the *MS* value used in the denominator of the corresponding *F* statistic as the s^2 estimate, together with its degrees of freedom.

Our two examples listed above represent two common empirical arrangements to which hierarchical ANOVA models are frequently applied. In the first setup (example 1), we are only interested in the differences at the highest hierarchical level (usually representing a fixed effect factor), while the other levels reflect the structure of our experimental design. Here we collect multiple samples of leaves from each plant to better estimate the average concentration of nitrogen in the leaves of this plant.

A similar design is frequently used in field experiments. For example, we might study the effect of animal grazing (e.g. comparing the effects of sheep and cattle) on plant community diversity, measured as species richness per square metre. There are some practical constraints for our study: we need to keep the animals in enclosures, but the enclosures must be large enough to ensure the animals behave normally (so we might need the enclosure size to be at least 1 ha). It is also obvious that we need replicated enclosures for each type of grazing, as the variation between grazing types will be compared with the variation among the enclosures with identical grazing type. We will also need to have multiple sampling plots within the enclosures to reliably estimate the plant diversity of each one. The power of the test we are interested in (at the highest hierarchical level) is determined primarily by the number of replicates and variation at the closest lower level (i.e. at the enclosure level). But the test power also decreases with an increasing error in the estimates of richness for individual enclosures, and this error is inversely dependent on the number of plots per enclosure. When planning such an experiment, we should consider the fact that the maintenance costs for a 1-ha enclosure are considerably higher than recording species richness at selected 1 m^2 plots. Hierarchical decomposition of variation, together with considerations of the relative expenses for replications at individual hierarchical levels, will enable us to plan our experiment with maximum efficiency.

Our example 2 above represents the type of hierarchical ANOVA use where we are more interested in decomposing the total variation across all hierarchical levels. This approach is often used with descriptive (observational) datasets and occurs most frequently in taxonomic (or biogeographical) studies.

11.2 Split-Plot ANOVA

In some cases, our studies combine hierarchical and factorial arrangements, with the simplest example being the *split-plot design*. This design can be derived from the simpler complete randomised blocks design if we consider an effect of an experimental factor (or multiple factors) at the block level.

11.2.1 Use Case Example

We investigated the effects of fertilisation on the structure of a grassland community in a long-term field experiment. Twelve plots were divided into two groups: with and without fertilisation. After a few years (when the changes in community composition stabilised), we wanted to find out whether the competitive effects that the surrounding vegetation has upon individual plants differs between the two plot types. To do so, we planted two individuals ('phytometers') of a test species in each plot – one in intact vegetation and another in an artificially created gap (with the nearest surrounding plants weeded out). We expected that the existence of a gap would suppress the competitive effects of the surrounding vegetation. We collected all planted individuals and measured their weight at the peak of the vegetation season.

For our analysis, we are interested whether the mean weight of individuals changes with fertilisation, how much the weight is affected by the surrounding vegetation, and also whether the effect of the surrounding vegetation differs depending on the fertilisation status of the plot. The first two questions are represented in our model by the main effects of the factors *gap* and *fertiliser*, while the last question is reflected by an interaction term between *gap* and *fertiliser* factors. The field design of our experiment is schematically outlined in Fig. 11.2.

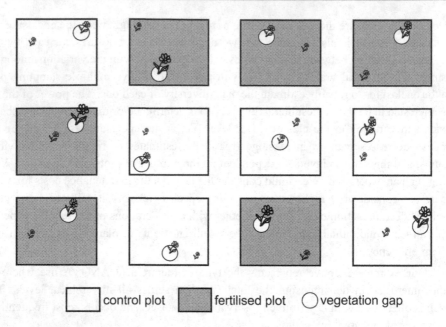

control plot   fertilised plot   ◯ vegetation gap

Figure 11.2 Arrangement of a field experiment producing a data structure suitable for a split-plot ANOVA model.

11.2.2 Analysis

Superficially, the experimental arrangement shown in Fig. 11.2 resembles the traditional factorial design with two factors (fertilisation and the presence of a gap). Here we are interested in both the main effects and their interaction,[2] again similar to a factorial design. But there is one important difference from the factorial arrangement: the two plants sharing the same plot are not mutually independent. When evaluating the effect of fertilisation, we do not have 24, but just 12 independent observations, despite our data being represented by a table with 24 rows. This must be reflected when decomposing the sum of squares and choosing the appropriate denominator for the F tests.

Aside from the two factor effects mentioned above, our model must also include the identity of experimental plots, which is described as a factor with a random effect. The factor at the level of 'blocks' (the fertilisation treatment in our example) is often called the *between-subject factor* or *main-plot factor* or *whole-plot factor*, while the factor varying within the blocks or plots (here the placement of an individual within or outside the gap) is called the *within-subject factor* or *split-plot factor*. When testing a whole-plot factor, the denominator of the F statistic is the MS for the plot effect, while for a test of a split-plot factor and for an interaction (if present in the model), the denominator represents the residual MS (which is actually the MS of the interaction of the plot effect with the within-plot effect).

In a split-plot design, the whole plots do not need to be experimental plots (that is why an alternative terminology uses *between-* and *within-subject* notation). As an example, we can study the density of stomata on the upper and lower surface of the leaf in relation to varying light intensity regimes in which the experimental plants grew. So the identity of the

---

[2] The existence of an interaction is likely the most interesting aspect of our analysis.

individual will be a random effect factor and we will also use the *light* and *surface* factors to represent the fixed effects. Or – as another example – we might have a set of experimental areas, some located on a chalk bedrock and others on a granitic bedrock, with each experimental area containing plots with three different types of management. In this case, the whole-plot factor will be the type of bedrock, while the split-plot factor is the management type. As we can see from those examples, either one of the factor types can be a manipulated or non-manipulated (observed) factor.

11.3 ANOVA for Repeated Measurements

Living objects change in time and that is why we need to measure them repeatedly when addressing particular research questions. In these cases, we obtain a time series of measurements for each object and the individual measurements made at the same object are clearly interdependent. This must be reflected in the ANOVA model that we use to evaluate such data. Usually, we call it a *repeated measurements ANOVA* (sometimes also a *repeated measures ANOVA*).

This model is perhaps most frequently used for evaluating the results of an experiment where we know the initial state of all observed objects before we start to manipulate them in our experiment (referred to as *baseline data*). We then apply experimental treatments to selected groups of objects and follow their further development – we want to demonstrate that the observed changes in values of the chosen characteristic(s) depend on the treatment being applied.

11.3.1 Use Case Examples

1. We grow a number of plants (one individual per pot) and after they achieve a certain size (so that we have some confidence they will survive through our experiment), we measure some characteristic on each plant (e.g. their height). So far they have not been treated in any particular way, so we can consider all the variation in height to be random variation. We then divide our plants into three groups (using a suitable random process) – one will be the control group, irrigated with water, another will have nitrogen added to the water, while the third group will have phosphorus added to the water. We then measure our plants three times in, say, 2-week intervals. We ask whether there are differences in growth (measured by height) resulting from nitrogen or phosphorus supplementation.
2. We can use a similar design when studying the effect of grassland management on the species richness of the plant community. We will create a set of permanent plots of a particular size (e.g. 2 × 2 m) in a homogeneous area and record the species present there, thus obtaining our data on species richness. We then divide the plots into three groups (using some random process) and start to manage them in different ways: we may stop mowing, mow the plots in June, or mow the plots in August. During the following few years we record the changing species composition (and so the species richness) in those plots.

11.3.2 Analysis

Our data should be evaluated with an ANOVA model that takes into account the interdependency of the observations of a particular object (plant or plot in our two examples above), taken at different times. We most often use the *split-plot ANOVA* model discussed earlier in this chapter, where each repeatedly investigated object becomes an instance of a *main-plot factor* and the predictor representing measurement time becomes a *split-plot factor*. This means that time is used (in a standard form of this analysis) as a categorical variable. As a result, we obtain significance values for the tests of three hypotheses: the first concerns the treatment (testing the difference of group averages calculated over all times), the second concerns the time (testing the differences among the time averages calculated over all groups), and the third concerns the interaction of time and treatment (testing whether the groups develop in the same way through time).

Our two examples in Section 11.3.1 represent an experimental design called the *Replicated Before After Control Impact* (*BACI*) *design*. In this design, it is essential that we know the state of all observed objects at the time before we start the experimental manipulation (and so the membership in a group of observations cannot have any effect on the response variable). We then follow if (and how) the groups start to differentiate depending on some treatment. We are therefore interested mainly in the test result for the interaction between the experimental treatment and time. If we can reject the hypothesis of no interaction, we can consider this as proof of the effect of our experimental treatment. The repeated measurements ANOVA model can also be used for other types of experimental design where the objects are followed through time, but in such cases the interaction of time and treatment does not necessarily need to be the most important term in the estimated ANOVA model.

The ANOVA for repeated measurements has its own assumptions which we should respect. Firstly, there is an assumption of *sphericity* (sometimes also called *circularity*). When checking for this assumption, we test whether the extent of dependency (variability of the difference in values) among all levels of the within-subject factor (typically the time) is of similar size for individual subjects. For a typical repeated measurements design, we study the variability in the response variable differences among individual times (not just the sequential ones) and ascertain whether it is similar across the measured objects with a statistical test. If we detect the assumption is violated, there are corrections for the repeated measures ANOVA model (namely Huynh–Feldt or Greenhouse–Geisser methods) that essentially reduce the number of degrees of freedom for the denominator of the corresponding F test statistic. As an alternative solution, we can use multivariate tests for the within-subject factor and its interactions, which are based on the multivariate analysis of variance (MANOVA) method and do not have such strong assumptions (but also provide generally weaker tests).

Like in a standard ANOVA, we can perform various multiple comparisons in a repeated measurements ANOVA. We do this after rejecting some of the null hypotheses in order to identify mutually different groups of observations. We can compare individual time periods and their differences among individual groups. We refer to this as *profile analysis*, and it is described in a chapter of Scheiner & Gurevitch (2001), written by Von Ende (2001).

Our description of ANOVA for repeated measurements only concerns its standard form where time is treated as a factor. We are therefore not concerned with the time intervals among the individual measurements, in fact we even ignore their order. However this information is important and interesting in many research problems. Typically, when we investigate the growth of organisms, we have some ideas about how the relationship between an organism's size and time might look. There are many extensions of the repeated measurements ANOVA model where the order and the intervals among individual measurements are important (see Von Ende, 2001 for examples of ecological applications).

11.4 Example Data

The example data in the first three columns of the *Chap11* sheet represent the results of the following greenhouse experiment. We followed the effect of soil type (variable *Soil* with two alternative levels called *sandy* and *clay*) on the average mass of plant seeds. There were three plants in each pot (identified by the *Pot* factor variable) and the value provided in the variable *Seedweight* represents the average weight of seeds for a particular plant.

The next four variables in the *Chap11* sheet (in columns *D* to *G*) represent data illustrating the calculation of variation components. These data come from the following study. We recorded benthic communities in mountain brooks, with species richness determined in each standardised sample. Three mountain ranges were compared, with three areas in each mountain range. In each area, three brooks were randomly chosen and each brook was represented by three randomly positioned sampling locations. There were no important differences in the surrounding landscape or altitude of the sampled locations, and we can consider the choice of areas, brooks and their parts as a result of random selection. Our task was to determine how species richness varies at different geographical scales. These results could then be used, for example, to make judgements about the extent to which species richness is limited by the dispersion of organisms.

The next four variables in the *Chap11* sheet (in columns *H* to *K*) represent the data illustrated in Fig. 11.2 and described in Section 11.2.1. The results are simplified, but correspond to a real experiment performed in an experimental grassland site at Ohrazení near České Budějovice, Czech Republic. In our simplified example, we have just 12 plots, six of them non-fertilised (*NF*) and six fertilised (*FER*). At each plot, two individuals of a test plant species were planted, one into an experimentally created gap in the vegetation (*GAP*), the other one into intact vegetation (*INT*). The first variable (*Plot*) identifies the plot, the second variable (*Fertil*) represents the fertilisation treatment, the third variable (*Microhab*) shows the microhabitat type, and the fourth gives the dry weight of an experimental plant (mg) at the end of the experiment.

Data which are suitable for repeated measurement analyses typically come from an experiment similar to that described in the first example of Section 11.3.1. We randomly assigned 18 plants into three groups (each with six plants), first measuring the height of all plants (baseline data in the variable *T0*) and we then started watering the pots either with water (*W*), or with water with added nitrogen (*N*), or with water with added phosphorus (*P*). Our data specify the applied treatment (variables *Treatm* as well as *Treatment*) and the plant height at the time *T0* and three times after the application of treatments (*T1*, *T2*, *T3*). The data are presented in two different ways, corresponding to formats required by different packages in R, either in columns *L* to *P*, or in columns *Q* to *T*. In the more expanded version of columns *Q* to *T*, the observations are sorted first by the plant identity, then by the observation time, but they might be sorted in any other way: the mutually correlated observations are identified by having the same value (level) of the variable *PlantID*.

11.5 How to Proceed in R

11.5.1 Hierarchical ANOVA

The simple type of hierarchical ANOVA (which is all that is required for our sample data) can be computed with the function *aov* using a special *Error* term in the model formula. This term specifies a factor which defines the groups of dependent observations (in our dataset this is the plant triple sharing a pot):

```
aov.1 <- aov( Seedweight ~ Soil + Error(Pot), data=chap11a)
summary( aov.1)

Error: Pot
          Df Sum Sq Mean Sq F value Pr(>F)
Soil       1 11.371  11.371   8.993  0.024 *
Residuals  6  7.587   1.264
---
Signif. codes:  0 '***' 0.001 '**' 0.01 '*' 0.05 '.' 0.1 ' ' 1


Error: Within
          Df Sum Sq Mean Sq F value Pr(>F)
Residuals 16  2.826  0.1766
```

The labels *Error: Pot* and *Error: Within* in the output of the *summary* function separate the variation decomposition into two error levels based on a factor specified with the *Error(Pot)* term. The upper level represents among-pot variation, in which we explain 11.371 by the *Soil* factor and 7.587 remains unexplained, and the lower level is within-pot variation (i.e. the variation of plant values around the per-pot averages) with sum-of-squares size 2.826.

The above summary does not deliver a test for the pot effect (our model just divides the total sum of squares into two hierarchically related components), but we can calculate an approximate test from the results shown by the *summary* function. The variation among pots not explained by the soil type is represented by the row *Residuals* in the *Error: Pot* section, while the variation within pots is in the *Residual* row of the *Error: Within* section. We must use the mean squares and corresponding degrees of freedom:

```
1-pf(1.264/0.1766,6,16)
[1] 0.0007644262
```

In doing this, however, we test the *pot* effect as if it were a fixed effect, but it would be more appropriate to test it as a random effect with a linear model with mixed effects. We first show how to fit a corresponding mixed effect linear model for our data with the package *nlme* (Pinheiro et al., 2018):

```
library( nlme)
lme.1 <- lme( Seedweight~Soil, random=~1|Pot, data=chap11a)
anova( lme.1)
            numDF denDF  F-value p-value
(Intercept)     1    16 869.9542  <.0001
Soil            1     6   8.9932   0.024
```

To test the random effect of *Pot*, we must also fit a model without a random effect. This can be done either with the *lm* function or with the *gls* function provided (for fitting general linear models) in the *nlme* package. We then compare the two models using the *anova* function, which performs a likelihood ratio test (LRT):

```
lm.1 <- gls( Seedweight~Soil, data=chap11a)
anova( lm.1, lme.1)
        Model df      AIC       BIC    logLik    Test  L.Ratio p-value
lm.1        1   3 56.94682  60.21995 -25.47341
lme.1       2   4 49.07231  53.43648 -20.53616  1 vs 2 9.874512  0.0017
```

We can see that the inclusion of the random effect of *Pot* significantly ($\chi^2_1 = 9.87$, $p = 0.0017$) increased the model likelihood (from -25.47 to -20.54) and so we accept the more complex *lme.1* model instead of the simpler *lm.1* model.

It is also easier to produce a plot with a fitted effect of *Soil* for the *lme.1* model than for a model based on an ANOVA with an *Error* term. We will use the package *effects* (Fox, 2003) to create the plot:

```
library( effects)
plot( allEffects( lme.1), main="",
      lines=list(col="black"))
```

The resulting plot is shown in Fig. 11.3. The input in the *lines* parameter simply ensures that the plot is produced in black and white.

The averages shown in the graph are also reflected in the regression coefficient estimates of the model's fixed effects:

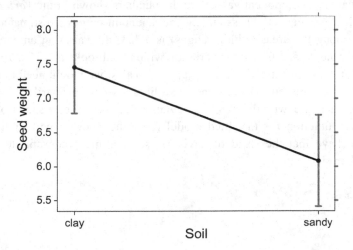

Figure 11.3 Estimated group means (with 95% confidence intervals) for the seed weight of plants grown in clay and in sandy soil.

```
fixef( lme.1)
(Intercept)    Soilsandy
   7.458333    -1.376667
```

The average value for the (reference) clay group is 1.377 mg higher than the value for the seed weight of plants from sandy soil (which is 6.082 mg).

11.5.2 Variance Components

The data used for this example were imported into the *chap11b* data frame. We can estimate the individual components of variation with one of the libraries for linear mixed effect models. We first demonstrate the required steps with the *nlme* library:

```
library( nlme)
lme.1 <- lme( Richness~1,random=~1|MntRange/Area/Brook,
              data=chap11b)
VarCorr( lme.1)
              Variance     StdDev
MntRange =    pdLogChol(1)
(Intercept)   28.6568539   5.3532097
Area =        pdLogChol(1)
(Intercept)   5.7231591    2.3923125
Brook =       pdLogChol(1)
(Intercept)   0.6090636    0.7804253
Residual      0.7777722    0.8819139
```

The variance component values are the numbers shown in the *Variance* column. So, the variation of species richness among the mountain ranges is estimated as 28.657, the variation among the areas (within ranges) is 5.723, the variation among the brooks (within areas) is 0.609, and finally the variation within the brooks is 0.778. To express the percentage contribution of individual geographical scales, we would need to use the sum of those values as a reference value. The *nlme* library works primarily with the square roots of those values (i.e. with the standard deviations), as can also be seen from an output of the *summary* function for the fitted model (only the relevant part of the output is shown). We believe that the standard deviation scale is more appropriate for judging relative variation size.

```
summary( lme.1)
Linear mixed-effects model fit by REML
...
Random effects:
 Formula: ~1 | MntRange
         (Intercept)
StdDev:     5.35321
```

```
Formula: ~1 | Area %in% MntRange
        (Intercept)
StdDev:    2.392313


 Formula: ~1 | Brook %in% Area %in% MntRange
        (Intercept)  Residual
StdDev:    0.7804253 0.8819139
...
```

We can even obtain the confidence intervals for the estimated size of the random variation[3] on the scale of standard deviations:

```
intervals( lme.1, which="var-cov")
Approximate 95% confidence intervals
 Random Effects:
  Level: MntRange
                   lower    est.    upper
sd((Intercept)) 1.874621 5.35321 15.28674
  Level: Area
                   lower    est.    upper
sd((Intercept)) 1.319976 2.392313 4.335805
  Level: Brook
                   lower    est.    upper
sd((Intercept)) 0.4867092 0.7804253 1.251391
 Within-group standard error:
    lower      est.    upper
0.7304182 0.8819139 1.0648314
```

We proceed in a similar way when fitting a linear mixed effect model with the *lme4* library (Bates et al., 2015), however we specify the random effects differently:

```
library( lme4)
lmer.2 <- lmer( Richness~1+(1|MntRange)+(1|Area)+(1|Brook),
                data=chap11b)
VarCorr( lmer.2)
 Groups    Name        Std.Dev.
 Brook     (Intercept) 0.78042
 Area      (Intercept) 2.39226
 MntRange  (Intercept) 5.35328
 Residual              0.88192
```

---

[3] To translate the interval limits to the scale of variances, we would need to square the output values (see the computation with *lme4* library).

If we want to compute the confidence intervals for the random effects only, then we can do the following (we squared the result to obtain confidence intervals for variances):

```
confint( lmer.2, parm="theta_", oldNames=F)^2
Computing profile confidence intervals ...
                            2.5 %      97.5 %
sd_(Intercept)|Brook    0.2010616    1.550909
sd_(Intercept)|Area     2.0185579   23.887322
sd_(Intercept)|MntRange 2.7974517  176.271594
sigma                   0.5454127    1.163184
```

Note here that the estimates are not shown from the upper to lower hierarchical level, but rather in the same order as shown in the *VarCorr* function output.

11.5.3 Split-Plot ANOVA

We will import the data for a split-plot ANOVA example from columns H to K and store the result in the *chap11c* data frame. As the categorical variable *Plot* (in column H) is represented by numbers, we must change its type into a factor:

```
chap11c <- transform( chap11c, Plot=as.factor( Plot))
```

We will log-transform the plant weights given that we expect the weights to be positively skewed, and also that their standard deviation is proportional to the mean. This also changes the null hypothesis for the interaction. The null hypothesis now represents an additivity of factors on the log-scale, which corresponds to multiplicativity on the original scale. In other words, the competition in the intact vegetation is (in the absence of an interaction) expected to decrease the plant weight by the same percentage in both control and fertilised plots. Note that it is much more sensible to test this null hypothesis than to test additivity on the original scale.

We can compute this simple split-plot ANOVA for a balanced dataset using the *aov* function with a special *Error* term (as in Section 11.5.1):

```
aov.2 <- aov( log( Weight)~Fertil*Microhab + Error(Plot),
              data=chap11c)
summary( aov.2)
Error: Plot
          Df Sum Sq Mean Sq F value Pr(>F)
Fertil     1 0.0136 0.01360    0.23  0.642
Residuals 10 0.5906 0.05906

Error: Within
            Df Sum Sq Mean Sq F value   Pr(>F)
Microhab     1  7.014   7.014  136.00 3.82e-07 ***
```

```
Fertil:Microhab  1   2.211   2.211   42.88 6.49e-05 ***
Residuals        10  0.516   0.052
```

Alternatively, we can use the *lme* function from the *nlme* package:

```
library( nlme)
lme.2 <- lme( log(Weight)~Fertil*Microhab, random=~1|Plot,
              data=chap11c)
anova( lme.2)
                numDF denDF   F-value  p-value
(Intercept)       1    10  1927.6610  <.0001
Fertil            1    10     0.2303  0.6416
Microhab          1    10   135.9949  <.0001
Fertil:Microhab   1    10    42.8747  0.0001
```

Both approaches provide identical results, but note that this might not always be the case, particularly if the data are not balanced. The main effect of fertilisation is negligible and non-significant, while the effects of microhabitat and its interaction with fertilisation are strong. We can display the estimates of fixed effects in order to interpret these results:

```
fixef( lme.2)
(Intercept)        FertilNF      MicrohabINT FertilNF:MicrohabINT
  2.9983352      -0.5594788       1.6883043            1.2141768
```

The plants growing in the intact community were significantly smaller (by 81.5%, as exp(−1.6883) = 0.185) than the plants grown in gaps, but that effect size applies only in the fertilised plots: for non-fertilised plots, the plants from the intact community are smaller by just 37.8% (as exp(−1.6883 + 1.2142) = 0.622).

11.5.4 ANOVA for Repeated Measurements

We will import the data from columns Q to T (as this is the usual arrangement for this type of repeated measurements data) into the *chap11d* data frame. As this type of analysis can be performed (at least when the assumption of sphericity is fulfilled) in the same way as a split-plot ANOVA, we will first analyse the dataset with the *aov* function, using the *Error* term in the model formula:

```
summary( aov( PlantH~Treatment*Time + Error(PlantID),
              data=chap11d))
Error: PlantID
          Df Sum Sq Mean Sq F value   Pr(>F)
Treatment  2 115.36   57.68   21.68 3.76e-05 ***
Residuals 15  39.92    2.66
---
Signif. codes:  0 '***' 0.001 '**' 0.01 '*' 0.05 '.' 0.1 ' ' 1
```

```
Error: Within
                 Df Sum Sq Mean Sq F value   Pr(>F)
Time              3  588.1  196.02  382.13  < 2e-16 ***
Treatment:Time    6   64.9   10.81   21.07 1.37e-11 ***
Residuals        45   23.1    0.51
---
```

Alternatively, we can perform the analysis using the *lme* function in the *nlme* package:

```
library( nlme)
lme.3 <- lme( PlantH~Treatment*Time, random=~1|PlantID,
              data=chap11d)
anova( lme.3)
               numDF denDF   F-value p-value
(Intercept)        1    45 2342.9006  <.0001
Treatment          2    15   21.6754  <.0001
Time               3    45  382.1300  <.0001
Treatment:Time     6    45   21.0740  <.0001
```

The results show significant main effects of both *Treatment* and *Time*, which confirm that the average height differs among treatments and that the plants change their height with time – presumably growing taller. But we also see a significant interaction term which suggests that the plant heights developed at different paces for different treatments. At this stage it is important to visualise the fitted model for an appropriate interpretation:

```
library( effects)
plot( allEffects( lme.3), confint=list( style="bars"),
      lines=list( col="black", multiline=T, lty=1:3))
```

The resulting graph is shown in Fig. 11.4. Obviously the treatment with added nitrogen (*N*) is responsible for the significant interaction term.

The results reported above are, however, correct only if the assumption of sphericity is matched, but we have not yet verified it for our model. To perform a repeated measurements ANOVA that offers a test of sphericity and also calculates the corrected tests for *within-subject* effects if the sphericity assumption is not met, we can use the *Anova*[4] function provided in the *car* package (Fox & Weisberg, 2011). It is slightly more difficult to specify the model there (particularly if we would have more within-subject factors).

The data must be imported in such a form so that the values for each observed object (here each plant) are in a single row and there are as many variables with the response data as there are sampling times (four in our case). We provided such data in columns *L* and *P* of the *Chap11* sheet and now we must import them into the *chap11e* data frame.

First we estimate a linear model (using the function *lm*) with the response variable represented by a matrix of plant height observations, with as many columns as there are

---

[4] Please note that the name of the function starts with a capital *A* here ...

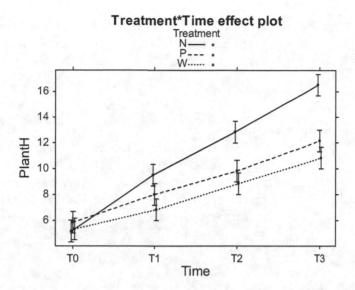

Figure 11.4 Visual summary of a repeated measurements ANOVA model displaying the change of plant height across time, with three variants of experimental treatments (W = control plants, P = added phosphorus, N = added nitrogen). In addition to the group averages (circles), 95% confidence intervals are also shown for each group, defined by the treatment and time combination.

measurement times and rows representing the repeatedly measured plants. These columns will be explained by our only *between-subject* factor, i.e. the *Treatm* variable:

```
lm.x <- lm( cbind( T0, T1, T2, T3) ~ Treatm, data=chap11e)
```

Next we must define a second data frame that describes the repeated measurements model structure, namely it describes the *within-subject* predictors. In our example, we have just one such predictor (*T.fac*) with four levels representing measurement times:

```
T.fac <- as.factor( c("T0","T1","T2","T3"))
time.frame <- data.frame( T.fac)
```

Finally, we fit and summarise the repeated measurements ANOVA using the *Anova* function (more technical parts of the output were omitted):

```
library( car)
Anova.1 <- Anova( lm.x, idata=time.frame, idesign=~T.fac)
summary( Anova.1)
Type II Repeated Measures MANOVA Tests:

...

Term: Treatm

...

Multivariate Tests: Treatm
                Df test stat approx F num Df den Df      Pr(>F)
Pillai          2 0.7429338 21.67536       2     15 3.7613e-05 ***
```

```
Wilks              2 0.2570662 21.67536       2    15 3.7613e-05 ***
Hotelling-Lawley   2 2.8900487 21.67536       2    15 3.7613e-05 ***
Roy                2 2.8900487 21.67536       2    15 3.7613e-05 ***


Term: T.fac
...
Multivariate Tests: T.fac
              Df test stat approx F num Df den Df     Pr(>F)
Pillai         1   0.98729 336.5769       3    13 1.4372e-12 ***
Wilks          1   0.01271 336.5769       3    13 1.4372e-12 ***
Hotelling-Lawley 1 77.67160 336.5769      3    13 1.4372e-12 ***
Roy            1  77.67160 336.5769       3    13 1.4372e-12 ***


Term: Treatm:T.fac
...
Multivariate Tests: Treatm:T.fac
              Df test stat approx F num Df den Df     Pr(>F)
Pillai         2  1.020901  4.86591       6    28 0.0016123 **
Wilks          2  0.101573  9.26333       6    26 1.8233e-05 ***
Hotelling-Lawley 2 7.639332 15.27866      6    24 3.7872e-07 ***
Roy            2  7.478091 34.89776       3    14 9.4508e-07 ***


Univariate Type II Repeated-Measures ANOVA Assuming Sphericity
            Sum Sq num Df Error SS den Df  F value     Pr(>F)
(Intercept) 6234.7      1   39.917      15 2342.902 < 2.2e-16 ***
Treatm       115.4      2   39.917      15   21.675 3.761e-05 ***
T.fac        588.1      3   23.083      45  382.130 < 2.2e-16 ***
Treatm:T.fac  64.9      6   23.083      45   21.074 1.372e-11 ***


Mauchly Tests for Sphericity
            Test statistic   p-value
T.fac             0.24092 0.0015789
Treatm:T.fac      0.24092 0.0015789


Greenhouse-Geisser and Huynh-Feldt Corrections
 for Departure from Sphericity
              GG eps Pr(>F[ GG] )
T.fac        0.70706  < 2.2e-16 ***
Treatm:T.fac 0.70706  9.435e-09 ***
              HF eps   Pr(>F[ HF] )
T.fac        0.8266454 7.616503e-27
Treatm:T.fac 0.8266454 6.514932e-10
```

The output first shows the tests from the multivariate analysis of variance (MAN-OVA) separately for each model term. The individual rows (*Pillai*, *Wilks*, *Hotelling–Lawley*, *Roy*) represent alternative test statistics suggested by different authors for multivariate

ANOVA tests and their transformations with an approximate F distribution under the null hypothesis (*approx F* column). When the effect degree of freedom (in the first *Df* column) is equal to 1, all variants provide identical results. If the *Df* value is larger, these approximations might be identical or they might differ (as we saw for the interaction test in our example). In this case, the F test based on Wilks' statistic (sometimes called Wilks' lambda) is most frequently used, but Pillai's test is believed to be more robust to violations of the MANOVA assumption.

These sections are followed by a standard output of the ANOVA for repeated measurements, assuming that the sphericity assumption is matched. But the test of sphericity then follows, which shows that our example data violate the sphericity assumption ($p = 0.0016$). Finally, we see two kinds of tests for *within-subject* factors (i.e. the main effect of time and its interaction with treatment) that correct for the violation. Even after those corrections, the tested effects remain highly significant.

11.6 Reporting Analyses

11.6.1 Methods

We evaluated the effect of soil type on average seed weight using ANOVA with pot as a random effect.

Or

... with the effect of pot nested within the effect of soil type.

The results of our experiment were evaluated using split-plot ANOVA, with the additional error level represented by plots, with the effect of fertilisation treated as a whole-plot factor, and the effects of microhabitat and its interaction with fertilisation treated as split-plot factors.

The effects of the experimental treatment on plant growth were evaluated using a repeated measurements ANOVA. We used the adjusted method of Greenhouse & Geisser (1959) for within-subject effects as the sphericity assumption was violated.

Or

... we used a multivariate test (based on Wilks' Λ statistic value; Mardia et al., 1976) for within-subject effects.

11.6.2 Results

Soil type significantly affected the average weight of seeds ($F_{1,6} = 8.99, p = 0.024$), with seeds from plants grown in sandy soils being on average 1.38 mg lighter (see Fig. X).

Figure X would show the group averages of seed weight, probably with confidence intervals.

We found a significant difference in plant weight between intact vegetation and vegetation gaps ($F_{1,10} = 135.995, p < 0.001$), with the biomass of plants in gaps being significantly larger. A significant interaction between microhabitat and fertilisation factors ($F_{1,10} = 42.875, p = 0.000065$) reflected the larger difference between intact vegetation and gap plants in the fertilised plots.

The growth of plants differs among the treatments, with the plants exposed to an increased supply of N growing faster and gradually increasing their gain (see Fig. 11.4).

11.7 Recommended Reading

Zar (2010), pp. 270–274 and pp. 307–315.

Quinn & Keough (2002), pp. 208–220 (hierarchical ANOVA) and pp. 301–338 (split-plot ANOVA and repeated measurements ANOVA).

Sokal & Rohlf (2012), pp. 277–318.

D. Bates, M. Maechler, B. Bolker & S. Walker (2015) Fitting linear mixed-effects models using lme4. *Journal of Statistical Software*, **67**(1): 1–48.

J. Fox (2003) Effect displays in R for generalised linear models. *Journal of Statistical Software*, **8**(15): 1–27.

J. Fox & S. Weisberg (2011) *An R Companion to Applied Regression*, 2nd edn. Sage, Thousand Oaks, CA.

S. W. Greenhouse & S. Geisser (1959) On methods in the analysis of profile data. *Psychometrika*, **24**: 95–112.

K. V. Mardia, J. T. Kent & J. M. Bibby (1976) *Multivariate Analysis*. Elsevier, London.

J. Pinheiro, D. Bates, S. DebRoy, D. Sarka & R Core Team (2018) *nlme*: linear and nonlinear mixed effect models. R package version 3.1-137. https://cran.r-project.org/package=nlme

C. N. Von Ende (2001) Repeated-measures analysis: growth and other time-dependent measures. In: S. M. Scheiner & J. Gurevitch (eds), *Design and Analysis of Ecological Experiments*. Oxford University Press, Oxford, pp. 134–157.

12 Simple Linear Regression: Dependency Between Two Quantitative Variables

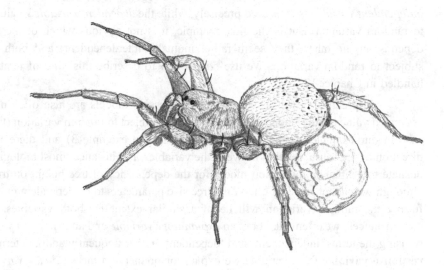

12.1 Use Case Examples

In Chapter 8 we compared the differences among groups of objects using a one-way ANOVA model. This task can also be described as modelling the dependency of one quantitative variable on another, qualitative variable; the qualitative variable represents the membership of objects within certain groups. Now we will focus on the relation of two (or more) quantitative (numerical) variables. These will most often be continuous variables on a ratio or interval scale. Here we give some examples of problems that can be addressed with a simple linear regression model.

1. We measure the diameter at breast height (*DBH*) and the total height for a number of trees of a particular species. We want to understand the relation among these two quantitative variables. We are likely to find that the taller a tree is, the larger its *DBH* value will be.
2. We study the dependency of the amount of floating woody debris (branches, logs) in lakes, on tree density on the lake shores. We expect that the amount of woody material will increase as tree density grows. We want to quantitatively describe this relationship.
3. We want to investigate how the body size of spider individuals grown in lab culture depends on their age (in days). We want to characterise the relation of size to age with a simple numerical model.

12.2 Regression and Correlation

All of the above examples deal with the relation of two numeric variables, but the examples differ with respect to the question behind the research. In examples 2 and 3 we can identify which of the two characteristics depends on the other one. For example, we can sensibly assume that the amount of branches and logs in a lake depends on tree density around the lake shore, but not the other way round. Similarly, the age of spiders is clearly not determined by their size, but rather their size changes with age. If we want to describe the dependency of one variable on some other variable(s), then we use a **regression model**. Here we assume that the *independent variable* is measured precisely, while the *dependent variable's* values are subject to random variation. But in the first example, it is not obvious which of the two variables depends on the other (they seem rather mutually interdependent) and both variables are subject to random variation. We use *correlation* to describe this kind of relation, which is handled in Chapter 13.

In practice, however, we find that regression models are also often used when the estimated values of the 'independent' variable are subject to random variation (this will be the case in our examples 1 and 2, and probably also in example 3) and there is no obvious direction of the causal relation between the variables. For instance, most biologists would not hesitate to estimate a regression model for the dependency of tree height on trunk diameter, although we cannot consider one of the tree size parameters to be dependent on the other, and further the random variation will be of a similar extent for both variables.[1] Under such circumstances, we often talk about an *explanatory variable* and an *explained variable* instead of using the terms 'independent' and 'dependent'. Other frequently adopted terms include the **response variable** for a variable we explain or predict and the *predictor variable*, or more simply just the **predictor** (or predictors, if there are multiple, as we will see in Chapter 14) for variables used for explanation. This is the terminology we will use in the current and proceeding chapters.

> If the predictor is a random variable then we understand the regression as a study of dependency of the response variable on the observed predictor values. The estimates of regression model parameters are not very good if the random variation in predictor values is of similar size (or even greater) than the random variation in the response variable (see also Section 12.8 in this chapter).

Drawing parallels between regression and correlation, we must also add that a correlation coefficient (described in Chapter 13) is significantly different from zero precisely when the linear dependency of one variable on the other is also significant.

12.3 Simple Linear Regression

The simplest kind of regression involving two variables is called a simple linear regression (or bivariate regression). This type of regression is called *linear* as we can describe the dependency between the two variables with a straight line. The word 'simple' refers to the simplicity of the predictors, where we have just a single variable (as opposed to a **multiple** linear regression, discussed in Chapter 14). The example data (plotted in Fig. 12.1)

---

[1] Such relationships among various parameters of organism size are often explored in the field of *allometry*.

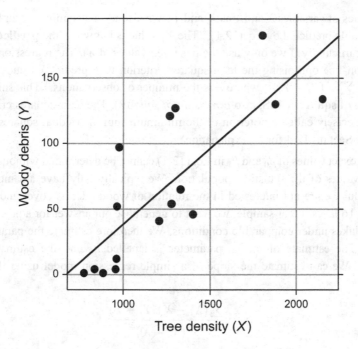

Figure 12.1 Dependency of the area of woody debris (floating branches and logs) on tree density near the shore line of 16 lakes.

represent our example 2 above, i.e. woody debris variation on lake shores (data from Christensen et al., 1996).

The predictor variable is usually labelled X and plotted on the horizontal axis, the response variable is usually labelled Y and plotted on the vertical axis. The equation of a simple linear model is then

$$EY = \beta_0 + \beta_1 X \qquad (12.1)$$

where EY is the expected value of variable Y, β_1 represents the straight line direction (usually called **slope**, as it relates to the angle between the regression line and the horizontal axis) and β_0 is the expected value of Y when X is equal to 0, i.e. the coordinate of the point where the regression line intersects the vertical axis (if the vertical axis is plotted at the zero position of the horizontal axis); this coefficient is therefore often called an **intercept**. The two β coefficients are generally called **regression coefficients**.

It is perhaps useful to point out that the value of β_1 specifies the amount of change of Y when the value of X increases by one unit, and so it depends on the units in which both variables are measured. Its value is therefore scaled in [Y units]/[X units]. On the contrary, the value of β_0 is in [Y units].

One could ask how we can construct a line which best approximates the plotted points. There are several possibilities (based on different criteria), but in statistical analyses the most common is to estimate the line using a **least-squares criterion**.[2] Let us label the

---

[2] A more general, widely used criterion is the *maximum likelihood* criterion; if the assumptions about the variables X and Y (required for testing hypotheses and described later in this chapter) are fulfilled, the estimates based on the maximum likelihood criterion are identical to those based on the least-squares criterion.

observed values of variables X and Y as X_i and Y_i. We also use the symbol $\hat{Y}_i$ for values of the response variable predicted by Eq. (12.1).[3] The $\hat{Y}_i$ value is known as the **predicted value** (or *fitted value*, particularly if we only use the observed values of X). The regression coefficients of a regression line optimising the least-squares criterion then predict Y values producing a minimal sum $\sum_{i=1}^{n}(Y_i - \hat{Y}_i)^2$, where n is the number of observations.[4] This sum is called a **residual sum of squares** (RSS, also *error sum of squares*). The least-squares criterion ought to be more precisely called a criterion of the minimum sum of residual squares (or squared residuals, see Section 12.4 for an explanation).

The exact values of β_0 and β_1 in Eq. (12.1) cannot be determined without knowing all the X and Y values of the statistical population. We typically only have a sample from that population. But we are not interested in the relation of woody debris cover and tree density just for those 16 lakes in our sample, we want to generalise our answer for a potentially much larger set of lakes under comparable conditions. We therefore estimate the parameters using our sample. The estimate of the β_0 parameter is labelled b_0 and the estimate of the β_1 parameter b_1. We can estimate the slope of a simple regression model using the following formula:

$$b_1 = \frac{\sum(X_i - \overline{X})(Y_i - \overline{Y})}{\sum(X_i - \overline{X})^2} \qquad (12.2)$$

but statistical software typically uses a different formula, one which is simpler to compute and gives identical results. It can be demonstrated that a fitted regression line passes through the estimated means of X and Y, i.e. through the point $[\overline{X}, \overline{Y}]$. The b_0 parameter is usually estimated by using this point $[\overline{X}, \overline{Y}]$ in Eq. (12.1). In this way, we can estimate the intercept value as

$$b_0 = \overline{Y} - b_1\overline{X} \qquad (12.3)$$

The value of b_1 (and thus the slope of the linear relationship) can be either positive or negative. The value of the denominator in Eq. (12.2) is always positive, but the sign of the numerator is positive only if positive deviations of Y from its average are matched with positive deviations of X (and negative Y deviations by negative X deviations), otherwise the numerator – and consequently the b_1 estimate – is negative.

The process of estimating a model's parameters, particularly its regression coefficients, is usually called model **fitting** (to data).

We have already mentioned that the estimates of regression coefficients are imprecise, they are therefore random variables. We generally need to find out how big the estimation errors might be. Therefore, we test hypotheses about the individual regression coefficients or about the whole regression model (represented by Eq. (12.1)). To perform such tests, our data should fulfil some specific assumptions. Beyond the obvious requirements that our sample was chosen from the sampled population in a random manner and individual observations are mutually independent, the most important assumption is that the predictor is not subject to random errors (it is not a random variable), while the response is a random

---

[3] In those predictions, we use the estimates of the coefficients β_0 and β_1, labelled b_0 and b_1, hence we do not use the symbol EY for the predicted values.

[4] We will omit the range of summation in other formulas within this chapter – it will always be assumed to range from 1 to n.

variable. Such an assumption is difficult to match for most real-world data. Usually, we must resort to the weaker assumption that the random variation in X is substantially smaller than the variation in Y.

Another assumption concerns the distribution of Y values, namely that for each value of X, the Y values come from a normal distribution (with its mean changing linearly with X) with a constant variance, i.e. not depending on the value of X. This assumption matches the assumption of variance homogeneity in ANOVA models. Alternatively, we can describe this assumption by rewriting the regression model as $Y_i = \beta_0 + \beta_1 X_i + \varepsilon_i$, with ε_i being a random variable with a normal distribution with mean 0 and variance not depending on X. This model also reflects the two assumptions for simple linear regression. The relationship is linear and the variability is constant, independent of the values of X (the homogeneity of variance assumption).

12.4 Testing Hypotheses

12.4.1 Introduction

In theory, the two variables (X and Y) can be completely unrelated in the sampled statistical population, but our sample might contain observations that demonstrate a dependency simply by chance. That is why we ask how probable it is to find a dependency of a given strength just as a consequence of chance during the sampling process. We are testing a null hypothesis claiming that in the sampled population, the values of the response variable Y do not depend on the values of the predictor X.

12.4.2 Test Based on Sum of Squares Decomposition

We typically use a decomposition of the total variation of variable Y into two parts in order to test the significance of a regression model: the variation explained by the model and the residual variation. These two parts are then compared using an F statistic, similar to tests in ANOVA models (see Section 8.4).[5] The decomposed variation is based on the sum of squared deviations from the mean, usually just called the 'sum of squares'.

The *total sum of squares* (SS_{tot})

$$SS_{tot} = \sum (Y_i - \overline{Y})^2 \tag{12.4}$$

describes the total variation of the variable Y. The *regression sum of squares* (SS_{reg}, also known as the *model sum of squares*)

$$SS_{reg} = \sum (\hat{Y}_i - \overline{Y})^2 \tag{12.5}$$

represents the variation of Y, which was explained by the fitted regression model. Finally, the *residual sum of squares* (SS_E, also known as the *error sum of squares*)

---

[5] The decomposition of the total sum of squares into explained and unexplained components is used both for ANOVA models (where the explanatory variables are factors) and for linear regression models (where we use numerical variables). Consequently, this created some confusion about the meaning of the term ANOVA (analysis of variance). It can mean either the ANOVA model or the decomposition of variation for almost any kind of statistical model. We therefore recommend the use of the term ANOVA in the form of unequivocal word combinations in the context of linear (or other) regression analysis, such as 'an ANOVA table of the regression model'.

$$SS_E = \sum (Y_i - \hat{Y}_i)^2 \tag{12.6}$$

corresponds to the Y variation unexplained by the model.[6] There is an important relationship between these three sums of squares:

$$SS_{tot} = SS_{reg} + SS_E \tag{12.7}$$

This additive relation is often used to calculate either SS_{reg} or SS_E from the other two sums of squares.

We also need to calculate degrees of freedom corresponding to individual estimated components of Y variation. They can be calculated as

$$DF_{tot} = n - 1 \tag{12.8}$$

for degrees of freedom corresponding to SS_{tot}, as

$$DF_{reg} = \text{number of estimated parameters} - 1 \tag{12.9}$$

for degrees of freedom corresponding to SS_{reg} (DF_{reg} is therefore equal to 1 for a simple linear regression model with two estimated parameters), and finally as

$$DF_E = DF_{tot} - DF_{reg} \tag{12.10}$$

for the residual sum of squares: DF_E is therefore equal to $n - 2$ for a simple linear regression. The degrees of freedom are additive, as for the sum of squares.

' *Mean square* (*MS*) values can be obtained (like in the ANOVA models) by dividing a sum of squares by its corresponding number of degrees of freedom, e.g. $MS_E = SS_E / DF_E$. If H_0 is true (i.e. when X and Y are independent), both MS_{reg} and MS_E are estimates of the variance of the dependent variable Y. If the values are dependent, MS_{reg} increases and MS_E decreases. The ratio

$$F = \frac{MS_{reg}}{MS_E} \tag{12.11}$$

can therefore be used as a test statistic for regression model significance, with assumed F distribution when H_0 is correct.

The sums of squares are also used to calculate the **coefficient of determination**, R^2:

$$R^2 = \frac{SS_{reg}}{SS_{tot}} = 1 - \frac{SS_E}{SS_{tot}} \tag{12.12}$$

The R^2 coefficient estimates the proportion of explained variation out of the total variation.[7] It is, however, a biased estimate, overestimating the size of this proportion compared with the sampled statistical population – see Section 14.2 for more on the corrected R^2_{adj} coefficient.

---

[6] If all the graph points representing observed values of X and Y lie directly on the estimated regression line, we would explain all the variation in Y by the fitted model and the value of SS_E would be zero.

[7] This is why R^2 is sometimes presented on a percentage scale, i.e. a value between 0 and 100; its traditional range is between 0 and 1, however.

12.4.3 Tests of Regression Coefficients

An alternative (and somewhat complementary, at least for more complex linear models) way of testing regression models is to test the individual regression coefficients (β_j) using a one-sample t test. In general, the t statistic for regression coefficient tests can be calculated as

$$t = \frac{(\text{coefficient estimate} - \text{hypothetical value})}{\text{standard error of estimate}} \quad (12.13)$$

Regression coefficient tests in statistical software usually show the results of a test for the null hypothesis that the regression coefficient value (in the sampled population) is equal to zero. When we test the β_1 coefficient of a simple linear regression model, the p-value of this test is identical to the p-value of the analysis of variance of the whole regression model. This is, indeed, logical: if $\beta_1 = 0$, the regression line is horizontal and the Y variable's values are not affected by the X variable's values. Unlike the regression model F test, we can also use a t test for testing a one-sided hypothesis or a hypothesis comparing the population value β_j with a hypothesised constant different from zero.

It is also possible to test H_0: $\beta_0 = 0$ – this corresponds to a null hypothesis that the regression line passes through the coordinate origin, i.e. that the value of the response variable Y is zero whenever the predictor X has zero value. However, it does not make much biological sense in most cases (Section 12.7 explains why).

> The majority of relationships between two variates in natural sciences do not have a linear shape, but the linear regression is frequently used. One reason for this is that with a sufficiently small range of predictor values, we can approximately characterise almost any kind of functional relationship with a straight line (a question remains, however, over what is considered 'a sufficiently small range'). Also, when we have no *a priori* idea about the shape of dependence, we usually resort to the simplest possible model, which is the linear relation. Additionally, many of the frequently occurring types of dependence (such as an exponential relationship) can simply be transformed into a linear form (i.e. linearised).

12.4.4 Test Power

In linear regression, we cannot simply interpret our failure to reject the null hypothesis as proof of the independence of Y on X. We must always take into account the power of the test. As for other tests of significance, the power of the test (at given significance level) increases with the number of observations and, naturally, also with the strength of the relationship (expressed by R^2). A more precise estimation of the test power is discussed in Chapter 13, where we deal with the related topic of linear correlation.

Usually we can increase the test power by increasing the range of predictor values. The values of the predictor(s) are determined by the experimenter in manipulative experiments, so we can (to some extent) decide its range. For example, in a fertilisation experiment, the test power (with the same number of replications) will likely be higher if the doses applied are evenly distributed between 0 and 140 kg N ha^{-1} than if the range were between 0 and 50 kg N ha^{-1}. As a matter of fact, by increasing the predictor range we usually increase the amount of both total and explained variability in the response variable; the total variability in biomass will be much larger if the range of fertilisation is between 0 and 140 kg N ha^{-1} than if it is between 0 and 50 kg N ha^{-1}, and a considerably larger proportion of total variability will be explained. Consequently we will get a higher R^2 value, leading to a stronger test. However, the range of the manipulated variable must correspond to our research question. For instance, if we use high fertiliser doses in semi-natural meadows, this might lead to significant relationships, but our experimental setting might then be highly unrealistic, not corresponding to anything truly present in nature. We must also take into account that increasing the range of values often increases the deviation of the relationship from a linear form.

12.5 Confidence and Prediction Intervals

The **confidence interval** (sometimes also called *confidence limits*) for the mean value of the Y variable's distribution for a particular value of X is defined so that the (unknown) mean value is located in the calculated interval with *a priori* set probability (typically 0.95). When you plot the confidence intervals across the whole range of the predictor X, i.e. around the whole plotted regression line, the confidence intervals form a *confidence band*.

The **prediction interval** (or *prediction limits*) is defined so that it includes any individual observation (for given value of X) with *a priori* set probability (again, typically set to 0.95). The prediction interval is therefore substantially wider than the corresponding confidence interval. Most statistical software draws the *confidence* band as its default. As such, you should not be surprised that most of the individual observations lie outside this band.

Also, a confidence region gradually shrinks with an increasing number of observations, while the prediction interval approaches a certain limit and cannot drop beyond that range. Both intervals are narrowest for X values near the mean of X.

12.6 Regression Diagnostics and Transforming Data in Regression

How do we know that the assumptions for linear regression models were fulfilled? The assumptions of representativeness of our sample and of the independence of observations rely on the way our data were collected, but here we focus on two specific assumptions: the linearity of the relation between Y and X and the independence of the variance of the response variable (Y) on the values of X.

The most quick-and-dirty approach would be based on inspecting a plot that presents the original observations together with the fitted regression line (as in Fig. 12.1). But a more precise approach (which is also easier to interpret) is to plot the **regression residuals** (i.e. the observed minus the predicted values, $Y_i - \hat{Y}_i$) against the predicted values $\hat{Y}_i$, as shown in Figs 12.2 and 12.3. In an ideal case, the residuals should lie in a band around the horizontal axis, as illustrated, e.g., in Fig. 12.2C.[8]

The two most common violations of simple linear regression model assumptions are illustrated in Figs 12.2 and 12.3. In the example in Fig. 12.3, the relationship between Y and X is not linear. For Fig. 12.2, the relationship of X and Y is linear and the residuals are spread symmetrically around the horizontal axis, but their absolute value increases with the predicted value of Y (Fig. 12.2B). In other, similar cases we can find that the absolute size of residuals decreases along the horizontal axis. If we regress the absolute values of those residuals against

---

[8] Note that if we fit a simple linear regression model for the dependency of regression residuals on the X values, the resulting line will have both b_0 and b_1 estimates equal to zero.

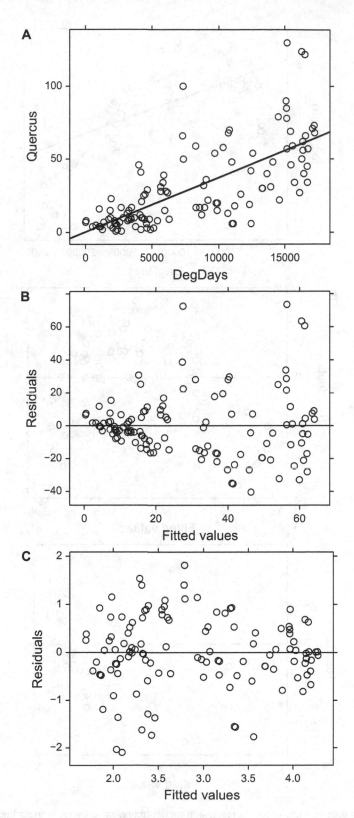

Figure 12.2 Example of a regression model for which the assumption regarding the independence of response variance on the fitted values is not met (part A). After plotting residuals against the predicted values (part B), we can see their increasing spread at higher predicted values. Transformation of the response variable could help. Part C shows the same kind of diagram as in B, but after a log-transformation of the response variable.

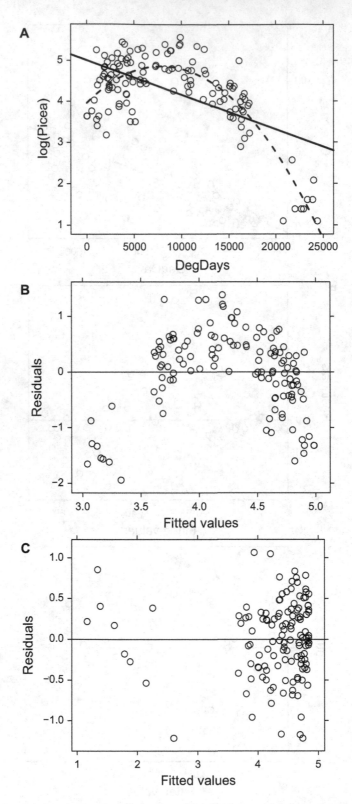

Figure 12.3 Example of a mis-specified regression model (represented by the straight line in part A). Regression residuals show (part B) that the dependency of *Picea* on *DegDays* is not linear, but rather quadratic (a quadratic model using the second-degree polynomial for the effect of *DegDays* is plotted in part A using a dashed line). Part C displays the regression residuals against the predicted values for this quadratic model. Both regression models presented in this figure use log-transformed values of the response variable (see also Fig. 12.2).

the values of the X variable, the resulting model will be significant (sometimes the squares of residuals are used instead of absolute values). The problems illustrated in Fig. 12.2 occur quite frequently, because for many response variables of this kind their variation coefficient is constant rather than the variance itself.

Plotting the residuals against predicted (fitted) values of the response variable is probably the simplest and most frequently used way to examine the appropriateness of a chosen model. But this is by no means the only tool available in the field of *regression diagnostics*. Another frequently used approach is to check the influence (measured e.g. by *leverage*) of individual observations on a fitted regression model. Observations (points in an *XY* diagram) lying far apart from a scatter of other observations exert the highest leverage. These are often called *outliers*. Our visual inspection can provide important hints about our data, particularly if we have additional information about individual observations. If we study e.g. a dependency of species richness on island size and we find that the island of Trinidad has the largest leverage, then we can consider the reasons behind this pattern. If we find that influential points are concentrated, e.g. at extreme values of the predictor, this might suggest an inappropriate choice of model. Sometimes we can even detect errors in our data in this way.

Although statistical software usually allows us to exclude such outlying observations, we consider this to be a dangerous approach, particularly when also performing significance tests on the reduced dataset. Therefore, do not exclude such observations unless you have other reasons for excluding them, unrelated to their outlying nature.

We can also use the regression residuals to check for the assumption of a normal distribution of residuals,[9] but we generally do not recommend that the reader goes much further than checking for a symmetrical shape in a frequency histogram.

Some deviations of our data from the assumptions of regression models can be cured by an appropriately chosen data transformation. The rules for transforming data in regression analysis match those for the transformations in ANOVA models (see Chapter 10). Transforming any variable of a regression model naturally changes the shape of the relationship. In some cases, this is a desired effect, but in others it might distort the linear character of the relationship. If the residuals are properly distributed around the mean for each value of the predictor, but the shape of the dependency of the response on the predictor is not linear, we can use any transformation of the predictor that helps to linearise the relationship as it does not change the statistical properties of the residuals. In contrast, when we transform a dependent variable, such a transformation changes the distribution of the regression residuals.

We very often use a log-transformation (or $\log(X + c)$, see Section 10.2) of the response variable. If, for the original values of X and Y, the standard deviation of Y is linearly dependent on its average, the Y variable has a log-normal, rather than a normal distribution, and the dependency of Y on X has an exponential shape, i.e.

$$Y = e^{b_0 + b_1 X} = e^{b_0} e^{b_1 X} \tag{12.14}$$

---

[9] We note that any checks for a normal distribution using the values of the response variable or of the predictors is a totally pointless exercise.

then, after log-transforming both sides of the above equation we obtain a linear dependency with a constant variance and normal distribution of variable Y. By log-transforming Eq. (12.14) (using the natural logarithm ln), we get

$$\ln Y = b_0 + b_1 X \tag{12.15}$$

We can use this approach to estimate the growth rate of an exponentially growing population. The change of population size with time is then characterised by the equation $N_t = N_0 e^{rt}$, where N_t represents the size of the population at times specified by the t index, t is time and r is the population growth rate. By log-transforming this relation (here we must use the natural logarithm), we obtain $\ln(N_t) = \ln(N_0) + rt$. The slope of the regression line using the natural logarithm of population size as the response variable and time (t) as predictor then represents the estimate of the growth rate r.

If we find a linear dependency of the standard deviation of Y on Y average, a log-normal distribution of Y, and the dependency has a shape corresponding to

$$Y = b_0 X^{b_1} \tag{12.16}$$

it is recommended to log-transform both variables (X and Y). Following this, Eq. (12.16) then becomes

$$\log Y = \log b_0 + b_1 \log X \tag{12.17}$$

We usually refer to this as a log–log transformation. Such a transformation is able to linearise most dependencies which are monotonic, have no inflection point and pass through the coordinate origin. Possible shapes of such dependencies are illustrated in Fig. 12.4.

Such shapes often match the dependency of species richness on the size of a sampled area (known as the *species–area curve*) or many allometric relationships (e.g. the dependency of tree volume on the diameter of its trunk). The *species–area* dependency is often presented as $S = c A^z$, where S is the number of species, A is the area of investigated plots and c, z are the two parameters estimated by the regression analysis. Before fitting a linear regression model,

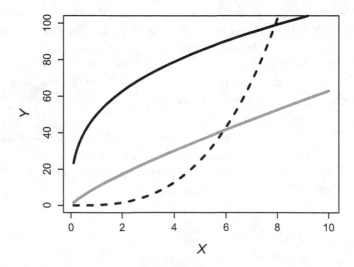

Figure 12.4 Various curves representing a $Y = b_0 X^{b_1}$ equation.

we log-transform the equation and obtain $\log(S) = \log(c) + z \log(A)$, i.e. we regress the log-transformed species richness on the log-transformed area values.

The transformation approach discussed in the above paragraphs is sometimes called *linearised regression*. When using it for our data, we must be alert to the fact that the transformations of the response variable and of the predictor(s) have some important differences. We can transform a predictor at will, as it is assumed to have no random variation (it is *error free*). But a transformation of the response variable changes not only the shape of the relationship between Y and X, but also the distribution of Y values and so too the constancy (homogeneity) of variance. Log-transformation of a response variable might improve the homogeneity of variance if the standard deviations of Y values depend linearly on Y mean for non-transformed data. But if the assumptions of linear regression were fulfilled for non-transformed data then they will not be met by transformed values.

Model parameters (regression coefficients) are estimated by the least-squares method. This means that we minimise the sum of squared residuals and at the same time the sum of residuals is equal to zero. But when we use a linearised regression, this rule holds for transformed data, but not for the data we obtain by a 'back-transformation'. For example, if we use log-transformed Y, then after back-transforming the predicted values (using the exponential function), the sum of positive residuals will be larger than the sum of negative ones; in this sense, our estimates are biased to some extent (as a matter of fact, such a regression model predicts a geometric, rather than an arithmetic, mean for the predictor values).

If the assumptions of a linear regression model are fulfilled (except for the linearity of the relation between Y and X) for non-transformed data and a transformation of the predictor X does not help (logarithmic transformation is not helpful e.g. in changing a non-monotonic relation to a linear one), we can use a polynomial or non-linear regression (see Chapter 16). In other cases, instead of using a linearised regression, it is often far better to employ GLMs (see Chapter 15). They allow for a wider scale of functional dependencies and estimate model parameters using the maximum likelihood method. In doing so, they can use our *a priori* expectations about the statistical distribution of the response variable. The use of GLMs has already replaced the linearised regression to a large extent.

12.7 Regression Through the Origin

For some types of data we already know in advance that the estimated regression line should pass through the coordinate origin. As an example, we might study how the number of rodents caught by the common kestrel depends on the rodent's population density (so-called *functional response*), assuming the functional response is of Type I, i.e. a linear relation for low densities. We also know that the straight line describing this dependency must pass through the coordinate origin (you cannot catch anything for zero density). We can then use a regression through the origin, i.e. with the b_0 regression coefficient explicitly set to 0: $Y = b_1 X$. The formulas for estimating this type of regression model can be found, for example, in Zar (2010, pp. 355–357).

We should, however, be careful about the mindless application of regression through the origin. The functional response seen for the kestrel to rodent density relation can in fact be of Type III, when the predator does not hunt the rodents at low densities and starts to respond

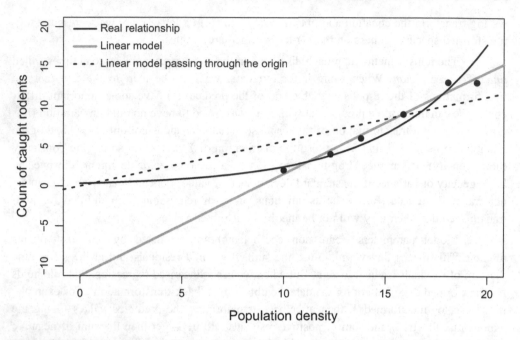

Figure 12.5 Dependency between the number of caught rodents and their availability (rodent population density). If we approximate the real relationship (shown as the solid black curve) with a linear model (solid grey line), the predictions in the observed range of densities are very good, but the predictions extrapolated for lower population densities are not realistic. We cannot solve this problem by forcing the linear model to pass through zero coordinates (dashed black line), as the resulting model does not do a very good job of describing the data.

to this prey only if its density exceeds a certain limit. Such a shape is shown in Fig. 12.5 by a solid black curve.[10] If our study area does not contain locations with very low densities, so we are restricted only to a limited range, the relation can be linear. But if we extrapolate for population densities close to zero, our model would predict a negative number of rodents being caught (see the solid grey line in Fig. 12.5). But if we force our linear model to pass through the coordinate origin, we obtain a very unrealistic straight line that does not fit the observed data very well (see the dashed line in Fig. 12.5). This is because our dependency is linear in the observed range of densities, but it is not linear in the extrapolated range (of lower densities). As a consequence, if the relationship is linear in the studied range of X values, we should describe it with a linear regression without restricting the intercept (b_0) value. We should be aware, at the same time, that our model cannot be used for extrapolating outside the observed range.

In general terms, it is good to realise that linear relationships are not the rule in nature, but the more complex shapes of a relationship can often be well approximated by a linear model in a restricted range of predictor values. If we decide to extrapolate with such a model then we can come to entirely wrong conclusions. Particularly for variables measured on the ratio scale where we must expect different behaviour for predictor values close to zero.

---

[10] We do not show, however, the saturating part of a Type III functional response for high prey densities.

The dangers of extrapolation must also be acknowledged when testing the regression coefficient b_0. If the predictor was measured on the ratio scale, but the studied range is distant from zero, it makes no sense to test whether the line passes through the coordinate origin, i.e. H_0: $\beta_0 = 0$. We have no way to verify that the relationship between Y and X stays linear throughout the whole range, starting at zero for X.

12.8 Predictor with Random Variation

Earlier we discussed that one of the assumptions of linear regression is that the predictor values are fixed with no random variability, however most of the data to which regression is applied do not fulfil this assumption.

> **If our task is not to use a regression model for predicting new values of a response variable, but rather to quantify the real relationship between variables X and Y (i.e. to correctly estimate parameter β_1), and the random variability of variable X is of similar or even larger size than for variable Y, it is not correct to use a classical least-squares method (also called model I regression). Such an estimate of the β_1 coefficient would be underestimated (shifted towards 0).**

But there are methods referred to as model II regression that take the variation of X into account. The most often used methods are the **major axis regression** (MA regression) and the **standard major axis regression** (SMA regression), sometimes also called the *reduced major axis regression*. An important limitation of these models is that most of their implementations can support only a single predictor variable X. The studies of allometric relationships represent a typical application of model II regression.

12.9 Linear Calibration

Sometimes it happens, particularly in ecological field research, that we need to know the values of some parameter, which can be potentially measured quite precisely, but such measurements are either too expensive, consume too much time, or destroy the subject we need to observe multiple times. So we need to resort to an alternative method, one that is typically less precise, but is cheaper and/or less time-consuming and/or non-destructive.

For example, we can determine the aboveground plant biomass very precisely by harvesting it and then drying and weighing the collected matter. Such a method is not only time-demanding, but also destructive as no biomass is left in the sampling plots. But there is an alternative method that is cheap, quick (so that we can perform multiple measurements) and does not do much damage to the vegetation. We let a disc descend on a pole from above the sampled vegetation until the vegetation stops it: we measure the height above the ground at which it was stopped. This method is routinely used for estimating e.g. the amount of biomass available for herbivores. The measurement has a relatively large estimation error and does not give us an estimate of absolute value of the biomass, just a relative one – the higher the stopping position, the more biomass per unit area we can expect.

So we need to calibrate our method. We do this by first estimating biomass values with the disc at multiple, randomly selected locations and then determining the biomass by a destructive harvesting method. Using a regression model (sometimes even a simple linear regression works), we obtain a function for transforming the height of disc arrest above the ground (used as a predictor X) into estimated biomass weight per unit area (used as a response variable Y). In this way we minimise the differences between predicted and observed values of biomass, not between the predicted and observed value of the disc arrest. There are multiple other examples of using calibration in biological field research. A nice one is the example where we estimate the dominance of organisms on the sea floor from a boat (an imprecise but quick method), but calibrate our measurements by diving on the sea floor and harvesting the organisms.

12.10 Example Data

The *Chap12* sheet contains the variables used to illustrate simple linear regression in its first two columns. These are the data from 16 North American lakes (Christensen et al., 1996), describing the relationship between tree density at lake shores (variable *TreeDens*, km^{-1}) and the cover of woody debris in the lakes (variable *WoodDebris*, m^2 km^{-1}). The purpose of modelling this relationship can be e.g. the prediction of the amount of woody debris in other lakes with a known density of trees.

Variables *W_body* and *W_brain* in columns *D* and *E* represent the body and brain weights of a set of mammal species. Our task is to verify a research hypothesis that the allometric ratio between log-transformed brain biomass and log-transformed body weight is equal to 2/3 for mammal species. This hypothesis is based on the expectation that body weight is proportional to body volume, while brain weight is proportional to body surface, as body surface innervation demands a large share of the neural capacity of mammal brains.

12.11 How to Proceed in R

Variables in columns *A* and *B* were imported into a data frame called *chap12a*, while those in columns *D* and *E* were imported into a data frame called *chap12b*.

12.11.1 Simple Linear Regression

We can estimate a simple linear model (i.e. to fit a straight line) using the function *lm* in the following way:

```
lm.1 <- lm( WoodDebris ~ TreeDens, data=chap12a)
```

A basic summary of a fitted linear model, containing (after a brief report on how the model was created and on the distribution of regression residuals) the estimates of regression coefficients, standard errors of those estimates and *t* tests of individual regression coefficients in a table, can be obtained by submitting the linear model object to the *summary* function:

```
summary( lm.1)
Call:
lm(formula = WoodDebris ~ TreeDens, data = chap12a)
Residuals:
    Min     1Q Median     3Q    Max
 -38.62 -22.41 -13.33  26.16  61.35


Coefficients:
              Estimate Std. Error t value Pr(>|t|)
(Intercept) -77.09908   30.60801  -2.519 0.024552 *
TreeDens      0.11552    0.02343   4.930 0.000222 ***
---
Signif. codes:  0 '***' 0.001 '**' 0.01 '*' 0.05 '.' 0.1 ' ' 1


Residual standard error: 36.32 on 14 degrees of freedom
Multiple R-squared:  0.6345,    Adjusted R-squared:  0.6084
F-statistic:  24.3 on 1 and 14 DF,  p-value: 0.0002216
```

The two lines of the *Coefficients* table present summary information about the estimates of two regression coefficients in the model. The b_0 (intercept) estimate is introduced with the word *Intercept*, while the slope of the regression (b_1) estimate is introduced with the name of the corresponding predictor variable (*TreeDens* in our model). The values of the two coefficients for our model *lm.1* tell us that we can estimate the amount of woody debris based on a known tree density near the shoreline (*TD*) using the equation $WD = -77.10 + 0.116 \times TD$. For example, a tree density value of 1000 trees km^{-1} predicts woody debris cover of $116 - 77.1 = 38.9$ m^2 km^{-1}.

Although we did not plot the fitted line yet, the positive estimate for the slope coefficient (+0.116) suggests that the relationship between tree density and woody debris cover is positive: the larger the density, the more debris we can expect. The nature of a linear model (with no variable transformations involved) implies that this relation can be described (without paying attention to the value of the intercept) e.g. as 'with an increase of tree density by 100 trees per km, the average woody debris cover increases by 11.6 m^2 per km of shore'.

The negative value of the intercept (-77.1) identifies a limitation of our choice of model: although a lake with no trees on the shore can be imagined, we can hardly imagine such a lake to have a -77.1 m^2 cover of woody debris. We should recall that the minimum value for our density predictor is a value of nearly 800 trees per km of shore, so that our prediction for a null density (resulting in an estimate of -77.1 m^2 km^{-1}) is an extrapolation far beyond the range of observed values. If we decided to use a line passing through the origin, the resulting regression line would not be a good predictor for the observed values.[11]

---

[11] Although not an appropriate approach here, we note that to enforce a model with the intercept coefficient set to 0, we would have to add -1 into the model formula (e.g. as *WoodDebris ~ TreeDens* -1).

A much better solution is to use a GLM of an appropriate type (see Chapter 15), in which we can specify the random distribution for the woody debris cover (such as one limited to positive values and with variation increasing with increasing predicted cover, e.g. gamma distribution). Even with a GLM, we cannot avoid the basic limitation of our dataset, namely that we have no observations in circumstances where the tree density is below 770 trees km^{-1}.

The column labelled *Std. Error* in the output of the *summary* function shows the estimates of standard errors of regression coefficient estimates and the ratio between the coefficient estimate and its standard error is then presented in the *t-value* column as a test statistic for testing a particular regression coefficient, as described by Eq. (12.13) and in the text that follows that equation. These partial tests that employ the t statistic are particularly sensitive to deviations from the assumption of homogeneity of response variance. The results of both tests presented above tell us that both coefficients are significantly different from zero.

The table describing fitted regression coefficients is followed by information about the coefficient of determination (including its adjusted version, see Section 14.2) and about the F test of the whole regression model. The logic of the F test is better seen from a detailed table of variance decomposition for the fitted linear model, which we can obtain by using the *anova* function:

```
anova( lm.1)
Analysis of Variance Table

Response: WoodDebris
          Df Sum Sq Mean Sq F value    Pr(>F)
TreeDens   1  32054   32054  24.303 0.0002216 ***
Residuals 14  18466    1319
---
Signif. codes:  0 '***' 0.001 '**' 0.01 '*' 0.05 '.' 0.1 ' ' 1
```

From the total sum of squares of the response variable (50,520, not shown in the *anova* output), our model explained (*TreeDens* line in the above table) 32,054 and 18,466 remained unexplained (*Residuals*). By dividing the sums of squares (*Sum Sq* column) by the corresponding degrees of freedom (*Df* column), we obtain mean squares (*Mean Sq* column). The ratio of model mean square (32,054) and residual mean square (1319) represents the F test statistic that is expected to originate from an F distribution with parameters 1 and 14, if the null hypothesis (that there are no linear effects of the predictors in the model – here just the tree density) is correct. For our data, it is highly unlikely ($p < 0.001$) that we make a mistake by rejecting H_0, so this result supports the existence of an effect of tree density upon woody debris cover.[12]

If we work with a simple linear regression that has just a single predictor, this F test does not provide information different from the t test of the regression coefficient b_1: the p-values of both tests must be identical (they are just displayed with different precision in the above outputs). For linear models with two or more predictors, the F test represents an

---

[12] It is good to take a moment to recall that all regression models have a descriptive nature, so the uncovered significant effect of density is a statistical incantation and it implies no causal effect, although in this particular example we do not doubt it.

evaluation of the whole model, but we can also use it to compare e.g. two models differing by the presence or absence of a particular predictor, this is referred to as a partial F test (see Section 14.6.3).

When we want to display the estimated regression model, we can do so easily for a simple linear regression. For example, we can use the following:

```
plot( WoodDebris ~ TreeDens, data=chap12a)
abline( lm.1, lwd=2)
```

When we decide we want to supplement the regression line with region(s) displaying 95% confidence intervals (or perhaps even 95% prediction intervals, see Section 12.5), the task becomes more difficult. We must calculate the intervals for a range of predictor values, ideally covering the range of the horizontal axis in the graph. This new variable (stored in the code below in a *chap12a.new* data frame, in a variable of the same name as the predictor used in the fitted model) is then passed (together with the fitted model and an appropriate value for the parameter *interval*) to the *predict* function:

```
chap12a.new <- data.frame( TreeDens=seq( 700, 2200, by=50))
lm.1.ci <- predict( lm.1, newdata=chap12a.new,
                    interval="confidence")
```

The function *predict* creates a matrix with three columns representing, respectively, the fitted value (for the line already present in the graph) and lower (*lwr*) and upper (*upr*) range of the confidence region:

```
summary( lm.1.ci)
     fit                lwr                upr
Min.   :  3.762    Min.   :-29.94     Min.   : 37.47
1st Qu.: 47.081    1st Qu.: 25.74     1st Qu.: 68.43
Median : 90.399    Median : 68.43     Median :112.37
Mean   : 90.399    Mean   : 60.42     Mean   :120.38
3rd Qu.:133.718    3rd Qu.: 98.76     3rd Qu.:168.68
Max.   :177.036    Max.   :125.35     Max.   :228.72
```

Similarly we can create the prediction interval:

```
lm.1.pi <- predict( lm.1, newdata=chap12a.new,
                    interval="prediction")
```

Now we can plot the estimated limits of confidence and prediction intervals into an existing plot as four multilines, using the *lines* function:

```
lines( chap12a.new$TreeDens, lm.1.ci[,"lwr"], lty=2)
lines( chap12a.new$TreeDens, lm.1.ci[,"upr"], lty=2)
lines( chap12a.new$TreeDens, lm.1.pi[,"lwr"], lty=3)
lines( chap12a.new$TreeDens, lm.1.pi[,"upr"], lty=3)
```

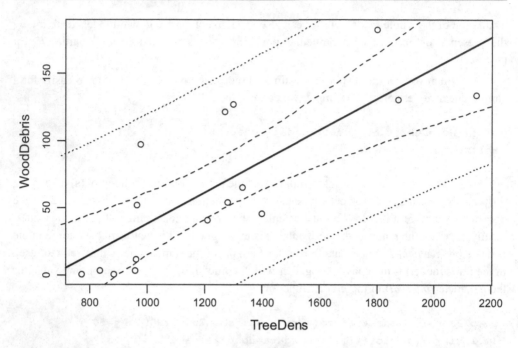

Figure 12.6 Plotted regression line with 95% confidence intervals (dashed lines) and 95% prediction intervals (dotted lines).

The resulting diagram is illustrated in Fig. 12.6.

If you simply need to plot the confidence intervals for the predicted means of the response variable then we recommend that you use the *effects* library. The way we use it below normally offers a separate plot for each independent predictor, but as we have just a single predictor in our model, it creates a graph representing the whole model (the second *plot* command produces a graph similar to Fig. 12.6, but without the prediction intervals).

```
library( effects)
plot( allEffects( lm.1))
plot( allEffects( lm.1, resid=TRUE),
        partial.residuals = list( plot=T, smooth=F,
                                    col="black"),
        confint=list(style="lines"), main="")
```

The diagrams of regression diagnostics can be created with the function *plot* (if we pass the object with the fitted model to it as its first parameter) or with the aid of the extraction functions *residuals* and/or *fitted*:

```
plot( lm.1, which=1, add.smooth=F)
plot( lm.1, which=3, add.smooth=F)
plot( residuals( lm.1) ~ fitted( lm.1))
```

12.11.2 Model II Regression

This type of regression model can be estimated e.g. with the library *lmodel2*, which typically must be added to your installation of R:

```
library( lmodel2)
lm2.1 <- lmodel2( log(W_brain)~log(W_body), data=chap12b,
                  range.y="interval",
                  range.x="interval", nperm=999)
```

The *range.** parameters are relevant just for the so-called *ranged major axis (RMA) regression*, which is used rarely. The *lmodel2* function estimates the classical linear model using the least-squares method (labelled in the results as *OLS*, i.e. ordinary least squares), but also three methods of Type II regression: MA regression, SMA regression and RMA regression. The *nperm* parameter represents the number of permutations used when testing the null model (see Section 7.4 for an explanation of the permutation test principle).

We do not use the *summary* function to see the fit results, but rather we print the returned object (the output text was reduced):

```
lm2.1

Model II regression

...
n = 54   r = 0.9753605   r-square = 0.951328
Parametric P-values:  2-tailed = 8.347005e-36
            1-tailed = 4.173503e-36
Angle between the two OLS regression lines = 1.364954 degrees


Permutation tests of OLS, MA, RMA slopes: 1-tailed, tail corresponding to
sign
A permutation test of r is equivalent to a permutation test of the OLS slope
P-perm for SMA = NA because the SMA slope cannot be tested


Regression results
  Method Intercept     Slope Angle (degrees) P-perm (1-tailed)
1    OLS -2.968594 0.7183359       35.69104           0.001
2     MA -3.072829 0.7309896       36.16642           0.001
3    SMA -3.118077 0.7364825       36.37100              NA
4    RMA -3.129393 0.7378562       36.42199           0.001


Confidence intervals
  Method 2.5%-Intercept 97.5%-Intercept 2.5%-Slope 97.5%-Slope
1    OLS      -3.372758       -2.564430  0.6731221   0.7635497
2     MA      -3.460514       -2.701784  0.6859464   0.7780527
3    SMA      -3.501951       -2.757048  0.6926552   0.7830829
4    RMA      -3.525572       -2.759170  0.6929129   0.7859504
```

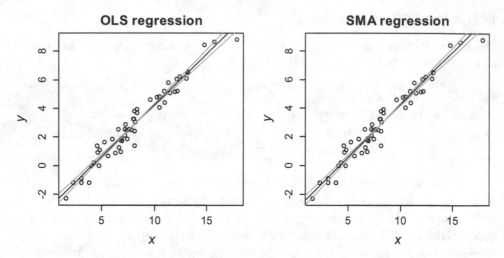

Figure 12.7 A comparison of two linear models fitted to the same data with the *lmodel2* function using two approaches: standard least squares method (*OLS regression* plot) and Type II regression called standard major axis (SMA) regression.

Estimated regression coefficients can be found for individual fitting methods in the columns *Intercept* and *Slope* of the *Regression results* table, together with the estimated significance of the slope (except the SMA method).[13] The *Confidence intervals* table shows the confidence intervals estimated for the intercept and slope estimates from the individual methods. These 95% confidence intervals show that the hypothesised value 0.6667 is not included in the confidence interval for the slope of any of the estimated Type II models, i.e. we can reject H_0: $\beta_1 = 2/3$ with $p < 0.05$. This package also allows us to create a graph with a fitted line of some chosen type – below we compare the classical Type I regression with the standard major axis regression results (Fig. 12.7):

```
par( mfrow=c(1,2))
plot( lm2.1, "OLS")
plot( lm2.1, "SMA")
par( mfrow=c(1,1))
```

12.12 Reporting Analyses

12.12.1 Methods

The relationship between shore tree density and the cover of woody debris was described using a linear regression model.

We tested whether the allometric relationship between mammalian brain and body weights conforms to the hypothesised 2/3 ratio, using a standard major axis (model II) regression on log-transformed weight values.

---

[13] The value of the regression coefficient is similar but lower for OLS than for a model II regression (the difference would be larger if the relationship was less strong).

12.12.2 Results

Woody debris relative area increases significantly with the shore tree density (R^2_{adj} = 0.608, $F_{1,54}$ = 24.3, p = 0.00022) at a rate of 11.6 m^2 km^{-1} of shore with each increase of tree density by 100 trees km^{-1} (see Fig. X).

Figure X would probably contain both the data points and the fitted regression line, possibly 95% confidence intervals also, with the fitted equation containing the estimates of parameters present in the figure caption (or in a separate table). The level of detail we use for describing model parameters would depend on the type of journal and also on the relative importance of this model in the context of the whole study.

Our estimates of the standard major axis regression model, including the 95% confidence interval for the slope (0.693, 0.783), suggest that the allometric coefficient is larger than the hypothesised 2/3 value.

12.13 Recommended Reading

Zar (2010), pp. 328–362.

Quinn & Keough (2002), pp. 77–105.

Sokal & Rohlf (2012), pp. 471–550.

D. L. Christensen, B. R. Herwig, D. E. Schindler & S. R. Carpenter (1996) Impacts of lakeshore residential development on coarse-woody debris in north temperate lakes. *Ecological Applications*, **64**: 1143–1149.

13 Correlation: Relationship Between Two Quantitative Variables

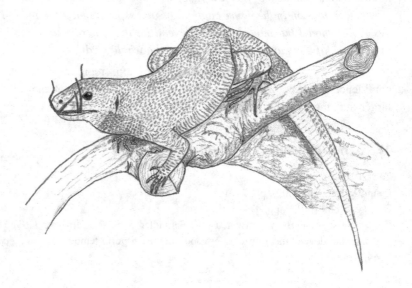

13.1 Use Case Examples

Calculating correlations among numerical variables is, to some extent, an approach complementary to relating them via linear regression. Therefore, we start with a use case identical with one of the Chapter 12 examples.

1. We measure the diameter at breast height (*DBH*) and total height of a number of trees of a particular species. We want to understand the relation among these two quantitative variables. We are likely to find that the larger the tree height is, the larger the *DBH* value will be. This time (see Section 12.1, first example) we do not want to predict, say, the tree height from its *DBH* value, but to measure the strength and direction of the relationship of these two parameters.
2. We quantified conductivity and calcium ion concentrations in 33 water samples from various brooks in the Šumava mountains. We want to quantify the strength of their relationship (degree of mutual dependency).

13.2 Correlation as a Dependency Statistic for Two Variables on an Equal Footing

In the linear regression model discussed in the preceding chapter, we assumed the functional relationship between the variables and were able to distinguish between dependent and

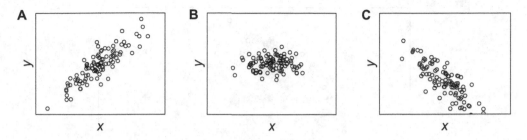

Figure 13.1 Simple linear correlation: positive correlation (A), negative correlation (C) and no correlation (B).

independent variables, or at least the response variable and the predictor. We also assumed that the predictor is not subject to random variation, or that such a variation plays only a minor role. In correlation analysis, however, we do not focus on the existence of a functional relationship of one variable to another, the two variables are merely *correlated* and both variables are expected to exhibit random variation.

We also assume (unless we use non-parametric correlations, see Section 13.4) that the two variables come from a two-dimensional normal distribution. This essentially means that variable Y has a normal distribution for each possible value of variable X, and X has a normal distribution for each possible value of Y. This assumption implies the linearity of the relationship between X and Y. A core measure of the strength of the relationship between the two variables is the **correlation coefficient** (sometimes also called the Pearson coefficient of linear correlation), which can be calculated as follows:

$$r = \frac{\sum (X_i - \overline{X})(Y_i - \overline{Y})}{\sqrt{\sum (X_i - \overline{X})^2 \sum (Y_i - \overline{Y})^2}} \tag{13.1}$$

with the summation proceeding across all available observations, i.e. $i = 1, \ldots, n$.

Despite the two variables having an equivalent role (there is no dependent vs. independent variable), the letters X and Y are used here as in the linear regression. The role of the two variables is entirely symmetrical, so the labels X and Y are assigned *ad hoc* to both variables. The expression in the formula's denominator is always positive. But if the positive deviations of X values from their mean are matched, for the most part, with positive deviations of Y values from their mean, or the negative deviations of X from its mean are matched with negative deviations of Y from its mean, most of the expressions summed up in the numerator will be positive,[1] and so the whole coefficient has a positive value. In the opposite situation, the resulting value will be negative. The meaning of positive and negative correlations is further illustrated in Fig. 13.1.

The values of a correlation coefficient r are always in the range from -1 to $+1$. The -1 value represents a deterministic negative dependency, while $+1$ a deterministic positive dependency. The r value equal to 0 implies that there is no linear relationship between the variables. Figure 13.2 illustrates a case where two variables have quite a strong dependency,

---

[1] This applies particularly if <u>large</u> deviations (in a specific direction) of one variable are matched with <u>large</u> deviations (in the same direction) of the other variable.

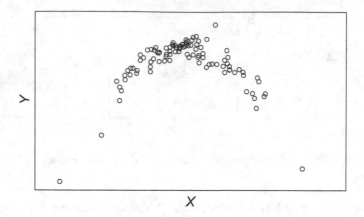

Figure 13.2 An example of research results where two variables are not independent, but their correlation coefficient is almost equal to zero ($r = 0.013$).

but not of a linear nature; their correlation coefficient has a value close to 0. We should note that for some values of Y, the X variable has a bimodal distribution, so the assumption of normality is strongly deviated. The correlation coefficient is therefore only a good measure of the relationship for data coming from a two-dimensional normal distribution, or distributions similar to it.

If we take the two variables used for calculating the correlation coefficient (r) and use them in a linear regression model (it does not matter which of the variables becomes X and which becomes Y), the coefficient of determination from that regression is equal to the second power of the correlation coefficient r (this is why we label it R^2).

What is the difference between a correlation coefficient and a regression coefficient from a simple linear regression based on the same couple of variables? A regression coefficient estimate (b_1) tells us how much the expected value of a response variable changes with a unit change of the predictor. The regression coefficient is therefore given in the units translating from predictor units to response units – for our woody debris example (see Chapter 12), this would be square metres of debris per individual tree. This also implies that the value of b_1 changes when we change the units of measurement. In theory, the b_1 coefficient may have values from minus infinity to plus infinity. On the contrary, the correlation coefficient r is a unitless number representing the strength of the relation, ranging from -1 to $+1$, and its value does not depend on the units chosen for our variables.

The value of the correlation coefficient is almost always computed for a sample of observations. We therefore consider the r-value as an estimate of the correlation in the sampled population, ρ. Consequently, we can test hypotheses about ρ, most often a null hypothesis that there is no correlation among the variables, $H_0: \rho = 0$. This hypothesis can be tested with a one-sample t test, using the following test statistic:

$$t = \frac{r}{s_r} \tag{13.2}$$

where s_r is the standard error of the r estimate, calculated as follows:

$$s_r = \sqrt{\frac{1 - r^2}{n - 2}} \tag{13.3}$$

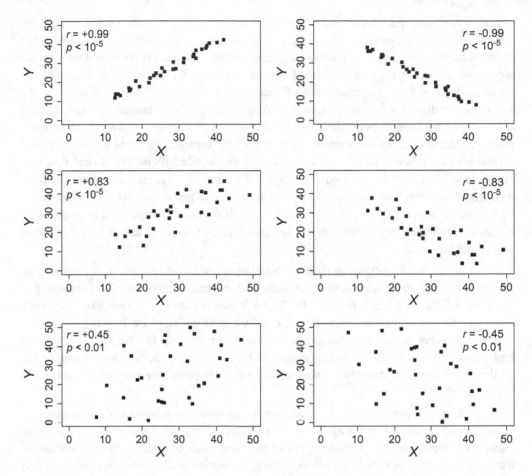

Figure 13.3 The strength of dependency between two numerical variables at different values of the linear correlation coefficient. All r estimates are calculated based on a set of 31 observations.

with r being the estimate of the correlation coefficient and n the number of observations. The t statistic of Eq. (13.2) is compared with a t distribution with $n - 2$ degrees of freedom. We can use both the one-sided and two-sided forms of the t test. For a given number of observations, we can also calculate critical values of r (see Table 13.1 in Section 13.3). It is worth noting that the achieved significance level (p) for the test of the null hypothesis $\rho = 0$ is identical with the p-value of the linear regression of one variable on the other. Figure 13.3 provides a sense of how a relationship between two variables might look for various values of correlation coefficients.

13.3 Test Power

Because the p-values are identical whether we test a regression line of Y and X or whether we test a linear correlation coefficient, the data properties affecting the test power are also identical. The power of the test increases with the strength of the relationship between X and Y (i.e. with the absolute value of the correlation coefficient ρ in the sampled statistical population) and with the sample size (n). While exploring correlation among variables, we sample a statistical population and none of the sampled variables can be affected by the experimenter, so we cannot (unlike in some cases where we are analysing by linear regression) increase the range of sampled values for any variable. However, as is also the case for regression, increasing the range of variable values will in many cases lead to an increased test power (which will be a consequence of increasing ρ, the correlation coefficient in the statistical population we plan to sample). We can change these ranges by changing our definition of a statistical population. For example, when we study the correlation between BOD (biological oxygen demand, a measure of organic pollution in water) and P (phosphorus) concentration, we can expect that the correlation coefficient (and thus also the power of the test) will be considerably higher if we include stagnant water bodies from the whole country rather than just the lakes of a single mountain range. This is because in lowland water bodies, depending on pollution levels, both BOD and P can potentially reach much higher values, increasing the range in our dataset compared with using data collected just from mountain lakes.

From this it follows that for a correlation coefficient value to be meaningful, we always need to clearly define the statistical population we sample. For example, the value of the correlation between BOD and P concentration will very likely be much lower in a set of mountain lakes (which are usually oligotrophic), and will be much higher in a set of all types of water bodies across a country. In the second case we have a much higher chance of rejecting the null hypothesis (with the same number of samples examined), so the conclusion that these two values are significantly positively correlated might seem rather trivial.

A very approximate, yet simple way to estimate the sample size (n) required to have a good chance of rejecting the null hypothesis that ρ is equal to 0 is to examine Table 13.1, which contains critical values of the correlation coefficient. When we increase the sample size, the expected value of the sample correlation coefficient r does not change. If we expect e.g. that the correlation in the sampled population (ρ) will be equal to 0.5 and we intend to perform a two-sided test with $\alpha = 0.05$, then a sample with size 15 ($df = 13$) has just a 50% chance of enabling us to reject the null hypothesis. We should realise that if the expected value of the correlation coefficient is equal to its critical value for a given sample size (e.g. for $n = 17$ we would assume $\rho = 0.48$), we have about a 50% chance that we reject the null hypothesis.

The approach described above is not completely correct from a statistical point of view, but it is sufficient for a rough estimate. There are more precise methods (one of them illustrated for R software in Section 13.8), but all of them are based on our expectation about the size of the correlation in the sampled population and this expectation is usually rather fuzzy. Typically, we arrive at it based on the results published to date, or it can be based on a pilot study.[2] Sometimes our expectation is based on a minimum value that we would still consider as biologically meaningful.

---

[2] This is probably the best solution: before our 'real' experiment or observation, we perform another one with more limited sampling and based on its results we can work out what results we can expect in a full-scale experiment or observation.

Table 13.1 *Critical values of the Pearson correlation coefficient r for a two-sided test of the null hypothesis ρ = 0. The value n represents the number of observations. We reject the null hypothesis if the absolute value of the correlation coefficient estimate exceeds the critical value*

n	5	6	7	8	9	10	15	20	30	50	100
α = 0.05	0.878	0.811	0.754	0.707	0.666	0.632	0.514	0.444	0.361	0.279	0.197
α = 0.01	0.959	0.917	0.875	0.834	0.798	0.765	0.641	0.561	0.463	0.361	0.256

13.4 Non-parametric Methods

If our data cannot be expected to come from a two-dimensional normal distribution, we can use a non-parametric method measuring the strength of the relationship between two variables. The most frequently used method for non-parametric correlation is probably the **Spearman correlation coefficient** (also called *rank correlation coefficient*). It is based on observation ranks within each of the two correlated variables. The easiest way to calculate it is to replace the original values within each variable with their rank and then to calculate the standard Pearson coefficient of linear correlation (see Eq. (13.1)).

Alternatively, we can use the following equation:

$$r_S = 1 - \frac{6 \sum_{i=1}^{n} d_i^2}{n^3 - n} \tag{13.4}$$

where d_i is the difference in rank between two compared variables. It is important to note, however, that data such as those corresponding to Fig. 13.2 will also lead to a Spearman r close to zero, as the non-parametric coefficients require a monotonic relationship between variables.

The *Kendall tau coefficient* is even more non-parametric than the Spearman r_S, as it is based just on the counts of identical vs. different rank numbers for the compared variables, it does not calculate rank differences.

13.5 Interpreting Correlations

When calculating either a linear regression or a correlation, users often ask 'how large must a correlation coefficient (or R^2 in regression) be to evidence a sufficiently close relationship or dependency?' Sometimes even the achieved significance level (*p*-value) is presented as a measure of strong dependency, which is, unfortunately, an incorrect idea. Statements like 'the relationship is very strong, as it is significant with $p < 0.0001$' are entirely misguided. In fact, we have only rejected – at the given level – a hypothesis that there is no relationship: when we analyse data with a large number of observations, even a relatively weak relationship will lead to a highly significant correlation (check the last row in Fig. 13.3 and also the last column in Table 13.1).

The strength of the relationship is measured solely by the value of the correlation coefficient (r) or the coefficient of determination (R^2). In a regression analysis, R^2 specified the proportion of variation of the response variable that we explained by the predictor (or even multiple predictors, see Chapter 14). Therefore, what we consider as a reasonably strong relationship depends on the particular context of our study. In some cases, we just want to quantify this strength and it is essentially pointless to test the r-value. As an example, when we compare two methods of determining nitrogen content in plant biomass, it makes little sense to test a null hypothesis that there is no dependency between the results of those two methods. Even more dangerous is to simply state that these two methods are equivalent because the calculated correlation coefficient is highly significant. In fact, a value of r equal to 0.90 would be considered insufficiently low in this context, whether it differs significantly from zero or not.

In contrast, if we study dependency of species richness per square metre on the amount of soil organic matter, it is appropriate to first test the null hypothesis and only then consider the strength of the relationship. In this context, even a low value of the coefficient of determination (or of r, with either positive or negative sign) will be of interest, if the relationship between two variables is significant.

Before calculating the correlation between two variables, we should always plot them on an XY diagram so we can visually verify the shape of their relationship. This shape should be linear when we use Pearson's r and monotonic (increasing or decreasing, but not necessarily in a linear way) for non-parametric correlation coefficients. For relationships that are not monotonic (see Fig. 13.2 as an example), we can estimate the strength of the relationship by fitting an appropriate type of regression model to our data (e.g. a second-order polynomial for data from Fig. 13.2) and then calculating the correlation between the fitted (predicted) and observed values of response variable Y (this is therefore a square root of the coefficient of determination R^2). As an example, for the data in Fig. 13.2 this value is $r = 0.940$.[3]

When we summarise the results of regression analyses in a research paper or project report, we usually present the coefficient of determination (R^2) – rather than the correlation coefficient (r) – as the measure of relationship strength. But there is a simple algebraic relationship between these two statistics (a second power or square root), so we (or our readers) can calculate one from the other. As a bonus, the value of a correlation coefficient is signed, so we can easily see whether the relationship is positive or negative. It is perhaps worth noting that there is an interesting psychological consequence borne from the seeming decrease in the proportion of adults able to quickly calculate the second power of a fractional value. Seeing $r = 0.3$ feels substantially better than $R^2 = 0.09$. So remember, if someone writes that there is a mild relationship ($r = 0.3$) between two phenomena, this means that the predictor variable explains just about 9% of the response's variation.

13.6 Statistical Dependency and Causality

We have already mentioned in this book (see Section 3.4) that a statistical relationship does not necessarily imply a causal effect. If we consider a correlation estimate, we look at both variables in a symmetrical way, so we can hardly consider a significant correlation as evidence of a causal relationship. This does not prevent us, however, from seeking the causes of observed correlations.

We might be a little more tempted to infer causality when we try to interpret significant results from a regression model. Here we have a response variable (often called a dependent variable) and a predictor, and often we think (perhaps intuitively) about a causal relationship between those variables. When are such considerations justified? Take, as an example, the results of a regression model (Fig. 13.4) where the response (dependent) variable is the number of murders per 100,000 citizens in individual states of the USA and our predictor is the number of days with freezing temperatures (per year).

An explanation that the murder rate is affected by the extent of freezing weather is quite brave, but if we rephrase our theory, claiming that hot weather encourages violent behaviour, while cold weather suppresses such activities, it seems quite plausible.

---

[3] But given the non-monotonic relationship, the sign of the correlation coefficient becomes irrelevant.

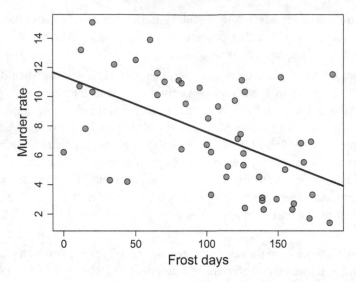

Figure 13.4 Relating the murder rate (number of killings per 100,000 citizens) in year 1976 across individual US states to the mean number of frost days in the state capitals (per year, averages from 1931–1960 period) using a simple linear regression.

Surprisingly, the content of Fig. 13.4 supports such a theory quite well. But when we inspect a broad suite of statistics from the USA, we find that the number of frost days also explains the mean income per citizen, the percentage of illiterate citizens, or the percentage of people with higher education. There is no causal effect: traditionally, the south states were poorer and wilder, so there is a cultural and economic north-to-south gradient across the USA, which is well correlated with air temperature and hence the number of frost days.

This illustrates that a significant correlation/simple regression can be the result of the existence of a third variable (or multiple variables) that affect both variables included in the statistical model. In this and many other cases, it is a common dependence of the two variables on a geographical gradient (or a spatial gradient, generally). Both the climate and the culture change along the north-to-south gradient: temperature decreases with latitude, cultural differences are due to a historical contingency. We can consider this north-to-south gradient to be a *confounding factor*. This leads to counter-intuitive correlations being occasionally presented as causal dependencies (referred to as *spurious correlations* in these situations). Typical examples also come from time series of human demographics, such as the strong and positive correlation between CO_2 concentration in the air and the population size in India (both increasing through time) or the relationship between the number of refrigerators and the number of divorces in the past 90 years for any economically developed country (again, both increasing through time).

So when may we consider a significant correlation or regression model to be evidence of a causal relationship? We believe this is justified only when the data for our model come from a manipulative experiment in which the predictor values were set (using the correct experimental design) by the experimenter. If we randomly choose 10 meadow plots, randomly assign the amount of fertiliser (from 0 to 9, say) to each plot, and then measure the amount of biomass produced after a reasonable time period, only then can we claim that a significant regression model is evidence of a causal effect of the fertiliser on the plant biomass.[4]

What we said about the interpretation of the regression model results extends to any study of the relationship between two (or more) variables, whether they are categorical or numerical. As an example, we can study the population size of a spider species on a set of islands and how it is affected by the presence of a carnivorous lizard on each island. We can compare, using a *t* test, the mean spider population size between the islands with and without the lizard. If we find a significant difference, this can be caused by the lizard predating on spiders or by a completely different, presumably unknown, factor that affects both the spider population size and the lizard presence. Or we can observe a causal relationship, but running in the direction opposite to the one we would expect: on islands where the spider density is low (for some not yet known reason), the lizard species is starving and eventually becomes extinct. Only if we manipulate the lizard population size, e.g. by focusing on islands without the lizard and randomly choosing half of them upon which we establish a viable lizard population,[5] can we speak about a causal effect, after we observe a differential decline of spiders on islands with newly established lizard populations.

> Only a manipulative, correctly established experiment can provide evidence for causality. If we cannot perform manipulative experiments relevant to our research theory, we can at best compare the agreement of our data with the hypothesised causality – see Chapter 17 introducing the structural equation models.

The experimental results in some real-life situations are inherently difficult or impossible to obtain, such as many ecological questions at the landscape or continental scale, most evolutionary studies, or many human-focused studies. Even the lizard–spider manipulative study above would face resistance by the local protection agencies. We must then remain content with a statistical relationship and support of possible causality effects with additional, indirect 'evidence'. There has been a long-standing debate in ecology as to what extent we should sacrifice spatial and temporal scales (where large-scale manipulations are not feasible or ethical and we must mostly rely on observational studies) to get an opportunity to manipulate the explanatory variable. Ecologists often seek situations in nature that resemble some correct experimental design, and call these situations 'natural experiments' (Diamond, 1986), but in such cases we are never able to completely exclude the possibility that a *confounding effect* is present, causing *spurious correlation*.

---

[4] As a side note, we should stress that to demonstrate such a causal effect it would be much more effective to measure the amount of vegetation biomass at each plot also before applying the fertiliser and then take the change in biomass as the response. In this way, we would eliminate (at least partially) the effects of inherent spatial variation in grassland productivity. Note, however, that such a precaution is <u>not</u> an alternative to random plot choice for applied fertiliser doses.

[5] We do not encourage our readers to do such manipulative experiments if they run against the nature protection policies or any other ethical concerns in the manipulated areas. We simply want to point out that without such randomly assigned manipulation, we cannot reliably talk about the causality.

13.7 Example Data

Variables *Conduct* and *Ca* in the *Chap13* sheet represent the conductivity measurement and calcium ion concentration in water samples taken from 33 brooks in a mountain range. We expect these two parameters to be positively correlated, and we wonder whether it is true and what is the strength of their relationship.

13.8 How to Proceed in R

13.8.1 Estimating Correlation and its Significance

The classical Pearson coefficient of linear correlation r and its non-parametric counterparts (distinguished by using the *method* argument with values 'spearman' or 'kendall') can be calculated with the *cor* function:

```
with( chap13, cor( Ca, Conduct))
[1] 0.5370242
```

The non-parametric Spearman coefficient can be calculated as follows:

```
with( chap13, cor( Ca, Conduct, method="spearman"))
[1] 0.5841063
```

If we need to test the significance for a null hypothesis H_0: $\rho = 0$ and/or compute the related 95% confidence interval for ρ, we can do so with the *cor.test* function:

```
with( chap13, cor.test( Ca, Conduct))

        Pearson's product-moment correlation
data:  Ca and Conduct
t = 3.5445, df = 31, p-value = 0.001272
alternative hypothesis: true correlation is not equal to 0
95 percent confidence interval:
 0.2375024 0.7432954
sample estimates:
     cor
0.5370242
```

If we know *a priori* that r must be positive (or it does not make sense to be negative, e.g. when correlating the results of two methods of determining N content, as discussed earlier), we can use a one-sided test. Even for our present example (correlation between calcium concentration and conductivity), such a test makes sense:

```
with( chap13, cor.test( Ca, Conduct, alternative="greater"))

        Pearson's product-moment correlation
data:  Ca and Conduct
t = 3.5445, df = 31, p-value = 0.0006358
alternative hypothesis: true correlation is greater than 0
```

```
95 percent confidence interval:
 0.2909983 1.0000000
sample estimates:
      cor
0.5370242
```

Graphs displaying the shape of the relationship between the two variables can be created with the help of the *plot* function (or *xyplot* in the *lattice* package); a matrix of pairwise *XY* graphs for a reasonably small set of numerical variables can be drawn with the *pairs* function (or with the *splom* function in the *lattice* package).

13.8.2 Test Power Analysis

We can also perform power analysis for a correlation coefficient test with the help of the *pwr.r. test* function in the *pwr* package (this must be added to your default R installation):

```
library( pwr)
```

The *pwr.r.test* function is a flexible tool which requires you to fill in all but one of its mandatory parameters: expected value of ρ (parameter *r*), threshold for Type I error probability (α, specified as the *sig.level* parameter), target Type II error probability (β, specified as a 1-complement with the *power* parameter) and sample size (parameter *n*). The omitted parameter is then estimated and given in the function output. Optionally, we can also use the *alternative* parameter to perform power analysis for a one-sided test.

As an example, imagine we need to use a two-sided test of correlation and reject the null hypothesis (at $\alpha = 0.05$) with probability 90% (this is then the test power), if the absolute value of the correlation coefficient is at least 0.5. We specify this description of the *pwr.r.test* function as follows:

```
pwr.r.test( r=0.5, sig.level = 0.05, power = 0.9)

     approximate correlation power calculation
(arctangh transformation)
              n = 37.03547
              r = 0.5
      sig.level = 0.05
          power = 0.9
    alternative = two.sided
```

The output tells us that to fulfil those requirements our sample should have at least 37 observations. If we need to estimate the required sample size when we *a priori* expect the correlation to be positive, we can modify the request to reflect the one-sided test:

```
pwr.r.test( r=0.5, sig.level = 0.05, power = 0.9,
            alternative="greater")

     approximate correlation power calculation
(arctangh transformation)
```

```
         n = 30.4909
         r = 0.5
 sig.level = 0.05
     power = 0.9
alternative = greater
```

As we have a more specific hypothesis to test, the sample size required drops to $n = 31$ (rounding 30.49 up, to stay on the safe side). Alternatively, we can estimate the power of our test for a situation where e.g. we have 100 observations, the (unknown) value of ρ is 0.2 and we are ready to reject H_0 whenever the achieved significance level is smaller than 0.05:

```
pwr.r.test( r=0.2, n=100, sig.level=0.05)
     approximate correlation power calculation
(arctangh transformation)
         n = 100
         r = 0.2
 sig.level = 0.05
     power = 0.5181042
alternative = two.sided
```

The result indicates that there is about a 52% chance that the correlation will be found to be significant (i.e. that we reject the null hypothesis).

13.9 Reporting Analyses

13.9.1 Methods

We quantified the correlation between conductivity and calcium concentration using Pearson linear correlation and tested for an expected positive correlation using a one-sided t test.

In natural sciences, however, the use of the classical correlation coefficient is rarely mentioned in the Methods section, as it is a commonplace statistic: we just give the estimate values in the Results section. However, it can be prudent to justify why we have chosen a one-sided test.

Due to a non-linear dependency between the two variables, we used the Spearman correlation coefficient to quantify the strength of the relationship between water conductivity and calcium ion concentrations.

13.9.2 Results

We confirmed a positive, medium-strength correlation between conductivity and calcium concentration ($r = 0.537$, $n = 33$, $p < 0.001$).

13.10 Recommended Reading

Zar (2010), pp. 379–418.
Quinn & Keough (2002), pp. 72–77.
Sokal & Rohlf (2012), pp. 551–602.
J. M. Diamond (1986) Overview: laboratory experiments, field experiments, and natural experiments. In: J. M. Diamond & T. J. Case (eds), *Community Ecology*. Harper & Row, New York, pp. 3–22.

14 Multiple Regression and General Linear Models

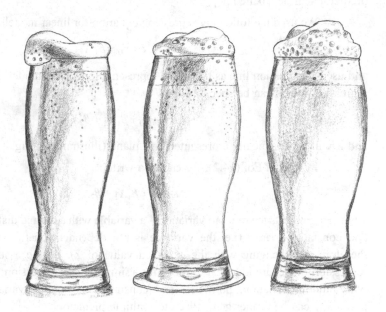

14.1 Use Case Examples

The models introduced in this chapter focus on the values of a single numerical response variable that is predicted with the help of two or more predictors. These predictors may either be all numeric or one or more may contain categorical information.

1. We want to describe how the peak aboveground biomass of smooth meadow grass (*Poa pratensis*) varies with the concentration of total soil nitrogen and phosphates across a range of managed meadows in our observational study. We want to judge the importance and direction of the effects of those two soil parameters and also compare their relative strength.
2. In a complementary project, we want to examine the response of aboveground biomass of *Poa pratensis* to a varied nitrogen supply in a greenhouse experiment. Here nitrogen is provided in two distinct concentrations that are better treated as a categorical predictor. We also want to account for the varying vitality of plant individuals, therefore we measure seedling size at the start of the experiment and use this as an additional predictor.

14.2 Dependency of a Response Variable on Multiple Predictors

In the regression models we have discussed so far, a single response variable was dependent on the values of a single predictor variable. Now we will move to cases where a single response variable depends on two or more predictors, i.e. to a **multiple regression model**. As an example, we can study the change in aboveground biomass of smooth meadow grass (*Poa pratensis*) with the concentration of soil nitrogen and phosphorus. Given the distributional properties of the original measurements (judged by visual summaries, see Section 1.8.1), we will work with all three numerical variables on a log-transformed scale. The predictors will generally be labelled X_1, X_2, etc., the response variable as Y. So the i-th observation for the first predictor will be labelled X_{1i}.

We used the following regression equation for linear models with a single predictor:

$$EY = \beta_0 + \beta_1 X \tag{14.1}$$

and used a regression line as the visual representation of that model. With two predictors, the regression model can be specified as

$$EY = \beta_0 + \beta_1 X_1 + \beta_2 X_2 \tag{14.2}$$

and it will be graphically represented as a plane (illustrated in Fig. 14.1).

Instead of Eq. (14.2), we can also write

$$Y = \beta_0 + \beta_1 X_1 + \beta_2 X_2 + \varepsilon \tag{14.3}$$

where ε represents the random variation – a variable with a normal distribution with zero mean and constant variance (i.e. the variance is not dependent on the values of predictors and therefore not changing with the expected value of Y). So the assumptions for a multiple regression model are identical to those for a simple linear regression: additivity of the effects with random variation, normality and constancy of random variation. The case of two predictors can be further generalised to multiple predictors:

$$Y = \beta_0 + \sum_j \beta_j X_j + \varepsilon \tag{14.4}$$

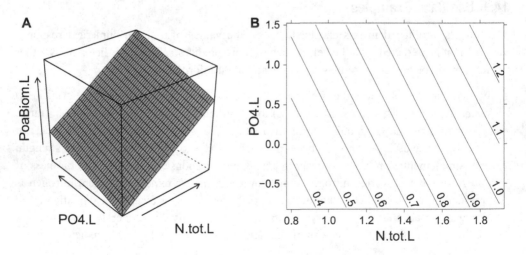

Figure 14.1 Dependence of the aboveground biomass of a meadow-grass species (*PoaBiom.L*) on the log-transformed total soil nitrogen (*N.tot.L*) and the log-transformed concentration of phosphate ions in soil (*PO4.L*). The three-dimensional regression plane is presented either using a perspective view (A) or as a contour plot (B).

The β_j coefficients are called **partial regression coefficients**. We do not know their true values, but we estimate them as the regression model parameters b_0 and b_j based on our data sample, so that the sum of residual squares is minimised. For each regression coefficient, the statistical software also calculates the standard error of the estimate. The ratio $t = b_j/SE(b_j)$ is used as a test criterion for a one-sample t test for a null hypothesis that the true value of β_j is equal to 0. If the null hypothesis is correct, the t statistic comes from a t distribution with $n - m - 1$ degrees of freedom, where m is the number of model predictors and n is the sample size (the number of observations). This test represents, for all coefficients except b_0, a test of a **partial effect** of predictor X_j.

The test for the β_0 coefficient is often pointless, particularly when it is based on an extrapolation, as we already illustrated for the simple regression. We test whether the value of the intercept coefficient is zero when all the predictors have zero values. In our example, where we are working with log-transformed data, we effectively test that the aboveground biomass of meadow grass is equal to 1 when the concentrations of soil nitrogen and phosphorus are also both equal to 1, with all variables in the original units of measurement. This is of course a very ridiculous hypothesis to test.

While the t tests on individual regression coefficients are used to examine partial effects of individual predictors, the F test based on variance decomposition is a global test of the null hypothesis that the regression model does not explain any significant fraction of the variation of the response variable. It therefore corresponds to a null hypothesis that all regression coefficients β_j (i.e. excluding β_0) are equal to zero. As in a simple linear regression (see Section 12.4.2), we again decompose the *total sum of squares* (SS_{tot}) into a *regression sum of squares* (SS_{regr}), sometimes also called the *model sum of squares*, and the *residual sum of squares* (sometimes also referred to as the *error sum of squares*, SS_E). The corresponding degrees of freedom (DF) are then $n - 1$ (total), m (regression) and $n - m - 1$ (residual). The individual mean squares are then calculated as $MS = SS/DF$. Like the simple regression model, the null hypothesis test uses the following ratio as its test statistic:

$$F = \frac{MS_{reg}}{MS_E} \tag{14.5}$$

The coefficient of determination is again calculated as

$$R^2 = \frac{SS_{reg}}{SS_{tot}} \tag{14.6}$$

The R^2 value is a biased estimate of the fraction of explained variation in the sampled statistical population. The smaller our sample size (n) and the more predictors (m) we use, the higher the R^2 value will be (see also Chapter 12). When we have $m + 1$ observations, then a combination of m predictors will fit the observed response values precisely. But even with $m + 2$ observations used to estimate a regression model using m predictors, the coefficient of determination will be very high even when the response is independent of the predictor values. The following adjustment for R^2 was recommended in efforts to counter this bias:

$$R^2_{adj} = R^2 - \frac{m}{n - m - 1}\left(1 - R^2\right) \tag{14.7}$$

The output from statistical software usually shows values for both R^2 and R^2_{adj}. We recommend reporting R^2_{adj} values only, although the correction is negligible when the sample size is much larger than the number of predictor variables.

When comparing the results of a global F test and of partial t tests for a model with two or more predictors, it might happen that some of the regression coefficients are significantly different from zero, while the global F test is non-significant. This usually indicates that our regression model contains redundant predictors that have low explanatory power. If the F test for the whole model is non-significant, relying on the significance of individual partial regression coefficients is not recommended: the probability of Type I error might reach α for each partial test.

Alternatively, it might also happen that the F test of the whole regression model is significant, but none of the partial regression coefficients are significantly different from zero. This is most often an indication of some mutual correlation among the predictors. Ideally our predictors – sometimes also called the independent variables – should be truly mutually independent. But this is rarely the case in real life: for our example, we can expect that microhabitats rich in total nitrogen will also be, on average, richer in available phosphates. It might therefore be difficult to decide which of the predictors really affects the response variable. In this and similar situations, we can also expect to obtain large values of the regression coefficient's standard errors.

The extent to which a predictor will influence a response variable can differ greatly, and sometimes certain predictors can be dropped from our regression model without much effect on its quality. We can perform such model reduction either in an interactive way (comparing the results of alternatively defined regression models) or using an automatic approach. Most statistical programs offer various procedures, usually called a **stepwise selection** (or *stepwise regression*), which use some *a priori* defined criteria to gradually add or gradually remove predictors from a starting model specification. This procedure is expected to select a predictor subset so that adding any new predictor does not lead to a significant decrease of the unexplained variation, but elimination of any of the predictors already present in the model would lead to a significant increase of the unexplained variation.

An alternative approach to model selection is not concerned with significance tests at all. Instead, a measure of model *parsimony* (a measure quantifying the balance between model simplicity and its ability to predict the response variable values accurately) is used to score all alternative models and then we pick the one with the best score. A commonly used parsimony measure is *Akaike's information criterion* (Akaike, 1974), often presented using its acronym AIC (see Section 15.6 for more details). Its peculiarity lies in the somewhat counter-intuitive scale: the smaller the AIC value, the better (more parsimonious) the model is. Occasionally, AIC (or other similar criteria) is employed in a stepwise selection, where we evaluate its change with the addition (or removal) of a particular predictor.

> As we change the set of predictors (explanatory variables), the values of their partial regression coefficients change as well. This change is large when the variable's correlation with other predictors is also large. However, the standard errors of coefficient estimates can also change, and therefore also the conclusions based on predictor tests. This is because a test of a partial regression coefficient actually ascertains whether the effect of the predictor provides a significant, unique contribution to the explained variation of the response within the given set of predictors.

We can illustrate how the meaning of the regression coefficient changes after we include another variable. We use a study of local larch species (*Larix olgensis*) in the forests of

Paektu Mountain in North Korea (Šrůtek and Lepš, 1994) for our illustration. In this study, the researchers wanted to examine changes in tree characteristics along an altitudinal gradient. One element of this was an investigation of how the tree shape changes with altitude. The researchers used the allometric equation to describe tree shape (for simplicity we use coefficient estimates b_j and omit regression residuals):

$$\log(H) = b_0 + b_1 \log(DBH) \tag{14.8}$$

where DBH is the tree diameter at breast height and H represents the tree height. We can consider a significant value of the coefficient b_2 in the following equation as evidence that the tree shape changes with altitude (variable Alt):

$$\log(H) = b_0 + b_1 \log(DBH) + b_2 Alt \tag{14.9}$$

As the b_2 estimate was negative (and significantly different from 0) in the above model, we can conclude that the tree shape changes with altitude: for the same diameter, the tree height decreases with altitude.

If, however, we find that the regression coefficient b_2 in the following equation:

$$\log(H) = b_0 + b_2 Alt \tag{14.10}$$

is significantly different from zero (most likely with a negative value), this merely tells us that the tree height changes (decreases) with altitude. This finding is rather trivial, tree size truly does decrease with altitude – not just the total height, but also the DBH parameter. Consequently, the two predictors are mutually correlated. The estimate b_2 in Eq. (14.9) will therefore be different from the estimate b_2 in Eq. (14.10), reflecting their different meanings.

14.3 Partial Correlation

Imagine that we are interested in the mutual relationships among four variables, we will call them $X1, X2, X3, X4$. Our first idea would be to calculate correlation coefficients pairwise for each couple of variables. Doing so for all variables, we obtain a so-called *correlation matrix* and the calculated coefficients of correlation can eventually be supplemented by significance levels (for a null hypothesis H_0: $\rho_{ij} = 0$). Note that these significances are estimated separately for each partial test and if we calculate the correlation matrix for a sufficiently large set of variables, we can expect some of the correlation coefficients to be significantly different from zero as a consequence of committing Type I error.[1] The correlation matrix can also serve as a starting point for some more complicated statistical methods (e.g. principal component analysis, PCA – see Section 22.2).

Nevertheless, calculating correlations for pairs of variables cannot account for variable interactions of higher orders. To describe these we can use **partial correlation coefficients**. They represent the mutual dependency of two variables under the assumption that the values of another variable (or variables) do not change. For example, $r_{12.3}$ represents the dependency of variables $X1$ and $X2$ if the variable $X3$ does not change.

To help grasp the meaning of a partial correlation, we can represent the $r_{12.3}$ calculation in a somewhat non-standard way. We first estimate a (simple linear) regression

---

[1] This means that we can find significant correlations among some variables even when there are none in the sampled statistical population, analogous to multiple comparisons in the analysis of variance.

of $X1$ on $X3$ and calculate the residuals of this model. Then we use the same procedure for a regression of $X2$ on $X3$. A standard correlation coefficient between the residuals from the first and second regression models is then the partial correlation coefficient $r_{12.3}$. Because the dependency among variables is conditioned just by a single variable (namely $X3$), we speak here about a partial correlation coefficient of the first order. If we need to condition the correlation on two variables, we would label it something like $r_{12.34}^2$ and call it a partial correlation of the second order. A partial correlation coefficient $r_{12.3}$ is significantly different from zero whenever we find a significant regression coefficient for $X2$ in a multiple regression predicting $X1$ using $X2$ and $X3$ or (equivalently) whenever we find a significant regression coefficient for $X1$ in a regression predicting $X2$ using $X1$ and $X3$. The partial correlation (or regression) coefficients are also an important part of structural equation models (see Chapter 17).

14.4 General Linear Models and Analysis of Covariance

General linear models represent an extensive group of statistical models that we can use to describe the dependency of a continuous numerical variable either on categorical predictors (this covers the ANOVA models), on numerical predictors (multiple linear regression models), or on a mixture of categorical and numerical predictors. In other words, ANOVA models and multiple regression models can simply be seen as special cases of the general linear model. They share common approaches of decomposing the total variation of the response variable (characterised by the total sum of squares) into parts explained by individual predictors (and eventually their interactions, if any) and the unexplained (residual) variation. Also, the effects of individual predictors are represented by single or multiple regression coefficients (although these are not usually shown for ANOVA models).

We have not yet discussed an example of a mixture of numerical and categorical predictors in the preceding chapters, so we want to mention it briefly now. Imagine we are studying how the gross primary production of forest communities depends on altitude. If we study this dependency over a sufficiently wide geographical area, however, we will meet different types of bedrock that will also undoubtedly affect the production, alongside the altitude (and other factors). As for the bedrock, it might be practical to distinguish just three broadly defined types: basic sediments (such as limestone), acidic rocks (such as granite or gneiss) and igneous rocks (such as basalt). Our model should therefore use two predictors: one categorical (bedrock type, with three levels) and one numerical (altitude).

This setup fits nicely with a specific kind of general linear model, traditionally called the **analysis of covariance** (ANCOVA). We typically use ANCOVA whenever we want to test the effects of one or multiple categorical variables, but we acknowledge that the response is also affected by a quantitative variable and we failed to eliminate this effect in our sampling or experimental setup. Taking an example from the field of experimental ecology, we might study the effect of competition on the yield of a plant species (10 plants grown in an environment without competition and 10 plants in a competitive environment). But the seedlings varied in size at the start of the experiment. Under such circumstances, it is always

---

[2] This is of course just an example of a second-order correlation: if we consider a group of four variables, there are six distinct values of such coefficients, including $r_{14.23}$ or $r_{34.12}$.

advantageous to record the initial size of each plant (before it could be affected by experimental conditions) and use this information as an additional predictor – **covariate**[3] (sometimes also called *covariable*) in the analysis of covariance. In many cases, this use of a covariate(s) decreases the unexplained variation and therefore leads to an increased test power for our main effect (the competition effect in our example). We can describe the work of the ANCOVA model as first 'subtracting' the effect of the continuous variable and only then testing the differences among the groups of observations.

We can alternatively imagine the pattern described by an ANCOVA model as a linear dependency of the response variable on the covariate(s), estimated for each group defined by a categorical predictor. In a standard ANCOVA model with a single numerical and single categorical predictor (the latter with k levels), the joint effect of both predictors can be visualised by a set of k parallel regression lines. They are parallel because their slope (representing the regression coefficient for the numerical predictor) is identical. The test for a categorical predictor effect then represents a test of the identity of the β_0 parameter across the k groups. Often, however, we cannot simply suppose that the lines are parallel. We can test this (either to justify the use of the simpler model with parallel lines or as a separate research question) by adding an interaction between the categorical predictor and the numerical covariate. The two models (with and without the interaction) can then be compared using a statistical test, e.g. a partial F test.

The following example represents another example of a typical use of ANCOVA. We compare the body weight of male ecologists in the age category 40–45 years in a group identified by excessively drinking beer with another group of male ecologists (in the same age range) where beer consumption is low or none. If we test the weight difference between the two groups using a two-sample t test (or equivalent one-way ANOVA model), we will probably obtain a very weak test because the size variability of the males here is large, so their weight is strongly affected by overall body size, which can be expressed e.g. using their height. It is therefore much better to know their height and use an ANCOVA model with the height serving as covariate. This increases the power of our test and the effect of beer drinking would be better identified. The covariate plays a minor role when interpreting the results, because the dependency of body weight on height is rather trivial.

14.5 Example Data

The example data for multiple regression are in the *Chap14* sheet, columns A to E. The *PoaBiom.L* variable represents the aboveground biomass of the smooth meadow grass (*Poa pratensis*) at the time of seasonal peak, the two previously mentioned characteristics of soil chemistry (*N.tot.L* and *PO4.L*) are supplemented by another two (*NH4.L* and *NO3.L*) in order to illustrate the stepwise selection method for our predictors. All soil characteristics (and the meadow-grass biomass) were log-transformed (this transformation is known to improve the linearity and homogeneity of variances for most measures of concentration, volume, surface or dimension), with the original data present in columns J to N (but you do not need to import the original data into R).

---

[3] We note that there are research fields where any kind of explanatory variable in almost any type of statistical model is called a *covariate*. Such use of this term is rarely seen in natural sciences, however.

Columns *F* to *H* of the *Chap14* sheet contain example data for the analysis of covariance and correspond to the example introduced at the end of the preceding section. We explain the weight of middle-aged male ecologists (*Weight*, kg) by excessive consumption of beer (the *Drinks* factor, with values *yes* or *no*), but we also use a numerical covariate *Height*, representing their body height (cm). Primarily, we want to test the effect of excessive beer consumption. The dependency of body weight on height is rather assumed.

14.6 How to Proceed in R

The two examples used in this chapter should be imported into separate data frames (we will use data frame *chap14a* for columns *A* to *E* and *chap14b* for columns *F* to *H*).

14.6.1 Multiple Regression

We fit a model of multiple linear regression with the *a priori* chosen predictors *N.tot.L* and *PO4.L* using the *lm* function as follows:

```
lm.1 <- lm( PoaBiom.L ~ N.tot.L + PO4.L, data=chap14a)
```

We will use the *summary* function to display the core results from the fitted model:

```
summary( lm.1)
Call:
lm(formula = PoaBiom.L ~ N.tot.L + PO4.L, data = chap14a)

Residuals:
     Min       1Q    Median       3Q       Max
-0.48315 -0.11565   0.03657   0.14820   0.29407

Coefficients:
            Estimate Std. Error t value Pr(>|t|)
(Intercept) -0.06650    0.17623  -0.377  0.70806
N.tot.L      0.61347    0.12402   4.947 1.66e-05 ***
PO4.L        0.13033    0.04645   2.806  0.00795 **
---
Signif. codes:  0 '***' 0.001 '**' 0.01 '*' 0.05 '.' 0.1 ' ' 1

Residual standard error: 0.1971 on 37 degrees of freedom
Multiple R-squared:  0.4841,    Adjusted R-squared:  0.4563
F-statistic: 17.36 on 2 and 37 DF,  p-value: 4.805e-06
```

Starting from the overall *F* test (in the last line of the above output, $F_{2,37} = 17.36$, $p < 0.001$) and progressing to the partial *t* tests in the *Coefficients* table (see the *t value* and *Pr(>|t|)* columns), we can conclude that both variables have partial effects on meadow-grass biomass that are worth presenting. The estimates of partial regression coefficients (see the *Estimate* column in the *Coefficients* table) are both positive, so we can conclude that both the nitrogen and phosphates have a positive relation with the meadow-grass aboveground biomass. But at the same time we should take the following points into account:

(a) These positive correlations are not necessarily a result of causal relationships (we are only observing plots where values of these two predictors were not experimentally manipulated). Perhaps the higher biomass at some plots (causally affected e.g. by a higher soil moisture, which we failed to measure) leads to a higher amount of decomposing dead biomass, which in turn leads to a higher concentration of nutrients.
(b) The regression coefficients represent partial effects of corresponding predictors, affected by the presence of the other predictor in our model (see the discussion earlier in this chapter). In some cases (not in this example dataset, as the correlation between *N.tot.L* and *PO4.L* is quite small), a regression coefficient of a predictor from simple regression (representing the independent effect of the predictor) might have the opposite sign (so implying an opposite relationship) to a coefficient of the same predictor from a multiple regression model.

Another problem we must deal with when interpreting the results of multiple regression is that we cannot directly use the values of regression coefficients across different predictors (here the b_1 and b_2 estimates for total nitrogen and phosphate concentration) when comparing the extent of their influence. This is because the coefficients also translate units of the corresponding predictor into the response variable's units. If we decide, for instance, to measure a predictor in grams per gram of dry soil (instead of milligrams per gram of dry soil), all predictor values would become a thousand times lower and so the coefficient estimate would be a thousand times higher.[4] We can use the *t* statistics in the *Coefficients* table to roughly compare the relative importance of individual predictors included in the model.

R software also offers alternative *F* tests for individual predictors, i.e. a decomposition of the explained sum of squares into predictor contributions. This decomposition is performed in a simple sequential manner, so the result will typically depend on the order we list our predictors in the model formula (see also the discussion in Section 10.7):

```
anova( lm.1)
Analysis of Variance Table
Response: PoaBiom.L
          Df  Sum Sq Mean Sq F value   Pr(>F)
N.tot.L    1 1.04284 1.04284 26.8523 8.03e-06 ***
PO4.L      1 0.30578 0.30578  7.8735 0.007952 **
Residuals 37 1.43694 0.03884
```

It seems obvious from the *anova* output that total N is more important, although both predictors clearly have important (and significant) effects. However, the overall size of the explanatory power of the first predictor in our model is uncertain due to the sequential decomposition of the explained sum of squares. When we change the order of predictors, the conclusions remain the same, but the way the variation is split clearly differs:

---

[4] In this discussion we ignore the fact our predictors were log-transformed: a multiplicative change of 1000× will become an additive shift using log(1000).

```
lm.2 <- update( lm.1,  .~ PO4.L + N.tot.L)
anova( lm.2)
Analysis of Variance Table
Response: PoaBiom.L
          Df  Sum Sq Mean Sq F value    Pr(>F)
PO4.L      1 0.39832 0.39832  10.257  0.002799 **
N.tot.L    1 0.95029 0.95029  24.469 1.663e-05 ***
Residuals 37 1.43694 0.03884
```

The existence of alternative results might be unsettling for some readers, but it can also be seen as additional illuminating information. The two predictors share part of the variation they are able to explain in the response values and the size of this part can be deduced from the implied change in the explained sum of squares (*Sum Sq* column):

```
0.39832-0.30578
[1] 0.09254

1.04284-0.95029
[1] 0.09255
```

If you prefer a decomposition invariant to the order of predictors, you can use the *Anova* function from the *car* package (Fox & Weisberg, 2011):

```
library( car)
Anova( lm.1)
Anova Table (Type II tests)
Response: PoaBiom.L
          Sum Sq Df F value    Pr(>F)
N.tot.L  0.95029  1 24.4694 1.663e-05 ***
PO4.L    0.30578  1  7.8735  0.007952 **
Residuals 1.43694 37
```

It is perhaps worth noting that the partial effects of both predictors are presented here as if they were always considered after the other predictor(s). This means that their shared explanatory power is ignored in this decomposition method (Type II sums of squares). The p-values are exactly the same as the p-values for the test of individual partial regression coefficients, reflecting the fact that a test of partial regression coefficients evaluates the null hypothesis that the corresponding variable does not contribute anything in addition to the other variables present in the model.

If you need to create a core graph for a regression diagnostic, where regression residuals are plotted against the fitted values of the response variable, you can use the function *plot* with the fitted regression object. This function is able to create up to six different types of diagnostic plots, but the plot type identity can be set with the *which* parameter:

```
plot( lm.1, which=1)
```

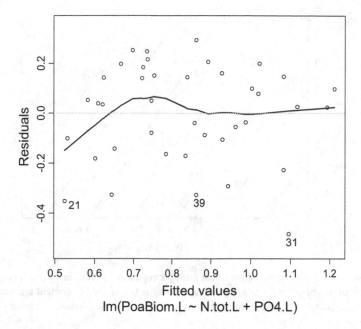

Figure 14.2 Output from the *plot* function applied to a regression model object created by the *lm* function. Model residuals are plotted against the fitted values of the response variable. A search for any remaining pattern is aided by a fitted smooth curve (using loess smoother).

The resulting diagram (Fig. 14.2) suggests that specifying the model as a linear dependency of log-transformed biomass on the log-transformed predictors was a reasonable choice. Further, Fig. 14.2 also shows that the variation of residuals is quite homogeneous across the range of predicted values.

14.6.2 Visualising Models of Multiple Regression

To plot a fitted model is more challenging than to create graphs of regression diagnostics given the fact that it uses two (or more) predictors and so it requires either a 3D display or the use of a contour plot. We demonstrate the creation of a contour plot below (as we believe this is a more useful display type), but the process is rather similar for creating a perspective 3D plot:

```
pred.vals <- expand.grid( N.tot.L=seq(0.8,1.8,by=0.05),
                          PO4.L=seq(-0.75,1.5,by=0.05))
```

The above command creates a sequence of values for each of the two predictors, roughly spanning their observed range, using the *seq* function. The *expand.grid* function then takes those sequences and creates a new data frame in which every value of one sequence is combined with every value of the other sequence:

```
pred.vals$fit <- predict( lm.1, newdata=pred.vals)
```

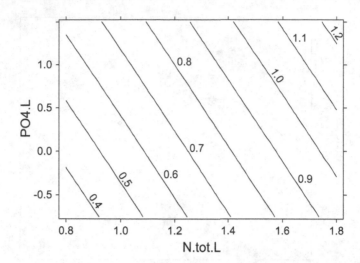

Figure 14.3 Contour diagram visualising a linear multiple regression model in which the log-transformed aboveground biomass of *Poa pratensis* is predicted from the log of total N content and concentration of phosphates in soil. These two predictors explain $R^2_{adj} = 45.6\%$ of the biomass variation.

The *predict* function takes the new predictor values (specified by the *newdata* parameter) and estimates the fitted response values, which we then store into a new *fit* variable in the existing *pred.vals* data frame. Finally, we call the function *contourplot* (from the *lattice* package; Sarkar, 2008), which draws our diagram (shown in Fig. 14.3):

```
library( lattice)
contourplot( fit ~ N.tot.L*PO4.L, data=pred.vals,
         cuts=10)
```

Visualisations of fitted multiple regression models which combine the effects of all the predictors are inherently limited by the dimensionality of our presentation media, as well as by our ability to comprehend complex visual patterns. But there is an alternative visualisation approach that effectively matches the nature of the model, where the partial effects of predictors are combined by summation given that their effects are **additive**. This model property effectively allows us to plot partial effects of each predictor separately, unless the predictors are combined in an interaction term in the model formula.[5] This approach for visualising partial effects is shown in the following text.

The *effects* package (Fox & Weisberg, 2018) is an appropriate tool for displaying partial effects of predictors and its use is illustrated in the following example code, with the resulting graph in Fig. 14.4:

```
library( effects)
par( mfrow=c(1,2))
plot( allEffects( lm.1), main="",
       confint = list( style="lines"))
```

---

[5] Using interaction terms is relatively rare in multiple regression models, particularly when data originate from an exploratory study.

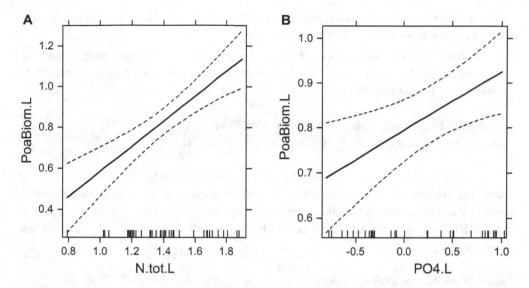

Figure 14.4 Partial effects of two predictors, total nitrogen (A) and phosphate concentration (B), in a model predicting *Poa pratensis* aboveground biomass, visualised using the *effects* package. 95% confidence regions for partial linear effects are shown as dashed lines.

The effect plots in Fig. 14.4 show the expected value of the response variable (plus its confidence region) for varying values of one of the predictors, while keeping the other predictor(s) at their mean values. The short vertical lines at the horizontal axes (so-called 'rug') represent the predictor values for individual observations in the dataset. Overall, the graph illustrates a positive response of meadow-grass biomass to both N and P concentrations and a higher confidence (narrower confidence band) in the predictive contribution of *N.tot.L*.

14.6.3 Stepwise Selection of Predictors

Our task here is to create the optimum linear model predicting meadow grass's aboveground biomass from the known predictors. This does not necessarily mean we need to use all the available data. We are simply trying to identify the best model, and this might possibly contain just a subset of the predictors at hand. The selection of predictors should be driven by a criterion of model optimality. The predictive ability would seem to be the right criterion to judge model performance. But it is not advisable to base our estimation of the predictive ability on reviewing the model predictions for the set of observations we have used to estimate the model parameters. It is almost guaranteed that the performance of our model for a new data sample will be worse. Therefore, standard measures of model predictive ability, such as the residual sum of squares or R^2, cannot be used to select the best model[6] and we use other criteria such as *model parsimony* (quantified e.g. with AIC) or add new predictors to our model based on their performance judged by standard statistical tests of their partial effects.

We build this optimal model predicting the biomass of *Poa* by selecting from the four available predictors. Because the predictors include two forms of nitrogen (nitrate and ammonium), and also the total nitrogen, it is clear that both nitrogen ions contribute to total

---

[6] Such criteria would always maximise the set of selected predictors.

nitrogen content and thus we can expect their positive correlation. This also suggests that not all of the predictors will likely be needed.

It is good to begin the selection process by first building a starting model (usually an empty one, referred to as a *null model*) and also a description of the maximum set of predictors for our model (called *scope*):

```
lm.0 <- lm( PoaBiom.L ~ +1, data=chap14a)
lm.scope <- ~ N.tot.L + PO4.L + NH4.L + NO3.L
```

If we prefer to build our model in a closely controlled manner (deciding each step for ourselves), we can use the *add1* function. This function evaluates changes in model quality caused by adding each of the candidate predictors separately. By default, the quality is judged in the *add1* function by the AIC criterion only, but we can ask for an additional parametric test using the *test* parameter:

```
add1( lm.0, lm.scope, test="F")
Single term additions

Model:
PoaBiom.L ~ +1
         Df Sum of Sq    RSS      AIC F value    Pr(>F)
<none>                 2.7856 -104.58
N.tot.L  1    1.04284 1.7427 -121.34 22.7392 2.728e-05 ***
PO4.L    1    0.39832 2.3872 -108.75  6.3405   0.01613 *
NH4.L    1    0.24334 2.5422 -106.23  3.6374   0.06408 .
NO3.L    1    0.12156 2.6640 -104.36  1.7339   0.19580
---
```

As you can see, the most reliable model improvement (by both an F test and the largest drop in AIC value) is the addition of total nitrogen concentration (*N.tot.L*). We will therefore add it to the model and continue with our inquiry, searching for further improvements using the new model object (*lm.1*):

```
lm.1 <- update( lm.0, . ~ . + N.tot.L)
add1( lm.1, lm.scope, test="F")
Single term additions

Model:
PoaBiom.L ~ N.tot.L
         Df Sum of Sq    RSS      AIC F value   Pr(>F)
<none>                 1.7427 -121.34
PO4.L    1   0.305777 1.4369 -127.06  7.8735 0.007952 **
NH4.L    1   0.054763 1.6880 -120.61  1.2004 0.280319
NO3.L    1   0.067331 1.6754 -120.91  1.4870 0.230403
---
```

The partial effect of phosphate concentration still remains significant, so we add it to our model as well. But a new call to *add1* suggests that the remaining two candidate predictors would not improve the present model, so we cease its extension:

```
lm.2 <- update( lm.1, . ~ . +PO4.L)
add1( lm.2, lm.scope, test="F")
```
```
Single term additions

Model:
PoaBiom.L ~ N.tot.L + PO4.L
        Df Sum of Sq    RSS     AIC F value Pr(>F)
<none>                1.4369 -127.06
NH4.L    1 0.0017191 1.4352 -125.10  0.0431 0.8367
NO3.L    1 0.0112441 1.4257 -125.37  0.2839 0.5974
---
```

Note that if we decided to use the AIC values for model selection, we would end up with exactly the same couple of chosen predictors. This is not always the case, although the ordering of candidate predictors is usually coherent across both criteria. The Akaike criterion tends to be somewhat milder and occasionally produces models with a larger number of predictors than a selection using parametric tests. This might not be the case with alternative criteria of parsimony.

We do not test any hypotheses when comparing multiple models using AIC. Rather, we select a model with the highest parsimony, i.e. with the smallest AIC value (in our case with the lowest negative value).

We will illustrate the use of AIC with an example of automated model selection using the *step* function. This function displays the selection progress and returns the selected model:

```
lm.3 <- step( lm.0, lm.scope)
```
```
Start:  AIC=-104.58
PoaBiom.L ~ +1

           Df Sum of Sq    RSS     AIC
+ N.tot.L   1   1.04284 1.7427 -121.34
+ PO4.L     1   0.39832 2.3872 -108.75
+ NH4.L     1   0.24334 2.5422 -106.23
<none>                  2.7856 -104.58
+ NO3.L     1   0.12156 2.6640 -104.36

Step:  AIC=-121.34
PoaBiom.L ~ N.tot.L
```

```
          Df Sum of Sq    RSS     AIC
+ PO4.L    1   0.30578 1.4369 -127.06
<none>                   1.7427 -121.34
+ NO3.L    1   0.06733 1.6754 -120.91
+ NH4.L    1   0.05476 1.6880 -120.61
- N.tot.L  1   1.04284 2.7856 -104.58


Step:  AIC=-127.05
PoaBiom.L ~ N.tot.L + PO4.L

          Df Sum of Sq    RSS     AIC
<none>                   1.4369 -127.06
+ NO3.L    1   0.01124 1.4257 -125.37
+ NH4.L    1   0.00172 1.4352 -125.10
- PO4.L    1   0.30578 1.7427 -121.34
- N.tot.L  1   0.95029 2.3872 -108.75
```

As you can see, the final model is identical to the one we chose by interactive stepwise selection.

14.6.4 Partial Correlation

We can compute partial correlations among variables using the *pcor* function in the *ppcor* library (Kim, 2015). For example, to compute pairwise partial correlations between all variables of the *chap14a* data frame (computed correlations always describe the relationship of two variables, excluding the effect of all remaining variables), we can proceed in the following way:

```
library( ppcor)
pcor( chap14a)
$`estimate`
            PoaBiom.L   N.tot.L       PO4.L       NH4.L        NO3.L
PoaBiom.L  1.00000000 0.4575827   0.3534303  0.02691278 -0.08576814
N.tot.L    0.45758269 1.0000000   0.2338523  0.58204942  0.47326235
PO4.L      0.35343029 0.2338523   1.0000000 -0.46915262 -0.24131528
NH4.L      0.02691278 0.5820494  -0.4691526  1.00000000 -0.08649805
NO3.L     -0.08576814 0.4732624  -0.2413153 -0.08649805  1.00000000

$p.value
            PoaBiom.L    N.tot.L       PO4.L        NH4.L       NO3.L
PoaBiom.L  0.00000000 0.004405606 0.03188581 0.874367149 0.61374662
N.tot.L    0.00440561 0.000000000 0.16360508 0.000157508 0.00309283
PO4.L      0.03188581 0.163605080 0.00000000 0.003398759 0.15019402
NH4.L      0.87436715 0.000157508 0.00339876 0.000000000 0.61072122
NO3.L      0.61374662 0.003092834 0.15019402 0.610721222 0.00000000
$statistic
```

```
              PoaBiom.L  N.tot.L      PO4.L       NH4.L       NO3.L
PoaBiom.L   0.0000000  3.044530   2.235178   0.1592758  -0.5092878
N.tot.L     3.0445299  0.000000   1.422944   4.2346877   3.1783283
PO4.L       2.2351782  1.422944   0.000000  -3.1428950  -1.4711167
NH4.L       0.1592758  4.234688  -3.142895   0.0000000  -0.5136545
NO3.L      -0.5092878  3.178328  -1.471117  -0.5136545   0.0000000


$n
[ 1]  40
$gp
[ 1]  3
$method
[ 1]  "pearson"
```

So, as an example, the partial correlation between meadow-grass aboveground biomass and total nitrogen concentration is +0.4576, after excluding the effects of phosphate, ammonia and nitrate ion concentrations. We can also see that this correlation is significant ($p = 0.0044$). The *pcor* function is also able to calculate alternative, non-parametric versions of correlation coefficients, namely Kendall's coefficient (using *method="kendall"*) or Spearman's coefficient (using *method="spearman"*).

We can also calculate a partial coefficient for a specific pair of variables, using the *pcor.test* function. For example, we can use the following command to calculate the partial correlation between meadow-grass biomass and phosphate concentration, excluding the effect of ammonium and nitrate ions:

```
with( chap14a, pcor.test( PoaBiom.L, PO4.L, chap14a[,4:5]))
  estimate      p.value  statistic  n  gp  Method1
0.5325974  0.0005770416   3.775641  40   2  pearson
```

14.6.5 Analysis of Covariance

The implementation of statistical model fitting in R does not make substantial distinctions between models where numerical variables, or categorical variables, or a mixture of those two types are used as predictors. A general linear model can be fitted either with the *lm* or the *aov* function.[7] So we can illustrate our example of a simple analysis of covariance (ANCOVA) using the *lm* function:

```
lm.5 <- lm( Weight ~ Height + Drinks, data=chap14b)
anova( lm.5)
Analysis of Variance Table
Response: Weight
          Df  Sum Sq  Mean Sq  F value     Pr(>F)
Height     1  1315.54  1315.54   36.219  0.0005325 ***
```

---

[7] Models fitted with *lm* vs. *aov* differ in the way they are summarised with the *summary* function. Further, additional error levels can be specified in the *aov* function using an *Error* term in the model formula.

```
Drinks      1   937.11   937.11   25.800 0.0014320 **
Residuals   7   254.25   36.32
```

We can conclude that an excessive consumption of beer affects individual weight in this cohort of ecologists, but the effect of body size is even stronger. As we have used the *lm* function to fit the ANCOVA model, we can easily obtain the corresponding regression coefficients:[8]

```
summary( lm.5)

...

Coefficients:
             Estimate Std. Error t value Pr(>|t|)
(Intercept) -154.1595    33.4987  -4.602 0.002478 **
Height         1.2690     0.1798   7.059 0.000201 ***
Drinksyes     20.3514     4.0066   5.079 0.001432 **
```

The regression coefficients suggest that there is a positive relation of weight to not only height but also beer consumption (what a surprise!). The factor variable *Drinks* is represented with a single regression coefficient because it has just two levels (*no* and *yes*, with the *no* level being the reference here). More generally, a factor predictor is represented by $k - 1$ regression coefficients, where k is the number of factor levels.

It might also be informative to check how the effect of excessive drinking is reported when no height data are available (or when we decide to ignore it). We can test the *Drinks* effect using a one-way ANOVA (or also with a two-sample *t* test):

```
summary( aov( Weight ~ Drinks, data=chap14b))
             Df Sum Sq Mean Sq F value Pr(>F)
Drinks        1  442.8   442.8   1.716  0.227
Residuals     8 2064.1   258.0
```

We find no significant effect of excessive beer consumption in this model. This is because the effect of beer is 'overshadowed' by body height variation, which is no longer filtered out by a covariate.

Because the *anova* function uses the sequential (Type I) decomposition of the model sum of squares, the order in which we enter the variables into the model specification matters. We should always fit first the variable effect which is considered trivial and which we want to filter out first. The above example also represents a situation where the use of a covariate really helps to demonstrate the effect of the factor we are interested in. This is because we can expect that the drinking of beer affects weight, but has no effect on the other predictor, i.e. body height. There are, however, cases where the two predictors would be mutually dependent. In the example where we studied the effect of altitude and bedrock on forest productivity (Section 14.4), the basalt bedrock can occur mainly at low altitudes, whereas the higher elevations would be formed by acidic rocks. In this and similar cases, we would not be able to

---

[8] If you used an *aov* function, you can extract regression coefficients from it using the *summary.lm* function (unless your model includes *Error* terms).

separate the effect of bedrock from altitude. Consequently, if we do not specify altitude as the first predictor in our model specification, the effect of bedrock will be significant, but it will become non-significant when we start with altitude as a covariate.

The ANCOVA model for the effect of beer drinking has two additive terms, i.e. body height and beer drinking. From this follows the expectation that the two implied lines for the dependence of body weight on height are parallel, and we only test whether one of them is shifted up by the size of the effect of beer consumption. If we are interested in whether the change of body weight with height is different between the two groups (excessive beer consumers vs. control group), we must fit a new model including an interaction between *Drinks* and *Height* and either compare it with the original model containing just the additive effects, or simply evaluate it using the *anova* function:[9]

```
lm.6 <- lm( Weight ~ Height * Drinks, data=chap14b)
anova( lm.5, lm.6)

Analysis of Variance Table

Model 1: Weight ~ Height + Drinks
Model 2: Weight ~ Height * Drinks
  Res.Df    RSS Df Sum of Sq      F Pr(>F)
1      7 254.25
2      6 177.25  1    76.995 2.6062 0.1576
```

The alternative computation suggested above is as follows:

```
anova( lm.6)

Analysis of Variance Table
Response: Weight
              Df  Sum Sq Mean Sq F value     Pr(>F)
Height         1 1315.54 1315.54 44.5304 0.0005483 ***
Drinks         1  937.11  937.11 31.7208 0.0013407 **
Height:Drinks  1   76.99   76.99  2.6062 0.1575710
Residuals      6  177.25   29.54
```

So our results suggest a non-significant interaction term. But the size of the F statistic is quite large (2.61), so we can expect that low power is the primary reason for the non-significance given the small number of individuals in the sample.

14.7 Reporting Analyses

14.7.1 Methods

We estimated the effect of total nitrogen and phosphate concentration in soil on the above-ground biomass of *Poa* using multiple regression. Both the response variable and the predictors were log-transformed to achieve additivity of their effects and to increase the homogeneity of variances in the response variable.

---

[9] This works because the effect of the interaction term is evaluated after taking both main effects into account.

Table X *Multiple linear regression model of the relationship of* Poa *biomass (g m^{-2}, log-transformed) to log-transformed total N content and PO$_4^{3-}$ concentration in soil (mg kg^{-1} dry weight soil before transformation). The partial* t *tests of individual predictors had* df = 37. *Letter* b *refers to a regression coefficient. The absolute term (intercept) estimate (b$_0$) was* −0.0665

Model term	b	SE(b)	t	p
Total N	0.613	0.124	4.95	<0.001
PO$_4^{3-}$	0.130	0.046	2.81	0.008

The model predicting *Poa* biomass was selected using stepwise selection based on the AIC (Akaike, 1974).

Or

... stepwise selection based on a partial *F* test and an acceptance threshold $\alpha = 0.05$ at each step.

The effect of beer drinking on the body weight of a group of ecologists was tested using ANCOVA with body height used as covariate.

We checked for a difference in body weight change with subject height between the drinking/non-drinking groups using an *F* test of the interaction between height and drinking status in a general linear model.

14.7.2 Results

The fitted regression model is summarised in Table X. Both the total N and phosphate concentrations had significant positive relationships with the aboveground biomass of *Poa*.

We found a significant positive effect of excessive beer drinking on body weight ($F_{1,7} = 25.8, p = 0.0014$) alongside a significant (positive) effect of body height ($F_{1,7} = 49.8, p = 0.0002$).

We found no evidence for a difference in body weight change with increasing height between the two groups of subjects ($F_{1,6} = 2.6$, n.s.).

14.8 Recommended Reading

Zar (2010), pp. 419–457.

Quinn & Keough (2002), pp. 111–142 (multiple regression, stepwise selection of predictors) and pp. 339–352 for ANCOVA.

Sokal & Rohlf (2012), pp. 665–671 (ANCOVA), pp. 603–702 (multiple regression).

H. Akaike (1974) A new look at the statistical model identification. *IEEE Transactions on Automatic Control*, **19**: 716–723.

J. Fox & S. Weisberg (2011) *An R Companion to Applied Regression*, 2nd edn. Sage, Thousand Oaks, CA. (2018) Visualizing fit and lack of fit in complex regression models with predictor effect plots and partial residuals. *Journal of Statistical Software*, **87**(9): 1–27.

S. Kim (2015) *ppcor*: partial and semi-partial correlation. R package version 1.1. https://cran.r-project .org/package=ppcor

D. Sarkar (2008) *Lattice: Multivariate Data Visualization with R*. Springer, New York.

M. Šrůtek & J. Š. Lepš (1994) Variation in structure of *Larix olgensis* stands along the altitudinal gradient on Paektu-san, Changbai-shan, North Korea. *Arctic and Alpine Research*, **26**(2): 166–173.

15 Generalised Linear Models

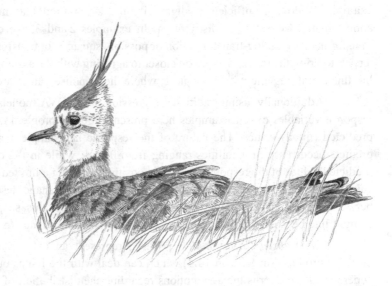

15.1 Use Case Examples

The following three examples from field biological research represent typical cases where we would use generalised linear models to analyse our data.

1. The presence/absence of smooth meadow grass (*Poa pratensis*) was recorded across 20 sites, together with measurements of the thickness of the upper soil horizon ($A1$). We want to explore if and how the probability of species occurrence changes with soil horizon thickness.
2. We investigated how the presence and size of breeding colonies of a particular wader bird species at multiple *a priori* chosen localities was affected by two categorical environmental characteristics: the presence of shrubs at the edge of the breeding colony (*yes* vs. *no*) and the presence and type of agricultural field in close proximity (*none*, *winter cereals*, *spring crop*). The presence/size of colonies were specified as a categorical variable (factor) with three levels (*absent*, *small*, *large*). Our task is to find out whether the two environmental characteristics affect the nesting choices of the bird species, and if so, how.
3. We manipulated the mowing and fertilisation regime on a grassland site using a field experiment based on 4 × 4 m plots, each with an individual factorial combination of the two manipulated factors. The effect of both factors was evaluated after five years using plant species richness (the count of the species present there). We want to determine whether plant richness varies due to management differences and also whether there is any interaction between the effects of the manipulated factors.

15.2 Properties of Generalised Linear Models

All three examples share a common property, namely that the nature of response variable's values (the presence or absence of meadow grass in example 1, the count of localities with a specific combination of the three factors in example 2, or the number of plant species in example 3) do not sufficiently align with the assumption that model residuals can be approximated by a normal distribution. In examples 2 and 3, we could apply some data transformation (e.g. log-transformation or possibly square-root transformation, see also Chapter 10) to bring the residual variation closer to agreeing with the assumptions of linear models, but this is not possible with example 1, where the response values are 0 or 1.

Additionally, using traditional regression or ANOVA models for the untransformed response variables of our examples here presents another problem concerning the range of predicted (fitted) values. The nature of the response in example 1 requires that the model predicts occurrence probabilities ranging from 0 to 1, while in the other two examples the predicted values of the response should be positive.[1] Having a limited range for our predicted values also affects the appearance of the simplest possible shape describing the relationship between the response variable and a numerical predictor: this shape cannot be a simple straight line because such a line has no limits on its Y coordinates (predicted values).

Generalised linear models (GLMs) represent an extension of the general linear model (introduced in Section 14.4) which can deal with the issues outlined above. The first generalisation concerns the assumptions regarding the distribution of random variability (i.e. the variability not explained by the model predictors), where we must choose one of the probability distributions belonging to the exponential family. An overview of the most frequently supported distributions can be found in Table 15.1.[2] Similar to classical regression and ANOVA models, where the assumption of a normal distribution for residuals is accepted even if it is just approximately fulfilled, we expect that the distributional assumptions chosen for a GLM are matched only approximately by the real data. Even so, there are ways of bringing our data closer to meeting the GLM assumptions (see Section 15.4 discussing overdispersion). Our choice of distribution type also implies some anticipated relationship between the conditional variance of the response variable (i.e. its variance for particular values of the explanatory variables) and its expected (predicted) mean value. As an example, for a Poisson distribution we assume that the variance of observed values around the predicted mean will have its value equal to the mean (see also Chapter 18).

The second generalisation offered by GLM concerns the shape of the relationship between the response variable Y and the explanatory variables (X_j). In a traditional model of multiple regression, we can describe such a relationship in the following way (see also Eq. (14.4) in the previous chapter):

$$EY = \beta_0 + \sum_j \beta_j X_j \qquad (15.1)$$

---

[1] We are predicting average counts of cases or species, so the average should be positive, even though specific observations may have a zero value.

[2] Note that the assumption of traditional linear models, requiring the random variation to have a normal distribution with zero average and constant variance, is one of the choices that is supported. In this way, the traditional general linear model (including not only regression, but also ANOVA models) is subsumed into the family of generalised linear models.

where EY is the expected value of the response variable and the right side of the equation is labelled – in the GLM context – η ('eta') and called a *linear predictor*. In GLMs, the extension of the possible relationships between expected values of the response and the linear predictor is most often presented on the left side of the equation, namely as

$$g(EY) = \eta \qquad (15.2)$$

The letter g represents the *link function*, which transforms the scale of the expected values of the response to the scale of the linear predictor η, which is a linear combination of the explanatory variables and so it can, in general, have any value on a real scale.

At first sight, the expression $g(EY)$ appears to be a formal representation of the transformation of the response variable values (as we did earlier, e.g. with a log-transformation, see Chapter 10), however there is a small yet important difference in its meaning. The transformation carried out by the link function is not applied to observed values of Y, but rather it concerns the expected values, predicted by the fitted model. So if we use a GLM for predicting the count of individuals (or number of localities in example 2 or number of species in example 3), which usually implies choosing the log link function (in combination with choosing a Poisson distribution to describe the random variation), the log-transformation concerns the mean of a Poisson distribution. This mean is always a positive value, so the usual problem with log-transforming observed zero counts does not apply here (see also Eq. (10.6) and the discussion below it).

For a given distribution type, we can select from a range of link functions, but among our options there is always one with optimal properties for that distribution type. It is called the *canonical link function* and is given for individual distributions in Table 15.1. When using GLMs, the canonical link function prevails as the best choice, except when handling the gamma distribution. There are two link functions that are used quite frequently for the gamma distribution, and this choice depends on the kind of data being analysed. The canonical inverse link function with a gamma distribution is an appropriate choice for response variables representing ratios of two independently changing variables (e.g. when we compare – by

Table 15.1 *Overview of the most frequently used distributions, types of response variables and canonical link functions for generalised linear models*

Distribution	Type of response variable	Range of EY	Canonical link function
Binomial	relative proportions (n cases out of N), $p = n/N$; presences and absences	$0 < p^{\text{a}} < 1$	logit: $\ln(EY/(1 - EY))$ where EY is p here
Poisson	number of events or cases	positive	log: $\ln(EY)$
Gamma	ratio of two variables measured on a ratio scale; weights, dimensions, concentrations	positive	inverse: $1/EY$
Normal	some physical measurements	any real number $(-\infty, +\infty)$	identity: EY

[a] p represents the expected value of Y for a binomial distribution, but for a response variable with a true binomial distribution (i.e. not just with 0s and 1s, which is often called the Bernoulli distribution), the predictor values are typically presented as $p \times N$, i.e. as the estimates of n values.

division – the biomass of two competing species). But if a response variable represents weight, volume, area, concentration or a single dimension, then the log link function is more appropriate.

A GLM which assumes a normal distribution with the identity link function represents the general linear models (including ANOVA, ANCOVA and multiple regression models). GLMs which assume a binomial distribution using the logit link function are sometimes referred to as *logistic regression*. In contrast, using the combination of a binomial distribution with the probit link function in GLMs has traditionally been called *probit analysis*.

At this point we remind the reader about a property of general linear models that is inherited by the GLMs: the explanatory variables can be either numerical or categorical (factors) and both types of explanatory variables can be combined in a single model.

15.3 Analysis of Deviance

In the classical linear regression and ANOVA models, model parameters are estimated using the least-squares criterion. Further, we evaluate the success of the fitted model by decomposing the total variability of the response variable (measured by the sum of squares or by a mean square) into two components: the part explained by the model and the unexplained (residual) variation. With generalised linear models, the model parameters are estimated using the *maximum likelihood* criterion. The way we decompose the total variation in the response is also similar to linear models, but instead of using sums of squares, we use *deviance*. More precisely, this term matches the unexplained (residual) sum of squares, but this does not prevent us from using it to decompose the total variation in our response variable: the total sum of squares matches the deviance of the *null model*, which represents a model without any explanatory variable (i.e. with $\eta = \beta_0$). The deviance of our actual GLM then matches the residual sum of squares and the variation explained by the model is the difference between those two deviances.

Unlike linear regression and ANOVA models, the analysis of deviance does not exclusively use the F statistic when testing overall model significance. The F test is only used for GLMs assuming gamma or normal distributions, but for models assuming binomial or Poisson distributions the F test is used only when overdispersion is detected (see the next section). For a standard binomial or Poisson distribution, we use the actual difference between the deviance of the null model and that of the tested model as a test statistic, thus representing the amount of explained variation. When the null hypothesis (no effect of GLM predictors) is correct, this test statistic is assumed to come from a χ^2 distribution with the number of degrees of freedom corresponding to the number of model degrees of freedom (i.e. the number of explanatory variables which were tested, if they are all of a numerical type).

When using analysis of deviance in lieu of a classical factorial ANOVA, we should remember that the null model for the test of factor interaction is one of additivity and is on the scale of the linear predictor. If we use the log link function, the null model represents multiplicativity on the scale of the original values. For example, when we study the effect of mowing and fertilisation on the number of species in example 3, we use the assumption of a Poisson distribution together with a log link function. Consequently, the null hypothesis for the interaction term is not that *the same number of species will be lost (or gained) due to fertilisation in the mown and unmown plots*, but instead that *the same proportion of species will be lost (or gained)*.

15.4 Overdispersion

If a binomial or Poisson distribution is appropriate to describe the random variability in a GLM, the variation of observed values around the mean (conditioned by the values of the explanatory variables) is fully determined by this mean value. The variance should be equal to the mean value for a Poisson distribution (see Section 18.2), and the variance around the mean value p is equal to $p \times (1 - p)$ for a binomial distribution (Section 18.5). However, the response variables encountered in biological research often have higher variability than this. There are several reasons for this, but one of the most frequent is the aggregation of observed cases (individuals) in space or time,[3] or we can have an incomplete model specification that omits an important explanatory variable. This *overdispersion* – if we ignore it when fitting a GLM – can lead to incorrect (underestimated) expectations of the Type I error probability in our tested hypotheses or (equivalently) to an underestimation of the true range for confidence intervals of our model parameters.

Most implementations of GLMs allow us to estimate both the regression coefficients and the extent of overdispersion in parallel by using the *quasi-likelihood* method. We can obtain a rough idea whether we should model the overdispersion in a GLM with an assumed binomial or Poisson distribution[4] by comparing the residual deviance of the estimated model with the residual degrees of freedom.[5] If the response variable values are not overdispersed, these two statistics should be of approximately identical size, but when overdispersion is present, the residual deviance is notably larger than the residual degrees of freedom. If our GLM is based on *quasi-likelihood* estimation, then we cannot test models which assume a binomial or Poisson distribution with a χ^2 test – we use the F test instead.

15.5 Log-linear Models

The log-linear models represent a quite distinct way of using GLMs. Here we can analyse more complex contingency tables, for instance when we are interested in the relationship of one factor (sometimes called the *response factor*) with two or more other factors (*explanatory factors*).

We usually start from a classical contingency table (see Section 3.3) and turn individual table dimensions (edges) into separate factor variables (with each factor level crossed with all the levels of the other factors). The frequencies within the table cells, which assume a Poisson distribution, then become a numerical response variable for our model. Note that the response variable in a log-linear model does not represent the response factor, as this factor is placed among the explanatory variables of the GLM, together with our explanatory factors.

---

[3] So if we observe, say, the count of individuals of a species in plots, the variability of the counts is larger than one would expect for a Poisson distribution (see also Chapter 18).

[4] The concept of *overdispersion* does not apply to GLMs with gamma or normal distributions.

[5] Our concern for overdispersion is not appropriate in a GLM with a binomial distribution if the response variable contains just 0s and 1s (Bernoulli distribution), as in our example 1.

Because the null hypothesis for tests on contingency tables implies a situation where the frequencies in table cells are not identical, but rather proportional to relative marginal frequencies, the null model differs from those used for other GLM types: its specification is not 'empty' (i.e. with only a β_0 regression coefficient), rather it contains the response factor and also all the explanatory factors and all interactions among the explanatory factors. To test the relation of the response factor to individual explanatory factors, we compare this unusual null model with another model in which we add the interaction between the response factor and the tested explanatory factor(s).

In the simplest case of a two-dimensional contingency table (with factors A and B, where we *ad hoc* label factor A as the response factor), we compare our null model (with the main effects of A and B) with a model including the interaction between A and B. This was already illustrated in Chapter 3, Section 3.7. But if we have multiple explanatory factors (and therefore a three-dimensional or even n-dimensional contingency table), there are multiple relationships to test and we should take care about the order in which we perform these tests. The usual recommendation is to test a higher-order interaction (say between the response and two explanatory factors) only after we have tested all the implied lower-order interactions (i.e. interactions between the response factor and each explanatory factor separately) and have found at least one of those first-order interaction terms to be significant.

15.6 Predictor Selection

Similar to normal multiple regression models, in generalised linear models we must sometimes decide which of the explanatory variables available to us should be used and which are redundant. One way of selecting the content of a model is to use *stepwise selection*, which we already introduced in Chapter 14. When we are deciding which explanatory variable to add (or remove) at a particular selection step, we can use a parametric test (based on an F or χ^2 statistic, see Section 15.3). In doing so, we compare the present model state with an alternative model, extended by the variable being tested (or alternatively simplified by its removal).

More recently, new approaches for model selection have increased in popularity and importance. These approaches do not employ a series of hypothesis tests or even the stepwise selection procedure. As a matter of fact, it is not certain that a directed stepwise selection always finds an optimum model or whether such an optimum model even exists. Quite often, we can find a group of alternative, partly overlapping model specifications which perform similarly in their ability to predict response variable's values. We can compare a range of candidate models without the need for significance tests, and we do this by scoring them with an information-theoretical criterion of *parsimony* (see also Section 14.2).

The idea of model parsimony reflects two conflicting interests we pursue when specifying a model for our data: (i) we want our model to be as simple as possible, but also (ii) we want the model to be as precise (best predicting response variable values) as possible. At first sight, we might believe that the most precise prediction for a chosen set of observations is achieved with the most complex model we can create. If we manage to create a model with as many parameters as there are observations in our data sample, we will predict the response values without any error. Clearly, this cannot be a correct solution of our problem. Not only is the model too complex to be useful for understanding the relationships under consideration, but it is also too dependent on the actual data sample we have collected. If we use such a model to predict the values of the response variable for a new sample from the same statistical population, its predictions will not be so good – the fitted model is *biased* towards the data sample used to estimate its parameters. In the interest of creating a model which performs well when working with new observations, during model selection we must balance its predictive ability with its simplicity, i.e. to seek a parsimonious model.

The most often used criterion of model *parsimony* is *Akaike's information criterion* (*AIC*), defined by Eq. (15.3):

$$AIC = D + 2k \tag{15.3}$$

where D is equal to -2 ln(model-likelihood)[6] and k is the number of model degrees of freedom (usually the number of model parameters). Thus, model parsimony is lower when the unexplained variability (D), or the number of model parameters (k), increases. We therefore prefer models with lower AIC values when comparing model performance. Further important information regarding the evaluation of statistical models using AIC and about other related procedures (e.g. model averaging) can be found in Burnham & Anderson (2002).

15.7 Example Data

We illustrate the use of GLMs with two data examples contained in the *Chap15* sheet of the example data file. The first dataset corresponds to example 1 from Section 15.1. The variable *PoaPrat* contains information about grass species presence (1) or absence at a locality, while the *A1hor* variable specifies the thickness (cm) of the upper soil horizon (A_1) of that locality. The corresponding data frame in the R code below is named *chap15a*.

The next four variables correspond to example 2 of Section 15.1 and represent the following contingency table, already reformatted into the shape needed for fitting a log-linear model. The division of the table (Table 15.2) into three rows (matching the levels of the response factor) and 2 × 3 columns (representing the levels of two explanatory factors) is described by the categorical variables *Colony*, *Shrubs* and *Cereal* in columns D to F of the sheet. The counts of observed cases (localities) are stored in the *Count* variable, column G. The data are stored in the data frame *chap15b* for the R code shown in Section 15.8.

Table 15.2 *Contingency table describing the frequency of locations with large, small and no colonies of a wader bird species in a research area (table rows) in relation to the presence of shrubs and the type of cereal crop (if any) in the proximity of the site*

	Shrubs	Yes			No		
Colony	Cereal crop	none	winter	spring	none	winter	spring
large		0	9	6	3	20	8
small		4	6	10	0	2	3
none		12	8	14	10	2	9

[6] Model likelihood is inversely related to the size of unexplained variation (model deviance).

15.8 How to Proceed in R

Generalised linear models can be estimated (fitted) using the *glm* function. The procedure is similar to fitting linear multiple regression models with the *lm* function, only this time we usually add one parameter called *family*. This parameter allows us to specify the assumed distribution type for random variation, and optionally also the link function, if we choose not to use the implicit canonical link function.

15.8.1 Simple Logistic Regression

For our first example, we use the binomial distribution with the logit link function chosen by default:

```
glm.1 <- glm( PoaPrat ~ A1hor, data=chap15a, family=binomial)
summary( glm.1)

...

Coefficients:
            Estimate Std. Error z value Pr(>|z|)
(Intercept)   4.2891     1.9877   2.158   0.0309 *
A1hor        -0.6956     0.3970  -1.752   0.0798 .
...

(Dispersion parameter for binomial family taken to be 1)

    Null deviance: 24.435  on 19  degrees of freedom
Residual deviance: 18.563  on 18  degrees of freedom
AIC: 22.563

...
```

The negative value of the regression coefficient estimate b_1 (-0.6956) shows that with increasing soil horizon A_1 thickness, there is a decreasing probability of the grass occurring there, but the test shown for this coefficient suggests the effect of *A1hor* is not significant. But the approximation of the *z-value* (which is a ratio between b_1 and the standard error of this estimate) by a normal distribution is not very good, and therefore we recommend ignoring the results of those tests. Instead, we advise using the tests based on a χ^2 (or, for some other types of GLM, on an *F*) test statistic. For a more complex GLM, this means we must compare our model with a simpler version in which the tested variable is missing, so we test the partial effect of that variable. But here our model has just a single explanatory variable, so the test is simple:

```
anova( glm.1, test="Chisq")

Analysis of Deviance Table
Model: binomial, link: logit
Response: PoaPrat
Terms added sequentially (first to last)

      Df Deviance Resid. Df Resid. Dev Pr(>Chi)
NULL                   19      24.435
A1hor  1    5.872       18      18.563  0.01538 *
...
```

Using this more appropriate test, the effect of *A1hor* is now significant, but not too strong; also note that the total variation in *PoaPrat* values dropped from 24.4 in the null model to only 18.6. Another difference concerns the use of the *anova* function. Here we must specify the type of test (either *Chisq* or *F*), otherwise no test is performed. This is because there are two mutually exclusive choices of the test statistic for GLMs (see Section 15.3). The concern about correctly using the *anova* function to evaluate a model with two or more predictors, which we have raised in Section 14.6.1 (regarding the sequential decomposition of the explained variation among the predictors), also applies to generalised linear models.

Now we will plot the fitted model,[7] starting with the original data and adding the fitted model line. Unlike the simple linear model, we cannot add this line using the *abline* function, but rather we must generate a set of regularly spaced predictor values and then use the fitted model to predict the corresponding probability levels. The resulting diagram can be seen in Fig. 15.1.

```
plot( PoaPrat ~ A1hor, data=chap15a, ylab="p(PoaPrat)")
A1hor.pred <- seq( 2, 12, length=30)
PoaPrat.pred <- predict( glm.1, type="resp",
                 newdata=data.frame( A1hor=A1hor.pred))
lines( A1hor.pred, PoaPrat.pred, lwd=2)
```

The graph nicely shows (Fig. 15.1) the effect of the logit transformation performed by the link function: although our model possesses exactly the same complexity as the straight line of a simple linear model, the dependency is shown as a curve that asymptotically approaches 0 on the right side and 1 on the left side (i.e. for shallow soils), exactly as we expect for a model predicting probability values.

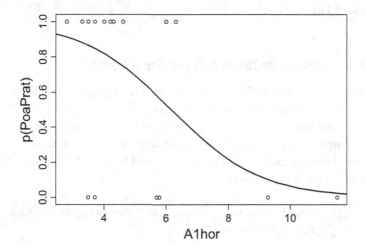

Figure 15.1 Simple dependency of the probability of *Poa pratensis* occurrence on the thickness of the upper soil horizon.

---

[7] Note that using the *plot* function directly with a fitted GLM object (e.g. using a *plot(glm.1)* command) does <u>not</u> display the fitted model, but rather a set of useful regression diagnostic plots, similar to that of a linear model (see Section 14.6.1).

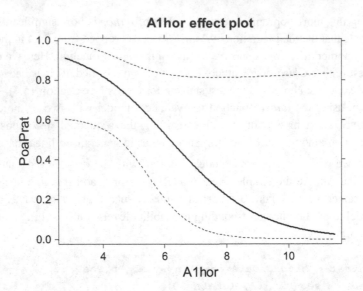

Figure 15.2 Generalised linear model describing the changing occurrence probability for *Poa pratensis* species as the thickness of upper soil horizon increases. This graph was created using the *effects* package.

Alternatively, we can plot the same model with the *effects* package (Fox & Weisberg, 2018). This visualisation method can be extended more easily into models with multiple explanatory variables, even when interaction terms are included. The resulting graph is shown in Fig. 15.2.

```
library( effects)
plot( allEffects( glm.1, resid=T),
      confint=list(style="lines"), type="response",
      lines=list(col="black"))
```

15.8.2 Analysing Contingency Tables with Log-linear Models

As we have already discussed in Section 15.5, we start fitting log-linear models from a rather unusual null (reference) model. This starting model contains, as its predictors, the main effect of the response factor (in our example this is the type of bird colony present at a site) and the main effects and mutual interactions of the explanatory factors. The response variable in this model is the cell frequencies. We set up the null model (with a Poisson distribution and an implicit log link function) as follows:

```
glm.x0 <- glm( Count ~ Colony + Shrubs * Cereal, data=chap15b,
               family=poisson)
```

We compare this model with alternative models, each extended by one of the two interactions between the response factor (*Colony*) and an explanatory factor:

```
add1( glm.x0, scope= ~ Colony * Shrubs * Cereal, test="Chisq")
Single term additions
Model:
```

```
Count ~ Colony + Shrubs * Cereal
Df Deviance     AIC     LRT  Pr(>Chi)
<none>                52.593 128.35
Colony:Shrubs  2    35.315 115.07 17.278 0.0001771 ***
Colony:Cereal  4    23.126 106.88 29.467 6.282e-06 ***
...
```

We use the *scope* parameter to specify the target model with a full interaction among all three factors for the *add1* function, but the function has its own rules regarding the sequence of testing interactions of different orders. Consequently, the test of the second-order interaction (i.e. the *Colony:Shrubs:Cereal* term) is omitted here, as well as of the *Shrubs:Cereal* interaction term, which is already present in the null model.

Both tested interactions have a significant effect ($p < 0.001$) and explain a relatively large fraction of the variability that was not explained in the null model.[8] The tests are based on χ^2 statistics (due to a specified *test* parameter in the *add1* function call), but in the *add1* output this test statistic is labelled *LRT* (*likelihood ratio test*), which it indeed represents. We also note that the *add1* function scores the three models under comparison with an information-theoretic statistic (AIC) value and this comparison confirms the appropriateness of adding both interactions to the model. The effect of the crop type seems to be larger than that of the shrubs, which is in agreement with the likelihood ratio test.

So we now extend our model by both first-order interactions and call *add1* again with the extended model to test the remaining second-order interaction:

```
glm.x1 <- update( glm.x0,
              . ~ . + Colony:Shrubs + Colony:Cereal)
add1( glm.x1, scope=~Colony*Shrubs*Cereal, test="Chisq")
Single term additions
Model:
Count ~ Colony + Shrubs + Cereal + Shrubs:Cereal +
        Colony:Shrubs + Colony:Cereal
                    Df Deviance    AIC    LRT Pr(>Chi)
<none>                6.2887 94.046
Colony:Shrubs:Cereal  4    0.0000 95.757 6.2887   0.1786
```

This interaction term, however, is not significant (and the AIC value even increases with its addition), so we can conclude that the shrubs and cereal crops within the neighbourhood affect the presence of colonies and their size independently. To provide readers of our research paper with a more specific ecological interpretation, we must work out the direction of the effects we have just revealed. For this, we start from the estimated values of our regression coefficients. These coefficients can be obtained with the extracting function *coef*:

---

[8] See the *Deviance* column: e.g. the *Colony:Shrubs* term explains $100 \times (52.593 - 35.315)/52.593 = 32.85\%$ of the variation unexplained by the *glm.x0* model.

```
coef( glm.x1)
              (Intercept)                 Colonynone
                0.8204104                  1.4503570
              Colonysmall                  Shrubsyes
               -0.7795212                 -1.1370845
             Cerealspring                 Cerealwinter
                1.4309762                  2.1359399
     Shrubsyes:Cerealspring     Shrubsyes:Cerealwinter
                0.3895751                  0.4602894
       Colonynone:Shrubsyes       Colonysmall:Shrubsyes
                1.3769864                  2.1807977
 Colonynone:Cerealspring   Colonysmall:Cerealspring
               -1.6228684                 -0.5541241
 Colonynone:Cerealwinter   Colonysmall:Cerealwinter
               -3.2074360                 -1.8020744
```

We used a different background to mark the regression coefficients that were already present in the starting null model, and hence their interpretation is of limited interest.[9] The next two coefficients represent the interaction between the *Colony* and *Shrubs* factors and they suggest (by their positive values) that the probability of a locality having no colony or (just) a small colony increases when there are shrubs in the proximity of the site. This might be explained, for example, by the utilisation of shrubs as elevated perch sites by birds of prey.

Please note that there is neither a regression coefficient for a combination of colony type with the *no* level of the *Shrubs* factor, nor a coefficient for the combination of shrub presence with a large colony. This is because the combinations of large colony and/or the absence of shrubs serve as the reference levels of factors, against which the other combinations are compared, and so they are already subsumed within the estimate of the β_0 coefficient, labelled here as (*Intercept*).

For the cereal crop interaction with colony type (last four coefficient estimates) we can see that the presence of spring crop, and even more so for the winter crop, decreases the probability of observing absent or small colonies, i.e. increases the probability of finding a large colony. This implies that this wader bird prefers localities where cereal crops are present.

15.9 Reporting Analyses

15.9.1 Methods

The change in the probability of *Poa pratensis* occurrence with A_1 soil horizon thickness was quantified and tested using a generalised linear model with an assumed binomial (Bernoulli) distribution.

[9] Their values reflect the relative frequencies of the various types of colonies and of the localities with different combinations of the shrubs and cereal crop types present there.

Or

... tested using logistic regression.

We tested the effect of the presence of a cereal crop field and shrubs upon the presence and size of nesting colonies using log-linear models and likelihood ratio tests.

15.9.2 Results

The probability of *Poa pratensis* occurrence decreases with increasing A_1 soil horizon thickness ($\chi^2_1 = 5.872$, $p = 0.0154$).

We can eventually add a graph here, representing the shape of the fitted model (similar to Fig. 15.1 or 15.2).

The presence of nesting colonies is significantly affected by the presence of cereal fields in the area ($\chi^2_4 = 29.467$, $p < 0.001$, with the absence of a field decreasing the probability that a colony is present), as well as by the presence of shrubs ($\chi^2_2 = 17.28$, $p < 0.001$, with the presence of shrubs decreasing the probability that a nesting colony is present). The effects of these two factors on colony presence and size are mutually independent ($\chi^2_4 = 6.29$, n.s.).

15.10 Recommended Reading

Quinn & Keough (2002), pp. 359–400.

K. P. Burnham & D. R. Anderson (2002) *Model Selection and Multimodel Inference. A Practical Information-Theoretic Approach*, 2nd edn. Springer, Berlin.

J. Fox (2008) *Applied Regression Analysis and Generalized Linear Models*, 2nd edn. Sage, Los Angeles, CA.

J. Fox & S. Weisberg (2018) Visualizing fit and lack of fit in complex regression models with predictor effect plots and partial residuals. *Journal of Statistical Software*, **87**(9): 1–27.

16 Regression Models for Non-linear Relationships

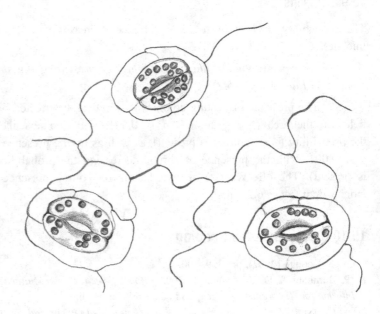

16.1 Use Case Examples

1. We want to describe the response of the population size of multiple insect species to the average height of vegetation. We measured the various population sizes across a range of sites differing in vegetation height. Taking vegetation height as an environmental gradient, we assume that the species have differing optima along this gradient and their population sizes gradually decline in both directions from those optima. The simplest possible model to describe such a relationship is a symmetrical unimodal curve.

2. We studied, under controlled conditions, how the carbon fixation rate (*FR*) of a plant species changes with increasing concentration of carbon dioxide in the atmosphere. We used seven different CO_2 concentrations, each with three independent plant replicates, and we measured their fixation rate under constant conditions (light intensity, temperature and air humidity). The relationship between CO_2 concentration and fixation rate is not linear, however, and cannot easily be linearised. The photosynthetic fixation starts at some minimum CO_2 concentration and increases up to a limit at which the photosynthetic capacity of the plant becomes saturated. We want to describe the data using a relatively simple statistical model with parameters matching the properties of the corresponding physiological process.

16.2 Introduction

Linear regression is one of the most frequently employed methods of studying the dependency of a response variable on explanatory variables. But at the same time, we can reasonably assume that many (if not the majority of) biological dependencies are not linear. So how can we study such non-linear relationships? We have already demonstrated some of the possibilities: we can try to linearise the relationship using variable transformations (Chapter 12) or use generalised linear models (Chapter 15). Whether we transform explicitly or use a generalised linear model, where each explanatory variable serves as a linear term (i.e. we do not use second and higher powers of the variables), the resulting relationships will always be monotonic, either increasing or decreasing across the whole range of values.

But there are multiple alternative approaches which allow us to model non-monotonic dependencies, including (i) polynomial regression, (ii) fitting non-linear models by the classical least-squares criterion or (iii) data *smoothing* methods, including loess model, splines or their more developed version called *generalised additive models* (GAMs). In this chapter, we introduce the first two groups, the polynomial regression and the non-linear least-squares method.

16.3 Polynomial Regression

When we find that the dependency of two variables in our regression analysis is non-linear, but the spread of values around the assumed regression curve is approximately constant, then there are several possibilities for how to proceed. One of the most popular options is the polynomial regression. When we work with just a single explanatory variable X, the model for a polynomial regression can be described as follows:

$$EY = \beta_0 + \beta_1 X + \beta_2 X^2 + \beta_3 X^3 + \cdots + \beta_m X^m \qquad (16.1)$$

The estimates of β_j regression coefficients in this *polynomial curve of the m-th order* are then labelled b_j. Figure 16.1 shows three alternative polynomial models (as well as a linear one) for the same pair of variables. The quadratic ($\beta_2 X^2$) or higher-order polynomial terms can also be combined with variable transformations (see the next paragraph) or become a part of the linear predictor in a generalised linear model (see Chapter 15) to describe a more diverse range of non-monotonic dependencies.

Polynomial curves often fit our data nicely, but it might be difficult (or even impossible) to interpret their individual coefficients, particularly for higher-order polynomials. Consequently, biologists will typically use a quadratic regression (based on a second-order polynomial) or – more rarely – cubic regression (based on a third-order polynomial). Modelling the relationship between <u>log-transformed</u> population size or fitness and environmental properties using quadratic regression leads to a well-known model referred to as a *unimodal response curve,* i.e. a symmetrical curve with one maximum, which we traditionally call species optimum (in the event where the b_2 coefficient is negative, see below). In this model, we can transform its estimated regression coefficients into two, more biologically meaningful parameters. The first is the *species optimum* representing a predictor value at which the response variable is predicted to have a maximum value (i.e. maximum

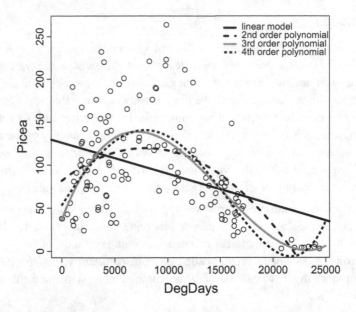

Figure 16.1 Fitting data using polynomial regression models of various complexity. The data represent the counts of spruce pollen grains obtained at different geographical locations, related to a climatic parameter called degree days (sum of positive daily averages of air temperature across a whole calendar year). The regression models here use the response variable without any transformation, but a log-transformation would also be suitable e.g. to limit the predicted values (on the original scale) to positive numbers. An unrealistic increase of the fourth-order polynomial curve for the highest values of the *DegDays* variable illustrates the undesirable properties of higher-order polynomial models.

population size or fitness). We can calculate the optimum based on the regression coefficient estimates as

$$x_{opt} = \frac{-b_1}{2b_2} \tag{16.2}$$

There is a limitation concerning the b_2 value, however. If the estimate is positive, x_{opt} does not represent a maximum for the response Y, but rather its minimum, i.e. the position of the lowest point of the fitted curve, not its 'summit'. Additionally, an estimated optimum cannot be trusted if it lies outside the range of observed predictor values.

The tolerance of the curve, x_{tol}, can be computed as

$$x_{tol} = \frac{1}{\sqrt{-2b_2}} \tag{16.3}$$

but again only if $b_2 < 0$. The estimated tolerance represents the width of a fitted unimodal curve and takes its name from the fact that unimodal response curves are frequently used to model species' niches.

Equation (16.1) reminds us of a multiple regression model. Indeed, the polynomial regression is a special case of multiple regression, using original values, squared values, etc. of a single predictor instead of multiple explanatory variables. As in multiple regression, we can test whether the individual regression coefficients are different from zero. We recommend starting with the simplest model (i.e. either a null model with no predictor or a linear model) and investigating whether the model is improved when we add the next higher polynomial term. If the effect of a quadratic term differs significantly from zero, this implies a non-linear dependency, which might be of biological interest. It is difficult to interpret the biological meaning of a significant cubic term: when we study the change of species abundance along an environmental gradient, a significant cubic term usually implies that the response curve is not symmetrical around the species' optimum. It is always dangerous to extrapolate regression-based relationships outside the studied range of predictors, and particularly so for higher-order polynomials. The predicted relationship can behave strangely already at the margins of the observed range of predictor(s).

> You should be aware that for a unimodal (quadratic) dependency with its minimum (or maximum) approximately in the centre of the explanatory variable (X) range, a linear regression on the same data might not be significant due to a strong quadratic dependency. We must therefore first plot our data and depending on the shape of the relationship between Y and X, decide about the models we should consider.

Multiple polynomial regression allows us to estimate the dependency of a single response variable on polynomials of multiple predictors, with the potential for different predictors to vary in their polynomial degree. This is often used to describe a range of trends in the spatial arrangement of response values, where we employ the polynomials of geographical coordinates of individual observations (*trend surface analysis*). The simplest possible model (ignoring a linear version) would be $EY = \beta_0 + \beta_1 X + \beta_2 X^2 + \beta_3 Y + \beta_4 Y^2 + \beta_5 XY$.

16.4 Non-linear Regression

In some applications, we know the expected shape of the dependency *a priori*, often described by a model using parameters with a research field-specific meaning. As an example, to describe the change of carbon fixation rate during photosynthesis in relation to carbon dioxide (CO_2) concentration, we often use the following asymptotic curve with an offset:

$$E(FR) = \beta_0\{1 - e^{-e^{\beta_1}(x - \beta_2)}\} \qquad (16.4)$$

where FR is the speed of carbon fixation rate, x represents carbon dioxide concentration in the air and the β_j parameters represent the asymptotic value of fixation rate (β_0), the log-transformed value of fixation rate increase with increasing carbon dioxide concentration (β_1) and the value of the offset (β_2), i.e. a minimum carbon dioxide concentration at which the carbon fixation starts. We can use non-linear regression to estimate the three parameters of this curve. If we use the least-squares criterion, the method looks for b_j estimates leading to a minimum sum of squared differences between the predicted and observed FR values. But unlike the standard linear regression, we need a numerical *approximation* to find the best parameter estimates. Various approximating methods are used, employing a set of steps representing a directed process of trial–correction–new trial–new correction, etc., to gradually find a combination of parameter estimates leading to the smallest sum of residual squares.

The greatest difficulty of this estimation procedure is that when seeking the truly minimal sum of residual squares, we might incidentally find a local minimum, yet the procedure is not able to detect that there is a better solution with a lower sum of residual squares. Most statistical software offering the non-linear least-squares regression therefore requires that the user specifies not only the model equation to be estimated, but also the initial (rough) estimates of its parameters. For specific functions, however, the software itself might have the ability to work out those initial estimates from the data.

Similar to a standard linear regression, even the non-linear regression assumes a constant value of unexplained variation in the response variable. This assumption is usually not met in the non-linear regression, however. Even in our example illustrated in Fig. 16.1, the unexplained variation seems to be larger near the species optimum, decreasing in both directions. In many cases, we can mend this issue by appropriately transforming the response variable. Another option would be to use a maximum likelihood criterion instead of the least-squares criterion and assume a different type of distribution for the unexplained variation.

16.5 Example Data

Our example data in the *Chap16* sheet (first two columns) represent the measurement of carbon fixation rate by a plant (variable *C.uptake*), depending on the carbon dioxide concentration in the air (variable *CO2*). The 21 plants were grown in one of seven different ambient CO_2 concentrations under identical temperature, soil humidity and light conditions. This type of experiment is often performed in a limited number of climaboxes and so the plants sharing the same climabox (e.g. with the same CO_2 concentration) are not fully independent observations. But let us assume that this is not an issue for our dataset. We will use these data to illustrate both a polynomial regression, and the estimate of a non-linear model using the least-squares criterion. The latter approach is undoubtedly more appropriate for this particular kind of data as it provides parameters that can easily be interpreted in terms of the observed process, in this case photosynthesis.

16.6 How to Proceed in R

16.6.1 Polynomial Regression

We can estimate and summarise the regression model with a third-order polynomial using the following commands:

```
lm.1 <- lm( C.uptake ~ poly( CO2, 3), data=chap16)
summary( lm.1)

...

Coefficients:
              Estimate Std. Error t value Pr(>|t|)
(Intercept)    27.0857     0.6458  41.944  < 2e-16 ***
poly(CO2, 3)1  24.4695     2.9592   8.269 2.32e-07 ***
poly(CO2, 3)2 -18.2268     2.9592  -6.159 1.05e-05 ***
poly(CO2, 3)3  10.0141     2.9592   3.384  0.00353 **
---
Signif. codes:  0 '***' 0.001 '**' 0.01 '*' 0.05 '.' 0.1 ' ' 1

Residual standard error: 2.959 on 17 degrees of freedom
Multiple R-squared:  0.8739,    Adjusted R-squared:  0.8516
F-statistic: 39.25 on 3 and 17 DF,  p-value: 7.362e-08
```

Before we start interpreting the fitted model, we should first look at how the polynomial was specified in the model formula and how the corresponding regression coefficients are labelled. Unfortunately, we cannot interpret the three estimated coefficients as representing the relative contribution of the linear, quadratic and cubic terms of the polynomial. This is because we specified the *orthogonal polynomial*, which transforms the values of those three explanatory terms so that they are linearly uncorrelated. This change offers a much more reliable estimation of the regression model, but using the regression coefficients to predict fixation rate is non-trivial. Instead, we should use an alternatively fitted model for the purpose of making predictions:

```
lm.2 <- lm( C.uptake ~ CO2 + I(CO2^2) + I(CO2^3), data=chap16)
```

However, this alternative model is now less appropriate for testing the significance of individual model parameters. We will use it, however, to plot the fitted regression curve. First, we must generate a regularly spread set of predictor ($CO2$) values and use them to predict the expected carbon fixation rate together with the standard errors of those estimates (so that a confidence region can be plotted). The resulting graph is shown in Fig. 16.2.

```
xpred <- data.frame( CO2=seq( 100, 1200, by=50))
lm.2fit <- predict( lm.2, newdata=xpred, se=T)
plot( C.uptake~CO2, data=chap16,
        xlim=c(0,1200), ylim=c(0,40))
lines( xpred$CO2, lm.2fit$fit, lwd=2)
```

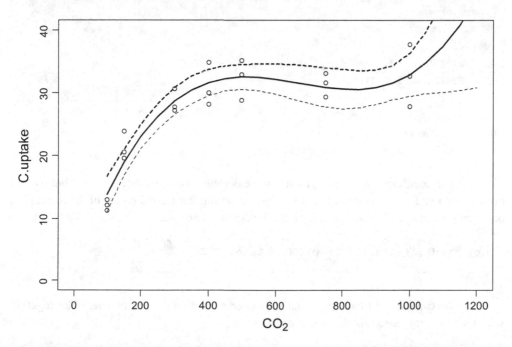

Figure 16.2 Third-order polynomial regression fitted to the data on the change of carbon fixation rate with ambient carbon dioxide concentration. Note that the prediction for $CO2$ values above 1000, i.e. outside the measured range, is already dubious.

```
lines( xpred$CO2, lm.2fit$fit-2*lm.2fit$se.fit, lty=2)
lines( xpred$CO2, lm.2fit$fit+2*lm.2fit$se.fit, lty=2)
```

16.6.2 Non-linear Regression

We can estimate the parameters of a non-linear regression model with relative ease using the *nls* function, which is available in the *nlme* package (Bates & Chambers, 1992). This is only easy, however, when our model represents one of the non-linear functions directly supported by the *nlme* package. This support takes the form of *self-starting functions* (their names begin with *SS*). These functions provide good initial estimates of the regression parameters and – during the model estimation – the known first-order derivative of the fitted function. If our model does not match one of the supported functions then our task suddenly becomes much more difficult. We must define our own support function that evaluates the estimated model function or its derivative, as well as the initial estimates for function parameters. Here, however, we will stick to illustrating the straightforward method only, because Eq. (16.4) is supported by the predefined *SSasympOff* function:

```
library( nlme)
nls.1 <- nls( C.uptake ~ SSasympOff( CO2, b0, b1, b2),
              data=chap16)
summary( nls.1)
Formula: C.uptake ~ SSasympOff(CO2, b0, b1, b2)

Parameters:
    Estimate Std. Error t value Pr(>|t|)
b0  32.0119    0.8756    36.56  < 2e-16 ***
b1  -4.5465    0.2533   -17.95 6.18e-13 ***
b2  53.4158   15.5749     3.43  0.00299 **
...
Residual standard error: 2.688 on 18 degrees of freedom
Number of iterations to convergence: 0
Achieved convergence tolerance: 6.864e-07
```

The coefficient of determination is not calculated for a non-linear model, but we can obtain its non-adjusted version quite easily by calculating the second power of the correlation between predicted and observed values of the response variable:

```
cor( predict( nls.1), chap16$C.uptake) ^ 2
[1] 0.8897759
```

We can use the following commands to create a graph of our two variables together with the fitted regression model (see Fig. 16.3):

```
xpred <- data.frame( CO2=seq( 100, 1200, by=50))
nls.fit <- predict( nls.1, xpred)
```

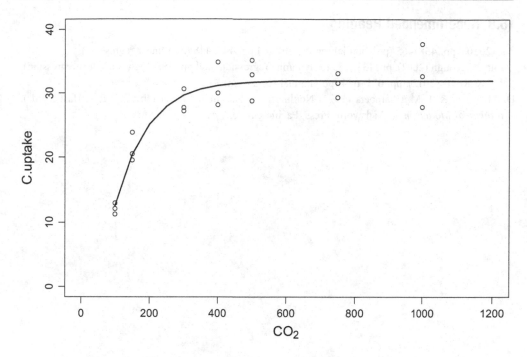

Figure 16.3 Fitted model of asymptotic growth with an offset for carbon fixation rate.

```
plot( C.uptake~CO2, data=chap16,
      xlim=c(0,1200), ylim=c(0,40))
lines( xpred$CO2, nls.fit, lwd=2)
```

16.7 Reporting Analyses

16.7.1 Methods

The non-linear nature of the change of C fixation rate with ambient CO_2 concentration was summarised using a third-order polynomial model.

We used a non-linear model of the asymptotic growth curve with an offset (see Eq. (16.3)) to describe the change of carbon fixation rate with increasing ambient CO_2 concentration, estimated by the least-squares minimising algorithm of Gauss–Newton (Bates & Chambers, 1992).

16.7.2 Results

We provide a description of the results for the non-linear regression only, but a presentation of the polynomial regression model results would be similar; we do not show the table or figure to which the text refers.

The estimated non-linear model of asymptotic growth (see Fig. X) explained about 89% of the variation in carbon uptake rate and its parameters are summarised in Table Y.

16.8 Recommended Reading

Zar (2010), pp. 458–465 (polynomial regression) and pp. 447–448 (non-linear regression).

Quinn & Keough (2002), pp. 133–135 (polynomial regression) and pp. 150–152 (non-linear regression).

Sokal & Rohlf (2012), pp. 671–684 (polynomial regression).

D. M. Bates & J. M. Chambers (1992) Nonlinear models. In J. M. Chambers & T. J. Hastie (eds), *Statistical Models in S.* Wadsworth Press, Pacific Grove, CA.

17 Structural Equation Models

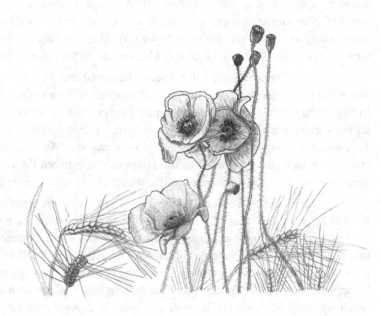

17.1 Use Case Examples

We performed a field fertilisation experiment (Pyšek & Lepš, 1991) where the richness of a weed community within a barley field was affected by the amount of fertiliser that was applied and by the crop cover. Our task is to disentangle the direct effect of fertiliser dose, the direct effect of barley cover and the indirect effect of fertiliser dose (affecting barley cover) on the richness of the weed community.

17.2 SEMs and Path Analysis

Structural equation models (SEMs) allow us to describe a system of three or more observed characteristics (variables, often representing some biological processes and state variables)[1] by defining a hypothetical model of causal relationships among those characteristics (which variable/process affects other particular variables). We can then estimate the model parameters and test this hypothetical model against the data we collect, comparing observed variable values and their correlations,[2] particularly the partial correlations (see Section 14.3).

---

[1] State variables describe the actual state of a dynamically changing system. For example, in ecosystem models, they might describe amounts or concentrations of resources, population sizes or growth rates, etc.

[2] Present-day models do not use correlations, however, but rather covariances, as we explain later in this chapter.

SEMs also enable us to describe systems in which we have a rough idea about some of the processes or events involved, but none of the measured variables explain those processes/events in a sufficiently precise way. Those general characteristics are then represented in our model as *latent variables* (also called *factors*),[3] which we might relate to a number of measured variables (often called *manifest variables* or *factor indicators*) that together characterise the latent variables to a certain extent, with each measured variable contributing to a latent variable in a unique way. This postulated definition of a latent variable then allows us to relate it to other variables present in the system, both measured and latent.

Latent variables are often used when applying SEMs in sociology, ethology or psychology (e.g. personality traits such as 'problem-solving ability' or 'extent of empathy'). In biological applications, however, simpler forms of SEM are used more frequently, in which all the variables are real, measured characteristics rather than representing abstract concepts. This simpler form was traditionally called *path analysis*. As with the more general SEM, it starts from an *a priori* model of causal relationships between the variables, estimates model parameters and tries to determine the likelihood of our model given the observed data.

Our example (Section 17.1) probably represents the simplest possible useful setup for a SEM, with three mutually interacting observed variables and no latent variable. Within the framework of a linear regression model, we would use the richness of the weed community (*NSP*) as a response variable and employ the amount of fertiliser (*dose*) and barley *cover* as two predictors. In this regression model, the correlation between the two predictors would be approached as a nuisance, making the interpretation of predictor effects less reliable. But when we use a SEM, we can learn more about the hypothesised causal effects. For our data, we can expect that the primary causal effect for weed richness is the changing cover of barley, which affects the weed community through competition for light and soil resources. However, the barley cover itself is also likely affected by fertiliser availability.

Finally, fertiliser can directly influence weed community richness by differentially changing the performance of individual weed species and their mutual competition. The fact that a single variable can act as both a predictor (even for multiple responses) and a response in the same model is one of the most important facets of SEMs in comparison with other statistical models. This example also shows one general phenomenon of experiments carried out on complicated biological and ecological systems. Even if we emphasise the importance of manipulative experiments for testing underlying mechanisms, we are never able to control for everything. When manipulating nutrient availability by fertilisation, we change some of the conditions affecting the target variable (*NSP* in our case). The use of a SEM might be very helpful in such situations.

The causal relationships among the variables in our example are summarised in Fig. 17.1. Drawing a conceptual graph (called a *path diagram*), such as the one in Fig. 17.1A, is an important step in all studies employing SEMs.

The causal relationships are displayed in Fig. 17.1 by thick arrows, the thinner arrows going from 'nowhere' (and labelled by the Greek letter λ) reflect the effects of unknown (unobserved) factors or purely stochastic behaviour, represented by the unexplained variation of the three variables we measured. According to the scheme in Fig. 17.1, variable

---

[3] Here the *factor* term is used in a sense different from categorical variables used e.g. in the ANOVA models.

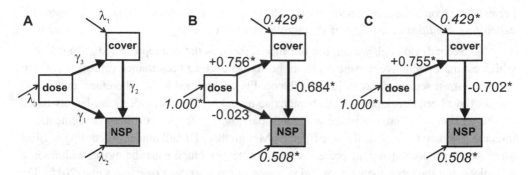

Figure 17.1 Path analysis model (SEM) for the effects of fertiliser dose (*dose*) and barley cover (*cover*) on the species richness of the weed community (*NSP*). (A) Schematic outline of the hypothesised causal model. (B) Parameter estimates for the model in part A (standardised coefficients, which are significant when followed by an asterisk). (C) Parameter estimates for a simplified model, excluding the non-significant direct effect of fertiliser dose on weed species richness (see Section 17.4).

dose is not causally affected by any of the other observed variables; we call such variables *exogenous*, while the remaining two (which are affected by *dose*, but also possibly affect other variables) are called *endogenous* variables. The Greek letter γ accompanying the arrows in Fig. 17.1A denotes the *path coefficients*. They represent partial regression coefficients, while the direction of the corresponding effect is given by its sign. In Fig. 17.1, the path coefficients are shown in a standardised form (calculated from variables that were standardised to zero mean and unit variance), so they also measure the relative effect strength of individual relationships.

The estimated values in Fig. 17.1B suggest (asterisks flag significant path coefficients) that the indirect effect of fertiliser increasing barley cover is strong and significant, while the direct fertiliser effect on the weed community richness is much smaller and not reliably different from zero (see also Section 17.4 describing the details of estimating and testing the models).

We must take several specific aspects of the SEM into consideration when assessing the quality of the estimated model. First, in models without latent variables, we are constantly facing an insufficient number of degrees of freedom when testing our model. The standard test for a fitted SEM (χ^2 test) compares the matrix of covariances[4] among observed variables with the matrix predicted by the fitted model,[5] and the number of compared values in these matrices depend on the number of variables, rather than on the number of observations. The path coefficients are also estimated using the variance–covariance matrix computed from the sampled data. Consequently, we have $k \times (k + 1)/2$ values (where k is the number of observed variables), which are used to estimate the SEM parameters (λ and γ values in Fig. 17.1). In our example, there are three variables and hence six covariance and variance estimates, but our path diagram in Fig. 17.1A requires the estimation of six coefficients. This means that we will have no residual degrees of freedom for a valid χ^2 test and our SEM will

---

[4] The *covariance* expresses the extent of the linear relationship between two variables, similar to the Pearson correlation coefficient (see Eq. (13.1) in Chapter 13). In fact, we can compute the covariance between X and Y variables by multiplying their correlation (r_{XY}) with the standard deviations of X and Y. The covariance of a variable with itself is the variable's variance.

[5] The null hypothesis being tested by the χ^2 test states that the observed covariances among the variables could be generated by the relationships described by our SEM (with its structure defined by the path diagram).

predict the covariance matrix perfectly (which is of course just an artefact). Such a model is called *just identified* in the field of structural equation modelling.

Second, although we can test our model (such as the one represented in Fig. 17.1C, which estimates only five parameters from the six variance and covariance values), the χ^2 test is not the most sensitive way of judging the quality of the fitted SEM. Therefore, multiple *fit indices* have been developed which characterise model fit. These fit indices are largely based on the χ^2 statistic discussed in the preceding paragraph, but some of them (incremental fit indices) compare the χ^2 statistic for a fitted SEM with that of a null model. According to SEM lore,[6] you must accompany the presentation of a fitted structural equation model with a set of fit indices, but the recommended set varies across different authors (see e.g. Kline, 2015). For the type of models under consideration in this chapter (with no latent variable), the null SEM is defined as having no causal relationship between the observed variables (for our example in Fig. 17.1 there would be just three λs, while the γ path coefficients would be set to 0).

Third, even when our model seems to fit well, we should be aware that alternative models of the same complexity (i.e. with a similar number of path coefficients) could have a similar (or even higher) quality. For example, if we reverse the direction of an arrow representing a causal effect (so e.g. instead of variable X_2 affecting variable X_3, variable X_3 will affect variable X_2 in an alternative model), the model quality represented by fit indices might not change depending on the model structure. With this particular example, the two alternative models cannot be directly compared using a statistical test because they are not hierarchically nested (one of them is not a subset of the other).[7] It is therefore essential to start with a model underpinned by an existing knowledge and/or by our specific hypotheses and to develop it further by gradual simplification or extension, depending on the results of SEM fitting and testing.

Finally, even though the number of independent observations in our dataset does not affect the number of degrees of freedom for the χ^2 test performed on the fitted SEM, it is important that the variance–covariance matrix is estimated with high reliability. The recommended sample size n is usually expressed by reference to the number of observed variables (k), with the n/k ratio suggested to be at least 10, but preferably around 20 or more (Kline, 2015).[8]

We believe that SEMs are under-utilised in the analysis of biological data. Some of the statistical models described earlier in this book (particularly the ANOVA and regression models) can be used to test hypotheses about the relationships among variables. Additionally, when our data originate from well-designed manipulative experiments, we can interpret the results of such tests as supporting or not supporting our ideas about causal relationships, but the nature of those models limits us to relatively simple types of relationships.

> When using structural equation models (SEMs), we often consider causal relationships, but we must be careful not to interpret a statistical (correlative) dependency as a causal dependency (Petraitis et al., 1996; Grace, 2006). You need your data to be based on experiments manipulating the hypothesised causes to prove a causal dependency.

---

[6] Some authors do not have much faith in such indices, see e.g. Shipley (2010).

[7] We can still compare the quality of non-nested models using e.g. the AIC (see Section 15.6).

[8] In this respect, our example data fare quite well, as the n/k ratio is about 41.

We manipulated only the fertiliser dose in our example. In order to demonstrate the direct effect of barley cover upon weed community richness, we would also need to add e.g. an experimental removal of barley biomass in all levels of fertiliser application. Nevertheless, the SEMs are also applied in studies where it is impossible to perform experimental manipulation. Depending on the circumstances we can – based on the results we obtain – speculate about the causality, although even SEMs cannot provide sufficient evidence for it under such circumstances. When we interpret our results, we must be aware of how much our final result is influenced by our *a priori* formulation of the possible causal relationships. In our example, these relationships are represented by Fig. 17.1A. For example, we expect that the cover of barley affects the weed community, but not vice versa (which is probably true as the weed community in our study is characterised by the number of species rather than e.g. its total cover). However, the final result is restricted by this decision. This is why the original model should always be presented together with the final one.

For additional information about using SEMs in biological research, we recommend the books of Shipley (2000) and Grace (2006), and for a more advanced treatment (in the context of social sciences) please check the textbook by Kline (2015).

17.3 Example Data

Our data represent the example described in Section 17.1. The variables in the *Chap17* sheet are the fertiliser dose (*dose*), cover of barley (*cover*) and species richness of the weed community (*NSP*).

17.4 How to Proceed in R

There are multiple packages implementing SEMs. Here we will demonstrate the use of the *sem* package (Fox, 2006).

We start with a null model that postulates no relationships among the three observed variables. You can imagine it as a simplification of the SEM described by Fig. 17.1A, but setting all its γ coefficients to 0. We will use the *specifyEquations* function to specify the model structure. Besides calling the function (in the second line of code), we must also enter the text following individual *N:* prompts. The specification is finished when we press the <Enter> key directly after the *4:* prompt:

```
library( sem)
sem.mod0 <- specifyEquations()
1: V(cover)=lam1
2: V(NSP) = lam2
3: V(dose)= lam3
4:
Read 3 items
```

We can fit the SEM using the prepared model specification and existing data with the *sem* function:

```
sem.0 <- sem( sem.mod0, data=chap17)
```

The *summary* function provides a brief summary of the fitted model. Its call is preceded by a change of the display precision, limiting the width of the text output:

```
options( digits=3)
summary( sem.0, fit.indices=c("AIC","RMSEA", "NNFI", "CFI"))
 Model Chisquare =  184    Df =  3 Pr(>Chisq) = 9.91e-40
 RMSEA index =  0.707    90% CI: (NA, NA)
 Tucker-Lewis NNFI =  0
 Bentler CFI =  0
 AIC =  190

Normalized Residuals
  Min. 1st Qu.  Median    Mean 3rd Qu.    Max.
 -7.72   -5.94    0.00   -1.19    0.00    8.31


 Parameter Estimates
    Estimate Std Error z value Pr(>|z|)
lam1 788.409  101.3618  7.78    7.36e-15 cover <-> cover
lam2   6.426    0.8262  7.78    7.36e-15 NSP <-> NSP
lam3   0.488    0.0627  7.78    7.36e-15 dose <-> dose
 Iterations =  0
```

Above we specified our choice of fit indices, but there are more available (see online help). As we already mentioned, the recommendations on indices vary, but most of them include *RMSEA* (root-mean-square error of approximation) and *CFI* (Bentler comparative fit index; Bentler, 1990). There are various rules of thumb specifying the desired values of those indices for a well-fitting SEM. For the *RMSEA* statistic, the recommended value is below 0.05, while a *CFI* value should be 0.95 or larger (Kline, 2015). We can clearly see that the null model does not match our data well. This is also evidenced by the χ^2 test, suggesting a large discrepancy between the covariance matrix implied by the null model *sem.0* and that based on the observed data.

We now continue by fitting the model described in Fig. 17.1A. The description of this diagram (often called a *path diagram*) is performed in the same way as it is for the null model above, but this time we start with the relationships among the variables, including three path coefficients:

```
sem.mod1 <- specifyEquations()
1: NSP = gam1 * dose + gam2 * cover
2: cover = gam3 * dose
3: V(cover) = lam1
4: V(NSP) = lam2
5: V(dose) = lam3
6:
Read 5 items
```

Next we estimate the model:

```
> sem.1 <- sem( sem.mod1, data=chap17)
```

We can now compare the summary of this path model with the earlier null model:

```
summary( sem.1, fit.indices=c("AIC","RMSEA", "NNFI", "CFI"))
Model Chisquare =  -3.22e-13   Df =  0 Pr(>Chisq) = NA
 AIC =  12
Normalized Residuals
     Min.    1st Qu.    Median      Mean    3rd Qu.      Max.
-8.99e-16  0.00e+00  6.07e-16  4.80e-16  7.95e-16  2.24e-15

R-square for Endogenous Variables
  NSP cover
0.492 0.571

Parameter Estimates
      Estimate Std Error z value Pr(>|z|)
gam1  -0.0850  0.35878  -0.237  8.13e-01 NSP <- dose
gam2  -0.0617  0.00892  -6.919  4.56e-12 NSP <- cover
gam3  30.3722  2.39449  12.684  7.24e-37 cover <- dose
lam1 338.4232 43.50933   7.778  7.36e-15 cover <-> cover
lam2   3.2613  0.41929   7.778  7.36e-15 NSP <-> NSP
lam3   0.4878  0.06271   7.778  7.36e-15 dose <-> dose
Iterations =  0
```

The model summary again starts with a χ^2 test, but you can see that the test statistic (measuring the discrepancy between the observed and expected variances and covariances) effectively has a zero value, but also the corresponding degrees of freedom are 0 because the model is fully saturated (or 'just identified'), as discussed in Section 17.2. Additionally, no fit indices are shown as they cannot be computed. The only exception is the AIC statistic, which suggests that this model is much better (more parsimonious) than the null model. At the end of the summary output, the individual model parameters are tested for a difference from zero. We can clearly see from the test results that only the γ_1 parameter is not significantly different from zero. Based on this finding, we can simplify our model by omitting the related direct effect of *dose* on weed community richness (*NSP*):

```
sem.mod2 <- specifyEquations()
1: NSP = gam2 * cover
2: cover = gam3 * dose
3: V(cover) = lam1
4: V(NSP)   = lam2
5: V(dose)  = lam3
6:
```

```
Read 5 items
```

```
sem.2 <- sem( sem.mod2, data=chap17)
```

We can formally compare our two candidate models by using a likelihood ratio test (LRT), and this is done with the *anova* function:

```
anova( sem.1, sem.2)
LR Test for Difference Between Models

       Model Df Model Chisq Df LR Chisq Pr(>Chisq)
sem.1          0     0.0000
sem.2          1     0.0561 1   0.0561       0.81
```

There is no significant difference between these two models, which shows that the inclusion of the direct effect of dose on species richness does not significantly improve the fit of the model. Therefore, based on the principle of parsimony, we prefer the simpler *sem.2* model. We can summarise that model again with the *summary* function:

```
summary( sem.2, fit.indices=c("AIC", "RMSEA", "NNFI", "CFI"))
Model Chisquare =  0.0561   Df =  1 Pr(>Chisq) = 0.813
 RMSEA index =  0    90% CI: (NA, 0.149)
 Tucker-Lewis NNFI =  1.02
 Bentler CFI =  1
 AIC =  10.1
Normalized Residuals
   Min. 1st Qu.  Median   Mean 3rd Qu.   Max.
-0.0977  0.0000  0.0000 -0.0217  0.0000  0.0000


R-square for Endogenous Variables
cover   NSP
0.571 0.492


Parameter Estimates
      Estimate Std Error  z value Pr(>|z|)
gam2  -0.0633   0.00585  -10.83  2.46e-27 NSP <- cover
gam3  30.3722   2.39449   12.68  7.24e-37 cover <- dose
lam1 338.4232  43.50933    7.78  7.36e-15 cover <-> cover
lam2   3.2628   0.41949    7.78  7.36e-15 NSP <-> NSP
lam3   0.4878   0.06271    7.78  7.36e-15 dose <-> dose
 Iterations =  0
```

We see that the AIC statistic improved (from 12.0 to 10.1), while the fit indices are now also presented, with both RMSEA and CFI reporting 'good' values (suggesting a well-fitting model). The estimates of path coefficients did not change much from the original model *sem.1*.

The estimates (*gam2*, *gam3*) are presented on their original scale, reflecting the scale of the predictor variables *cover* and *dose*, respectively. Further, the estimates of random (unexplained) variation in *cover* and *NSP* (parameters *lam1* and *lam2*) are shown on the scale of corresponding variables. But we must first standardise these parameters in order to compare their relative importance, as we have done in Figs 17.1B and C. We can obtain these standardised coefficients in the following way:

```
coef( sem.2, stand=T)

  gam2   gam3   lam1   lam2   lam3
-0.702  0.755  0.429  0.508  1.000
```

Comparing the standardised values of *lam1* and *lam2* with the amount of explained variation for these two endogenous variables shown by the *summary* function above ($R^2 = 0.571$ for *cover* and $R^2 = 0.492$ for *NSP*) reveals that these two standardised coefficients represent the proportion of unexplained variation in the respective endogenous variables.

We can also obtain confidence intervals for the coefficients by using a bootstrap method, but they refer to the original (non-standardised) scale:

```
boot.sem2 <- bootSem( sem.2, R=1000)

 1000 bootstrap replications
...
```

To display the bootstrap result, we use the *summary* function on the returned object *boot.sem2*:

```
summary( boot.sem2)
Call: bootSem(model = sem.2, R = 1000)
Lower and upper limits are for the 95 percent perc confidence interval
        Estimate       Bias Std.Error     Lower     Upper
gam2     -0.0633 -5.76e-05   0.00632   -0.0762   -0.0498
gam3     30.3722 -1.34e-01   2.07525   25.9309   34.2257
lam1    338.4232 -3.10e+00  41.14179  253.5958  419.3666
lam2      3.2628 -6.51e-02   0.45390    2.3233    4.1535
lam3      0.4878 -2.29e-03   0.04876    0.3970    0.5837
```

We can also display the path diagram including the estimated coefficients, but for that we must make sure that the *DiagrammeR* package (Iannone, 2019) is also installed in R (it is not automatically installed with the *sem* package):

```
library( DiagrammeR)
pathDiagram( sem.2, style="traditional",
              edge.labels="values",
              edge.colors=c("black", "red"))
```

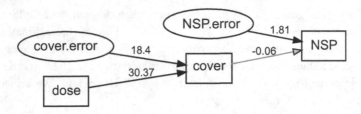

Figure 17.2 Diagram of the estimated SEM model.

The resulting diagram is shown in the default web browser. The *edge.labels* parameter value ensures that the coefficient estimates are used to label the arrows ('edges'). Note that these values are quite different from those seen in Fig. 17.1C, as here the *pathDiagram* function uses non-standardised path coefficients. The distinction between arrows with positive and negative coefficient estimates is done using black and red colour, respectively, but in our illustration (in Fig. 17.2) the red is replaced by grey.

Finally, we illustrate what happens if we change our mind and claim a different structure for the causal effects in the studied system. We may believe, for example, that the weed community richness is directly affected by the fertiliser dose only and that the barley cover is also affected by the dose, but also by the richness of the weed community. For this, we would fit a SEM as follows:

```
sem.mod3 <- specifyEquations()
1: NSP = gam1*dose
2: cover = gam2*NSP + gam3*dose
3: V(cover) = lam1
4: V(NSP) = lam2
5: V(dose) = lam3
6:
Read 5 items
```

```
sem.3 <- sem( sem.mod3, data=chap17)
summary( sem.3, fit.indices=c("AIC","RMSEA","NNFI","CFI"))
 Model Chisquare = -1.07e-13   Df =  0 Pr(>Chisq) = NA
 AIC =  12


 Normalized Residuals
     Min.   1st Qu.    Median      Mean   3rd Qu.       Max.
 -7.95e-16  0.00e+00  0.00e+00  3.23e-16  0.00e+00  2.70e-15


 R-square for Endogenous Variables
  NSP cover
 0.292 0.692


 Parameter Estimates
    Estimate Std Error z value Pr(>|z|)
 gam1  -1.960   0.2777   -7.06  1.67e-12 NSP <- dose
 gam2  -4.591   0.6636   -6.92  4.56e-12 cover <- NSP
```

```
gam3  21.373    2.4084     8.87   7.04e-19 cover <- dose
lam1 242.495   31.1763     7.78   7.36e-15 cover <-> cover
lam2   4.551    0.5852     7.78   7.36e-15 NSP <-> NSP
lam3   0.488    0.0627     7.78   7.36e-15 dose <-> dose
 Iterations =  0
```

This again generates a fully saturated model, as we saw for the *sem.1* model. If we examine the AIC values, then we can see that the quality of the *sem.3* model seems identical with that of the *sem.1* model, and all the estimated path coefficients are shown to be significantly different from zero. In contrast, the amount of explained variation for *NSP* dropped substantially (from $R^2 = 0.492$ to $R^2 = 0.292$).[9] If we try to extend the model by adding *cover* as another cause of *NSP* values then the estimation fails, as our model has now become overdetermined:

```
sem.mod4 <- specifyEquations()
1: NSP = gam1 * dose + gam2* cover
2: cover = gam3 * NSP + gam4*dose
3: V(cover) = lam1
4: V(NSP)   = lam2
5: V(dose)  = lam3
6:

Read 5 items
```

```
sem.4 <  sem( sem.mod4, data=chap17)

Error in sem.default(ram, S = S, N = N, raw = raw,
       data = data, pattern.number = pattern.number,  :
The model has negative degrees of freedom = -1
```

If, in contrast, we try to simplify the *sem.mod3* model by removing the effect of *NSP* on barley cover (removing the effect of *dose* would go against commonsense here), the resulting model is identified as a poor fit for our data, both by the χ^2 test and the fit indices:

```
sem.5 <- sem( sem.mod5, data=chap17)
summary( sem.5, fit.indices=c("AIC","RMSEA","NNFI","CFI"))

 Model Chisquare =  40.3   Df =  1 Pr(>Chisq) = 2.14e-10
 RMSEA index =  0.57   90% CI: (0.428, 0.727)
 Tucker-Lewis NNFI =  0.35
 Bentler CFI =  0.783
 AIC =  50.3
```

---

[9] The amount of explained variability for cover increased slightly (from $R^2 = 0.571$ to $R^2 = 0.692$), but given that the primary task of this study was to understand factors affecting weed species richness, this improvement is not so important.

```
Normalized Residuals
  Min. 1st Qu.  Median   Mean 3rd Qu.   Max.
-2.990  0.000   0.000  -0.664  0.000   0.000


R-square for Endogenous Variables
 NSP cover
0.292 0.571


Parameter Estimates
    Estimate Std Error z value Pr(>|z|)
gam1  -1.960   0.2777   -7.06  1.67e-12 NSP <- dose
gam3  30.372   2.3945   12.68  7.24e-37 cover <- dose
lam1 338.423  43.5093    7.78  7.36e-15 cover <-> cover
lam2   4.551   0.5852    7.78  7.36e-15 NSP <-> NSP
lam3   0.488   0.0627    7.78  7.36e-15 dose <-> dose
Iterations =  0
```

17.5 Reporting Analyses

17.5.1 Methods

To model the direct and indirect effects of fertiliser dose on weed species richness, structural equation models (SEMs; Shipley, 2000) were used and estimated in the *sem* package (Fox, 2006) for R software. The original model of causal relationships is shown in Fig. 17.1A. The model was simplified based on the results of Z approximation-based tests of path coefficients, eliminating non-significant effects from the model. The quality of the final model was evaluated using fit indices.

17.5.2 Results

The resulting SEM is shown in Fig. 17.1C. This model represents an adjustment of our original hypothesis, because the direct effect of fertiliser dose was not supported ($\gamma_1 = -0.09$, $Z = -0.24$, n.s.). The covariances among the variables predicted from the model do not differ from those estimated from the data ($\chi^2 = 0.056$, $p = 0.81$) and the fit indices suggest high model quality ($RMSEA = 0$, $CI_{95} = (0, 0.149)$, Bentler $CFI = 1.0$, Tucker–Lewis $NNFI = 1.02$).

17.6 Recommended Reading

Quinn & Keough (2002), pp. 145–150.

Sokal & Rohlf (2012), pp. 625–644.

P. M. Bentler (1990) Comparative fit indexes in structural models. *Psychological Bulletin*, **107**: 238–246.

J. Fox (2006) Structural equation modeling with the *sem* package in R. *Structural Equation Modeling*, **13**: 465–486.

J. B. Grace (2006) *Structural Equation Modeling and Natural Systems*. Cambridge University Press, Cambridge.

R. Iannone (2019) *DiagrammeR*: graph/network visualization. R package version 1.0.1. https://CRAN
.R-project.org/package=DiagrammeR

R. B. Kline (2015) *Principles and Practice of Structural Equation Modeling*, 4th edn. Guilford Press,
New York.

P. S. Petraitis, A. E. Dunham & P. H. Niewiarowski (1996) Inferring multiple causality: the limitations of
path analysis. *Functional Ecology*, **10**: 421–431.

P. Pyšek & J. Lepš (1991) Response of a weed community to nitrogen fertilization: a multivariate
analysis. *Journal of Vegetation Science*, **2**: 237–244.

B. Shipley (2000) *Cause and Correlation in Biology. A User's Guide to Path Analysis, Structural
Equations and Causal Inference*. Cambridge University Press, Cambridge.

18 Discrete Distributions and Spatial Point Patterns

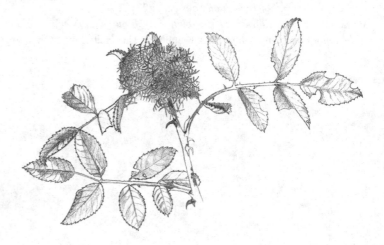

This chapter deals with two of the most commonly encountered discrete distributions (as defined in Section 1.6.1) in biological data: the Poisson distribution and the binomial distribution. We will also discuss the basics of spatial point pattern analysis, given that the Poisson distribution has such a close relationship with random distribution tests for objects or events across space (or time).

18.1 Use Case Examples

1. We counted ticks attached to the body of 86 mice caught in a study area. We ask whether the ticks are distributed across mice in a random manner. If so, all mouse individuals will have the same probability of receiving a tick and the presence of a tick neither increases nor decreases the probability of another tick selecting the same mouse.
2. We established 100 equally sized recording quadrats in the locality of an endangered orchid species, *Epipactis palustris*. The number of orchid individuals was counted in each quadrat. We ask whether the individuals are distributed randomly, independently of each other.
3. Among 120 randomly chosen individuals of dog rose (*Rosa canina*), 56 were found to have galls of a specialist gall-wasp (*Diplolepis rosae*). We want to estimate the percentage of infested rose individuals in the sampled area, together with the corresponding 95% confidence interval.

18.2 Poisson Distribution

The Poisson distribution characterises the counts of random, mutually independent events in a unit of time or space. We can reasonably expect e.g. the counts of bacteria in a unit volume of water to have a Poisson distribution, unless those bacteria occur in clumps. We will primarily use the Poisson distribution to describe this type of bacterial count data if we examine small water volumes and/or if the bacterial density is low. This is because at high mean values, the shape of the Poisson distribution approaches the normal (Gaussian) distribution.

The number of independent island colonisations observed during a period of time can serve as another example. Let us assume that a species occurs on a nearby continent, but it is generally absent on remote islands. This species has, however, a constant probability that its diaspore can be transferred from the continent to the islands (such transfer does not necessarily mean a successful colonisation). If we can assume that the individual transfer events are mutually independent, the number of (observed) transfers over a period of tens (or hundreds) of years will come from a Poisson distribution. Similarly, assuming that individual large earthquakes are mutually independent, the count of their occurrence on a continent across a 10-year period will also come from a Poisson distribution.

The values of a random variable with a Poisson distribution are whole, non-negative numbers, so the zero value is also included, causing difficulties when we attempt to log-transform such variables (see Section 10.2). The probability that this random variable x will have a particular value X for a random draw from a Poisson distribution can be computed as

$$P(x = X) = \frac{e^{-\lambda}\lambda^X}{X!} \tag{18.1}$$

where $X!$ is a factorial of X (e.g. $4! = 4.3.2 = 24$, $6! = 6.5.4.3.2 = 720$, etc.), and λ is the only parameter of the Poisson distribution – the mean value and variance of a Poisson distribution are both equal to λ. When we add two mutually independent random variables $x1$ and $x2$, both coming from Poisson distributions, the result will also have a Poisson distribution. So if the number of earthquakes in a particular geographical area per 10 years has a Poisson distribution, then their counts over centuries will also have a Poisson distribution (if we expect that the subsequent decades are not dependent).

Figure 18.1 shows the shape of a Poisson distribution for a range of λ parameter values. You can see that this distribution is positively skewed, particularly for low values of λ. For higher λ values it starts to resemble the normal distribution. The skewness of a Poisson distribution decreases with increasing λ (being proportional to $1/\sqrt{\lambda}$) and it is thus sometimes claimed that for $\lambda > 10$, the approximation by the normal distribution is reasonably good.

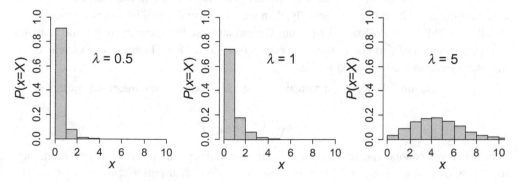

Figure 18.1 Frequency histograms for random variables x coming from Poisson distributions with different λ parameters.

We most often encounter the Poisson distribution in either of the following two situations when working with biological data:

1 If a particular variable under investigation is known to have a Poisson distribution (or its distribution can be approximated in that way), this implies that the distribution is positively skewed and its variance is not independent of the mean value. Both aspects break the model assumptions when we use such a variable as the response variable in regression or ANOVA models. The recommended solution is either to square-root transform the response (see Section 10.4) or – preferably – use a generalised linear model (Chapter 15) with an assumed Poisson distribution.

2 We need to determine whether events of a particular type take place independently, at random spatial positions or randomly across some observed period of time. This can be done by comparing their counts with a Poisson distribution. This approach is frequently used in ecology and in parasitology (see our use case examples 1 and 2 in Section 18.1). We typically count the individuals present in/adhered to the experimental units. If there are no natural experimental units, we must divide the space (most often just a plane) or temporal line into plots or time intervals of a particular size (scale) before counting. If we conclude that the counts match a Poisson distribution reasonably well, then this implies a random distribution of individuals across the units.

Comparisons with the Poisson distribution are frequently based on a χ^2 goodness-of-fit test (Chapter 2). First we estimate the λ value using a sample mean ($\bar{X}$) and then we can estimate the probabilities for individual count values using Eq. (18.1). We then multiply the expected probabilities by sample size to calculate the expected frequencies. We can compare these with the observed frequencies using the goodness-of-fit test. Categories with low expected frequencies are usually merged with the neighbouring ones. The number of degrees of freedom for the reference χ^2 distribution is equal to the (final) number of categories being compared minus two. Alternatively, we can compare our counts with a Poisson distribution using the Kolmogorov–Smirnov test (see Section 4.6.2).

18.3 Comparing the Variance with the Mean to Measure Spatial Distribution

There is an alternative approach which is frequently used to evaluate whether observed counts adhere to a Poisson distribution, and it is based on the mean value being equal to the variance in a Poisson distribution. If we compare these statistics, both of which are estimated from our data sample, and they differ substantially, then we can reject the null hypothesis which states that the variable has a Poisson distribution. We can also use the variance/mean ratio to judge the spatial pattern of particular objects or events (see Table 18.1). Examples of various types of spatial patterns are illustrated in Fig. 18.2.

We use the following test statistic to test the equality of the mean and variance:

$$\frac{s^2}{\bar{X}}(n-1) \tag{18.2}$$

If the observed counts represent a sample from a population with a Poisson distribution, then the test statistic in Eq. (18.2) comes from an approximate χ^2 distribution with $n-1$ degrees of freedom (where n is the sample size, i.e. the number of studied experimental units – plots, hosts – not the number of observed objects or events!). We reject the null hypothesis at an α

Table 18.1 *Types of spatial pattern, with the corresponding statistical properties and ecological causes (applicable mainly to population ecology studies)*

Spatial pattern type	Corresponding statistical distribution of observed counts	Variance/ mean ratio	Dependency among occurrences of individuals/ events	Ecological processes most often responsible
Regular (uniform)	e.g. binomial or uniform	<1	presence of one individual in a unit reduces the probability of occurrence of others	within-species competition, territorial behaviour
Random	Poisson	1	occurrence of individuals mutually independent	
Aggregated	contagious (e.g. negative binomial, Neyman)	>1	presence of one individual in a unit raises the probability of occurrence of others	reproductive strategies, environmental heterogeneity

level on two occasions: when the calculated statistic is smaller than the $\alpha/2 \times 100\%$ quantile of the χ^2 distribution (i.e. the estimated variance is significantly smaller than the mean, and the objects are distributed, to some extent, in a regular manner), or when the value of the test statistic is larger than the $(1 - \alpha/2) \times 100\%$ quantile (i.e. the variance is larger than the mean, corresponding to an aggregated spatial pattern of objects). We can alternatively perform a one-sided test when asking e.g. whether the variance is significantly higher than the mean. In such a case, we test the null hypothesis that the variance is equal to or smaller than the mean, the critical value is then the $(1 - \alpha) \times 100\%$ quantile of the χ^2 distribution.

Each of the statistical tests of spatial randomness (i.e. χ^2 goodness-of-fit test comparing count frequencies with a Poisson distribution, and the χ^2 test based on statistics from Eq. (18.2)) has its strong and weak points. The sample variance can be equal to the mean even when the statistical distribution is quite different from a Poisson distribution. When this occurs, the deviation will be apparent in the goodness-of-fit test. In contrast, comparing the variance and mean shows the direction in which the spatial pattern deviates from randomness and also allows for a one-sided test.

> **When we demonstrate that the sample variance is larger than the mean, we usually state that the events (or individuals) are aggregated. On the contrary, if the variance is smaller than the mean, we speak about some regular or uniform pattern of events (individuals).[1]**

An aggregated spatial pattern of events/objects can be caused either by their interdependency or by sampling units (such as the mice on which the ticks were counted) differing in the probability that the event/object occurs there. For example, an aggregated occurrence of ticks on mice can be the result of either a particular mouse being more attractive to the ticks, or

---

[1] Be careful to differentiate between statistical distribution and spatial pattern. Individuals located in space have a particular spatial pattern (or spatial arrangement, or also sometimes spatial distribution, which might be misleading). But once we start to count them within sampling units, we obtain a random variable with a particular statistical distribution. The relationship between these two characteristics is reported in Table 18.1 and also in Fig. 18.2.

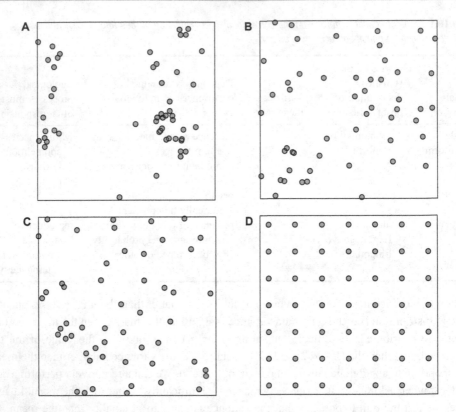

Figure 18.2 Different types of spatial pattern for individuals (or events) in a continuous space: (A) aggregated, (B) random, (C) little more regular, (D) fully uniform on a rectangular grid.

because particular habitats are more infested and so a mouse moving through such a place has a higher probability of hosting multiple ticks. Similarly, plant individuals can be spatially aggregated, either thanks to their dispersal (offsprings are located close to their parents) or due to the presence of areas with particularly favourable conditions for establishment and growth.

The last example of plant individuals nicely illustrates two important aspects of spatial point patterns that we must distinguish when studying the randomness of point locations. The essential property of spatial randomness is the independence among the points or events. But the tests outlined assume that a random pattern has an additional property, namely a constant density of points across the study area. Only the combination of both properties creates what is called *complete spatial randomness* (CSR), which is the property that the above statistical tests check for. But we can also find real-world spatial patterns (such as the plant individuals in our above example) where the locations of individuals are mutually independent, but the density of their occurrence (parameter λ of the Poisson distribution) varies across space, e.g. due to changing environmental conditions. This represents a pattern resulting from *inhomogeneous Poisson processes* (Baddeley et al., 2015).

In population ecology studies, we usually find that populations of most species have an aggregated distribution in space. The counts of individuals per sampling unit then correspond to a 'contagious' statistical distribution, most frequently approximated by the negative binomial or Neyman Type A statistical distributions.

When we find a more regular, or even uniform, spatial distribution of individuals in a population, we usually interpret it as a consequence of competition between neighbouring individuals. Likewise, we suspect competition is at play when we see the intensity of aggregation decreasing through time. It is advantageous to use *Lloyd's index of patchiness* (Lloyd, 1967) when studying these biological patterns:

$$\frac{\frac{s^2}{\overline{X}} - 1}{\overline{X}} + 1 \tag{18.3}$$

If the individuals present in sampling plots die out independently of the local density (of the number of individuals present), the value of Lloyd's index does not change. But if the individuals from more densely occupied units have a higher mortality, the value of Lloyd's index decreases. This statistic is therefore suitable for the detection of density-dependent thinning processes. But if we want to indisputably prove such processes, then we must experimentally manipulate the population density.

Oftentimes sampling units are naturally defined when studying the spatial patterns of individuals (ticks on mouse specimens, mites in the tubes of bracket fungi). But when we study such patterns in continuous space (e.g. plant individuals within a locality), we must decide upon the size of the sampling units. Obviously, this decision affects the results of our analyses. If the individuals are not distributed in a random manner and form groups of a particular size, then our conclusions will depend on the sampling unit size, and how it relates to the typical clump size. There is a range of methods called *spatial pattern analysis* that became particularly common in ecological research. These methods attempt to determine the size of individual groups and estimate the intensity of aggregation at different spatial scales. The data for such studies are often collected using quadrats arranged into rectangular grids or into linear transects. However, these methods are used less and less, becoming of mostly historical importance.

18.4 Spatial Pattern Analyses Based on the K-function

Nowadays, spatial pattern analyses are most often based on mapped point data, where the position of each individual is characterised by its coordinates, usually within a rectangle plot (similar to the data in our example 2). The *K-function analysis* counts the number of neighbours for each individual and compares it with a value expected for a spatial pattern with known properties.[2] The observations considered as neighbours are defined based on a chosen maximum distance value. A larger number of neighbours than is expected signifies the presence of clumping on the corresponding spatial scale, and a smaller number than expected indicates some regularity. When we vary this distance limit, we obtain a function describing the distribution of observations at different spatial scales. The expected value of the *K-function* for a random spatial pattern increases with the second power of the distance, but more often we use its linearised form called the *L-function*.

---

[2] Typically with complete spatial randomness, i.e. originating from a homogeneous Poisson process. However, an inhomogeneous Poisson process has recently become more commonly used as a null model.

But the change of neighbour count with increasing distance, represented by the K- (or L-)*function*, summarises only one of the important properties of spatial point patterns. This is why other types of spatial functions were developed, such as the *F-function* (cumulative function of distances from randomly chosen coordinates to the nearest observation) or *G-function* (cumulative function of distances from existing observations to their nearest neighbour). We can also use the *J-function*, calculated from the previous two functions using the formula $J = (1 - G)/(1 - F)$. A value of 1 for the *J-function* corresponds to a random spatial distribution (on the corresponding spatial scale), a value of <1 suggests an aggregated (clumped) distribution and a value of >1 reveals a more regular spatial distribution of observations.

Testing deviations from the null model is usually based on simulations, where we generate the selected null model distribution of individuals many times (e.g. 1000 times) and calculate the K-function (or other function) for each of the simulated patterns. This provides the distribution of K-function values for each spatial scale, from which we can then estimate 0.025 and 0.975 quantiles (e.g. as the 25th and 975th observation value), and these form the so-called 95% envelope (or we can chose any other, e.g. 99% envelope, in a similar manner). Empirical values outside this envelope are then considered as contradicting the null model.

There are also extensions of the methods for K- and other spatial functions, which take into account not only the observation positions, but also the properties of individual observations (*point marks*). The use of these extensions is called *marked point pattern analysis*. For example, we map the positions of individual trees in a forest patch, and we also know the species identity and size of each tree. This allows us to test very specific hypotheses about spatial relationships among the individuals of different tree species or among the individuals of different size classes, etc. Recently, there has been a massive upscaling of plots where all individual trees are mapped (areas of up to 50 ha). In fact, these are becoming standard target plots in forest research, yielding huge datasets (small datasets generally do not permit trustworthy analyses of this type). These datasets enable us to reliably estimate spatial pattern characteristics and use various null models, however as you can imagine, their analyses can become computationally challenging (50 ha plots often contain hundreds of thousands of individuals belonging to hundreds of species). You can find additional information about more advanced models in the excellent book of Baddeley et al. (2015). A very light introduction to spatial statistics can be found in Diggle (2013).

18.5 Binomial Distribution

Let us assume we perform n independent trials (or observations) and the results of each can be evaluated by assigning the case into one of two categories, often referred to as *success* vs. *failure*, although such labels can be controversial at times. For example, we can sample n individuals of a rodent species (randomly and independently chosen from a reference population) and observe whether they are females or males. Alternatively, we can apply different treatments to plants and observe whether they survive.

The number of successes (labelled x) is then a random variable with a *binomial distribution*. This distribution is characterised by two parameters: p is the probability of success in a single trial (for a single case) and n is the number of trials (observations).

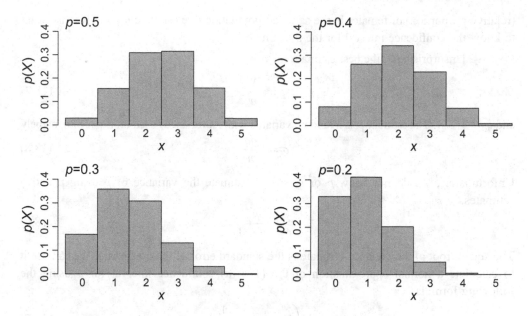

Figure 18.3 Binomial distributions with $n = 5$ but with different p parameter values (q is always equal to $1 - p$).

The probability that a random variable x, with a binomial distribution, will achieve a particular (integer) value X is then

$$P(x = X) = \frac{n!}{X!(n - X)!} p^X q^{n-X} \tag{18.4}$$

where q is the probability of failure ($q = 1 - p$). The mean value of a binomial distribution is

$$\mu_x = np \tag{18.5}$$

and its variance is

$$\sigma_x^2 = npq \tag{18.6}$$

If $p = q = 0.5$, then the binomial distribution is symmetrical, otherwise it is asymmetrical (see Fig. 18.3). When the value of the p parameter is very small and n is relatively large, the binomial distribution approaches the Poisson distribution discussed earlier in this chapter. When the value of p is not too close to 0 or 1 and n is sufficiently large, the binomial distribution approaches a normal distribution.

One of the frequent uses of a binomial distribution in biology[3] is estimating and comparing the relative proportions of events. For instance (and in addition to example 3 given in Section 18.1), we can estimate the proportion of females in a bat population. We catch n bat individuals and find that X of those individuals are females. We ask what is the percentage

---

[3] Another important area is predicting the probability of an event based on the values of a set of numerical and/or categorical predictors, using GLMs (see Chapter 15) or their various extensions (generalised additive models, GAM or generalised linear mixed-effect models, GLMM).

(relative proportion) of females in the sampled population (we estimate p), and we also want to know the confidence interval for the p estimate.

Unsurprisingly, the best estimate for p is

$$\hat{p} = \frac{X}{n} \tag{18.7}$$

and $\hat{q} = 1 - \hat{p}$. The estimate $\hat{p}$ is a random variable with its variance based on Eq. (18.6), namely

$$\sigma_{\hat{p}}^2 = \frac{pq}{n} \tag{18.8}$$

Unfortunately, we do not know p or q, so we estimate the variance of p using p and q estimates:

$$s_{\hat{p}}^2 = \frac{\hat{p}\hat{q}}{n-1} \tag{18.9}$$

The square root of the variance estimate is the standard error of the $\hat{p}$ estimate. We can use it to calculate a normal approximation of the $(1 - \alpha)$ confidence interval for p using the following formula:

$$\hat{p} \pm \left(Z_{\left(1-\frac{\alpha}{2}\right)} s_{\hat{p}} + \frac{1}{2n} \right) \tag{18.10}$$

where $Z(1 - \alpha/2)$ is a $100 \times (1 - \alpha/2)\%$ quantile of the standard normal distribution, $N(0, 1)$. Table 18.2 provides a rough guideline as to when it is reasonable to use such a normal approximation: the more the p estimate differs from 0.5, the larger n must be.

If we do not trust the normal approximation, we proceed by using the following formulas (confidence intervals are then non-symmetrical, but this matches the non-symmetrical shape of the binomial distribution; see Fig. 18.3):

$$CI_{low} = \frac{X}{X + (n - X + 1)F_{\left(1-\frac{\alpha}{2}\right),v1,v2}} \tag{18.11}$$

where $F_{(1 - \alpha/2),v1,v2}$ is a $100 \times (1 - \alpha/2)\%$ quantile of an F distribution with the following degrees of freedom: $v1 = 2(n - X + 1)$ and $v2 = 2X$.

$$CI_{high} = \frac{(X + 1)F_{\left(1-\frac{\alpha}{2}\right),v'1,v'2}}{n - X + (X + 1)F_{\left(1-\frac{\alpha}{2}\right),v'1,v'2}} \tag{18.12}$$

where the degrees of freedom are $v'1 = 2(X + 1)$ and $v'2 = 2(n - X)$.

Table 18.2 *Guidelines for when it is appropriate to use a normal approximation for the confidence interval of a binomial distribution parameter p*

$\hat{p}$	$n \geq$
0.5	30
0.4 or 0.6	50
0.3 or 0.7	80
0.2 or 0.8	200
0.1 or 0.9	600

Beside the construction of confidence intervals, we can also compare the proportions of p between groups. For example, if location A had 15 females out of 60 individuals and location B had 10 females out of 50 individuals, we can ask whether the relative proportion of females differs between the populations of the two locations. In most cases, however, it is easiest to use a contingency table and a χ^2 test (Section 3.1.2) or, if the observed frequencies are low, the Fisher exact test (Section 3.1.5).

Sometimes we ask how large a sample must be to estimate the p parameter with a particular precision. If we wish the standard error of the $\hat{p}$ estimate to be equal to w, the required sample size is then

$$n = \frac{pq}{w^2}$$
(18.13)

Note that with the computed sample size n, the mean value of the standard error will be w. So for our collected sample, the standard error will be larger than w with probability 0.5 and smaller than w with the same probability.

So if we assume that approximately 20% of individuals in a population have a particular mutation, and we want to estimate their percentage with a standard error below 1% (so that the 95% confidence interval for p will then be approximately equal to our estimate ± 2%), we need to sample and examine $n = (0.2 \times 0.8)/0.01^2 = 1600$ individuals. This estimation procedure for n is rather rough, but sufficient in many cases, particularly if our ideas about the p-value are derived from a 'best professional guess'. If we need to estimate the required sample size more precisely, and consequently the width of the confidence interval for p, then it is better to use power analysis of binomial proportion, introduced at the end of Section 18.7.

18.6 Example Data

We caught 86 mice in our study area and counted the number of ticks on their bodies. The *NumTicks* variable specifies the count of ticks per individual mouse, while the corresponding value of the *NumMice* variable represents the count of mice found to have that particular tick count. What can we say about the distribution of ticks across mouse individuals?

We studied the distribution of individuals of an endangered orchid species, recording their coordinates in a rectangular sampling area of 100×100 m. The *xPos* and *yPos* variables specify the coordinates of individual plants. We want to characterise the spatial pattern of orchid individuals (by testing whether the pattern deviates from randomness).

Finally, we analyse the data from example 3 in Section 18.1, but there are no data needed from the spreadsheet: 56 out of 120 rose brushes were infested.

18.7 How to Proceed in R

We first expand the number of ticks on individual mice, which is provided in a condensed form in the variables *NumMice* and *NumTicks*:

```
nPar <- with( chap18a, rep( NumTicks, NumMice))
length( nPar)
```
```
[ 1]  86
```

We can compare tick counts with a Poisson distribution using the Kolmogorov–Smirnov test:

```
ks.test( nPar, "ppois", mean( nPar))

        One-sample Kolmogorov-Smirnov test
data:  nPar
D = 0.2047, p-value = 0.001482
alternative hypothesis: two-sided
Warning message:
In ks.test(nPar, "ppois", mean(nPar)) :
  ties should not be present for the Kolmogorov-Smirnov test
```

While the function output suggests there is strong evidence against the null hypothesis that there is agreement with a Poisson distribution, it also warns that the tied values represent a problem for this test, so we should take its results with caution.

Alternative ways of comparing with the Poisson distribution are available in the *fitdistrplus* package (Delignette-Muller & Dutang, 2015):

```
library( fitdistrplus)
fit.pois <- fitdist( nPar, "pois")
```

After we fit our data to some selected distribution (here Poisson), we can see the results (particularly the estimate of the λ parameter and its standard error) using the *summary* function:

```
summary( fit.pois)
Fitting of the distribution ' pois ' by maximum likelihood
Parameters :
        estimate Std. Error
lambda 2.453488  0.1689051
Loglikelihood:  -221.0932   AIC:  444.1865   BIC:  446.6408
```

A graphical summary is useful for comparing the distribution of our data with that expected for a Poisson distribution:

```
plot( fit.pois)
```

On the resulting graph (Fig. 18.4), we can see that there is a higher than expected frequency of both zero and high tick counts compared with a Poisson distribution with the same mean value.

We can also test if our data conform to a Poisson distribution by employing a χ^2 statistic-based goodness-of-fit test:

```
gofstat( fit.pois)
Chi-squared statistic:  50.89291
Degree of freedom of the Chi-squared distribution:  4
Chi-squared p-value:  2.350246e-10
```

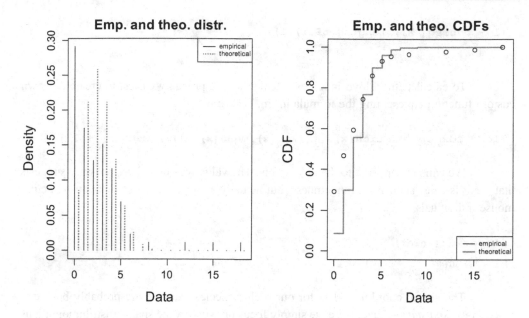

Figure 18.4 Graphical summary showing how much the distribution of the mouse ticks data agrees with a Poisson distribution.

```
Chi-squared table:
       obscounts  theocounts
<= 0  25.000000    7.395405
<= 1  15.000000   18.144541
<= 2  11.000000   22.258710
<= 3  13.000000   18.203829
<= 4  10.000000   11.165721
>  4  12.000000    8.831793


Goodness-of-fit criteria
                                    1-mle-pois
Akaike's Information Criterion       444.1865
Bayesian Information Criterion       446.6408
```

We again conclude that there is a strong discordance of tick counts with the Poisson distribution.

We now compute the χ^2 statistic directly by comparing the variance with the mean (based on Eq. (18.2)):

```
X2 <- var( nPar) * (length( nPar)-1) / mean( nPar)
X2
```

```
[1] 324.9716
```

We can now compare it with the reference χ^2 distribution (the 0 value is the estimated significance level, although it is not altogether very precise):

```
(1 - pchisq( X2, length( nPar)-1))
[1] 0
```

To calculate the Lloyd index of patchiness, it is probably easiest to create our own custom function representing the formula in Eq. (18.3):

```
lloyd.idx <- function(x) { ((var(x)/mean(x))-1) / mean(x) + 1 }
```

We can now apply it to the tick counts. The value we obtain here not only suggests that there is a deviation from randomness, but actually an aggregation of ticks on particular mouse individuals:

```
lloyd.idx( nPar)
[1] 2.150686
```

The spatial coordinate data for our orchid species example are probably best analysed in the *spatstat* package. Here we simply focus on whether the spatial distribution aligns with a model based on complete spatial randomness. However, the *spatstat* library contains a wide range of functions for analysing point patterns, including those which estimate and test *K*-, *L*-, *F*-, *G*- and *J-functions*. In addition, the *spatstat* library has functions for building statistical models that allow us to explain point pattern deviations from randomness (both in the direction of aggregation and towards regularity) using measured predictors, such as some environmental characteristics:

```
library( spatstat)
ppp.orch <- with( chap18b,
                  ppp( x=xPos, y=yPos, c(0,100), c(0,100)))
```

We first created an object of the spatial point pattern type. This was done with the *ppp* function, passing to it the *X* and *Y* coordinates from the *chap18b* data frame, together with a simple definition of a rectangular area which represents the sampled space (the range of *x* and *y* coordinates in an implied rectangle). Next we use the *quadrat.test* function to overlay the sampled area with a rectangular grid of quadrats and then count the observations falling into individual quadrats. The counts are compared with the expected frequencies using a goodness-of-fit test.

```
quadrat.test( ppp.orch)

        Chi-squared test of CSR using quadrat counts
        Pearson X2 statistic
data:  ppp.orch
X2 = 41.429, df = 24, p-value = 0.02988
alternative hypothesis: two.sided
Quadrats: 5 by 5 grid of tiles
Warning message:
Some expected counts are small; chi^2 approximation may be inaccurate
```

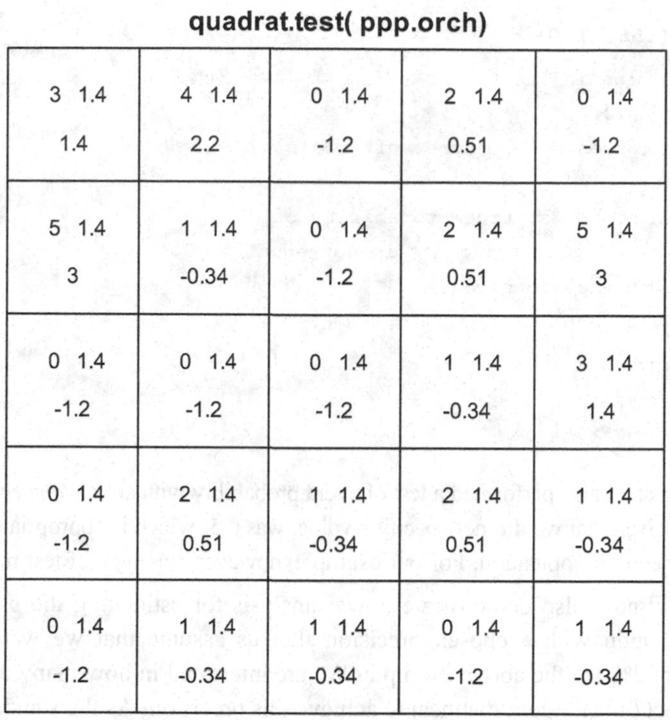

quadrat.test(ppp.orch)

3 1.4	4 1.4	0 1.4	2 1.4	0 1.4
1.4	2.2	-1.2	0.51	-1.2
5 1.4	1 1.4	0 1.4	2 1.4	5 1.4
3	-0.34	-1.2	0.51	3
0 1.4	0 1.4	0 1.4	1 1.4	3 1.4
-1.2	-1.2	-1.2	-0.34	1.4
0 1.4	2 1.4	1 1.4	2 1.4	1 1.4
-1.2	0.51	-0.34	0.51	-0.34
0 1.4	1 1.4	1 1.4	0 1.4	1 1.4
-1.2	-0.34	-0.34	-1.2	-0.34

Figure 18.5 Graphical summary of the quadrat test where the spatial pattern of orchid individuals was tested for complete spatial randomness.

As we can see, the results of the test suggests a mild deviation from the null hypothesis, so there appears to be a non-random distribution. But we should treat the results with caution, given the warning regarding low values for expected counts. Actually all the expected frequencies are 1.4, as can be seen from the following visualisation of the quadrat test (Fig. 18.5):

```
plot( quadrat.test( ppp.orch))
```

Each square represents a single quadrat of the grid defined by the *quadrat.test* function and gives the observed count (upper left corners), expected count (upper right corners, 1.4 everywhere) and also the contribution of a particular quadrat to the resulting χ^2 statistic (square root of $(O - E)^2/E$ in the lower part of each square). Note that the program decides the size of the quadrats by itself, and this decision affects the result.[4] An analysis using the methods within the K-function family would be more informative as it would suggest scales of spatial aggregation, however the present dataset is too small for most of these methods.

Next we use the *binom.test* function to estimate the p parameter and its confidence interval for the relative frequency of gall-infested dog rose shrubs:

---

[4] The number of columns and rows to divide the area can be specified by the *nx* and *ny* parameters, which are both set to 5 by default.

```
binom.test( 56, 120)

        Exact binomial test
data:  56 and 120
number of successes = 56, number of trials = 120,
                                p-value = 0.523
alternative hypothesis: true probability of
                        success is not equal to 0.5
95 percent confidence interval:
 0.3750729 0.5599445
sample estimates:
probability of success
          0.4666667
```

The function also performed a test of event probability with an *a priori* chosen value. The implicit setting, given that we did not specify a value, was 0.5, which is appropriate e.g. for testing the gender balance in a population. For our example, however, this type of test makes no sense.

We will now also demonstrate power analysis for estimating the p parameter of a binomial distribution with a chosen precision. Let us assume that we want to achieve a standard error of 2% for the above example. We are interested in how many dog rose bushes we need to select (in a random manner) to achieve this precision. As the standard error of 2% leads to a confidence interval spanning c. 4% either side of the estimated p,[5] we can replace our original question by asking what number of observations allows us to distinguish (at significance level $\alpha = 0.05$) the observed proportion of 46.7% from a proportion 4% smaller, i.e. 42.7%. We use the *pwr* package (Champely, 2018) to perform this calculation:

```
library( pwr)
pwr.p.test( h=ES.h( 0.467, 0.427), sig.level=0.05,
            power=0.8)
proportion power calculation for binomial distribution
      (arcsine transformation)
            h = 0.08047572
            n = 1211.928
    sig.level = 0.05
        power = 0.8
  alternative = two.sided
```

Hence we need to observe at least 1212 rose bushes if we require at least an 80% chance that we correctly reject the 4% difference, from our proportion of 45.7%, at a significance level no larger than 0.05. Please note that if you apply the 4% difference in the alternative direction (i.e. by specifying the h parameter as *ES.h*(0.467, 0.507)), you get a slightly different recommendation ($n = 1225$), due to the p estimate variation changing with the p-value. But in practical terms, the recommended sample size is virtually identical.

---

[5] At least under the normal (Gaussian distribution-based) approximation, where the confidence interval is symmetrical around the p estimate.

18.8 Reporting Analyses

18.8.1 Methods

The randomness of the distribution of ticks across mice was tested by comparing the observed counts with a Poisson distribution using a χ^2 goodness-of-fit test. The nature of the observed point pattern was summarised using Lloyd's index of patchiness (Lloyd, 1967).

We estimated the confidence interval for the frequency of gall-wasps across dog rose bushes in the studied area using the method of Clopper & Pearson (1934).

18.8.2 Results

The distribution of ticks among host individuals was significantly aggregated ($\chi^2_4 = 50.9$, $p < 0.001$, Lloyd index value $L = 2.151$).

The average rate of infestation of rose bushes was 46.7%, with a 95% confidence interval (37.5%, 56.0%).

18.9 Recommended Reading

Poisson and binomial distributions

Zar (2010), pp. 518–604.

Sokal & Rohlf (2012), pp. 59–87.

S. Champely (2018) *pwr*: basic functions for power analysis. R package version 1.2-2. https://cran.r-project.org/package=pwr

C. J. Clopper & E. S. Pearson (1934) The use of confidence or fiducial limits illustrated in the case of the binomial. *Biometrika*, **26**: 404–413.

Spatial pattern analysis

A. Baddeley, E. Rubak & R. Turner (2015) *Spatial Point Patterns: Methodology and Applications wih R*. Chapman & Hall/CRC, Boca Raton, FL.

M. L. Delignette-Muller & C. Dutang (2015) *fitdistrplus*: an R package for fitting distributions. *Journal of Statistical Software*, **64**(4): 1–34. http://www.jstatsoft.org/v64/io4/

P. J. Diggle (2013) *Statistical Analysis of Spatial and Spatio-Temporal Point Patterns*, 3rd edn. Chapman & Hall/CRC, Boca Raton, FL.

M. Lloyd (1967) Mean crowding. *Journal of Animal Ecology*, **36**: 1–30.

19 Survival Analysis

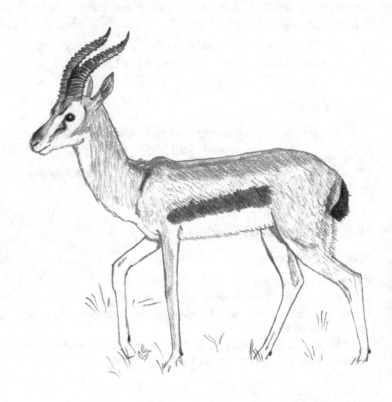

19.1 Use Case Examples

The methods of survival analysis were developed primarily in medical research, but they are occasionally applied to biological data concerning the survival (time to death) of individuals, but also to the temporal dynamics of other processes: how long it takes for a seed to germinate, how long it takes for prey exposed in the field to be taken by a predator, etc. Here we present two examples focusing on the death of individuals.

1. We studied the survival of seedlings in an experimental grassland. Seedlings of three species were planted in two locations in a meadow, differing in soil moisture. The seedlings were then monitored for 10 weeks. For each specimen, we know either the day when it was found dead or disappeared, or whether the seedling survived throughout the whole observational period. We want to know whether the survival (or death) rate differs between the three plant species and whether the survival rates differ between the two locations in the meadow. Additionally, we ask how many seedlings should be planted so that we see a sufficient number of them surviving throughout an eight-week experiment.

2. A large number of individuals of an antelope species were followed over an extended period of time (almost three years), with some of them having a radio transmitter attached to their neck. Additionally, we know how old each individual was at the start of the experiment (in years) and also their initial weight. Some of the antelopes died during the investigative period and we know the day of this determination, while others survived or disappeared from the area. We are interested in the effect that the attachment of a radio-collar might have on the animal's chances of survival (does the chance increase or decrease, and if so, to what extent?), but we are aware that the individual's weight and/ or age might also affect their survival.

19.2 Survival Function and Hazard Rate

Statistical models of survival describe the lifetime of individuals or duration of events. We can use these models to predict this length of time according to the objects' membership in a particular group, e.g. male/female, or by using models with multiple explanatory variables.

An important feature of the data typically underlying survival analysis models is that, for some cases (individuals), we do not know their lifespan precisely – they might outlive the observation period or we might even start by observing objects of an unknown age. The seedlings in our example 1 were all planted at a known age, but some of them lived longer than the 10 weeks they were observed. We call these *censored observations* and they correspond to *right censoring*. If we start our observations on individuals of an unknown age, they would represent *left censored* observations (if the date of their death was known). The third possibility, which is supported by few analytical methods, occurs when we know neither the starting nor the terminal date of a lifetime (*interval censored* observations).

For a group of observations on survival times, the usual way of summarising them graphically is the *survival function* (S_t), illustrated in Fig. 19.1 for our example 1 data (using all seedlings in the dataset).

The survival function is represented in Fig. 19.1 by a solid line descending in a staircase-like fashion from the top left to the bottom right corner. It shows the probability that, for a particular seedling age,[1] a seedling will live up to that age. The estimated probability can be read on the vertical axis. Survival function values, estimated for the times when a change in the number of surviving (living) seedlings was observed (i.e. at the time of field visits), were calculated using the *Kaplan–Meier method*, together with standard errors of those estimates. These standard errors are then converted into confidence regions in Fig. 19.1. The $S(t)$ estimates can be calculated for a particular time t using the following formula:

$$\hat{S}_{KM}(t) = \prod_{t_i < t} \frac{r(t_i) - d(t_i)}{r(t_i)} \tag{19.1}$$

where $r(t_i)$ is the number of individuals still living at time t_i (i.e. being at risk in that time), $d(t_i)$ is the number of observed deaths among those $r(t_i)$ individuals, taking place at time t_i (or earlier, but after the time of the previous visit) and the Π symbol represents multiplication. The estimate is based on a traditional rule that the probability of surviving over two time intervals,

---

[1] Presented on the horizontal axis, and assuming incorrectly that the seedlings were planted at age 0.

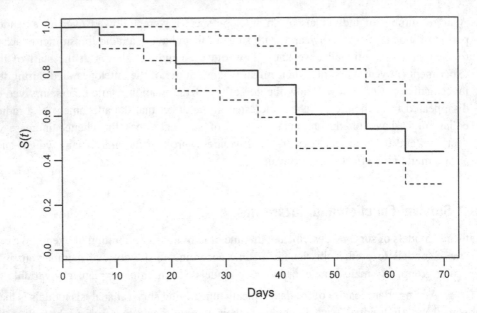

Figure 19.1 Survival curve for the seedling survival experiment, combining both locations and all plant species. The dashed lines are the limits of the 95% confidence region.

e.g. years, can be calculated as a product of the probability that you survive the first year and the probability that you survive the second year (provided you are alive after the first year).

When we describe the distribution of lifespan values t for a population of observed individuals with a cumulative distribution function $F(t)$ (see Section 1.6.2), its value will represent – for a given lifespan length t – the probability that a randomly chosen individual will live t time units or less, i.e. that it, at the latest, dies at age t. The $F(t)$ function therefore increases from 0 to 1, from left to right (if time t is on the horizontal scale), and it has a simple relationship with the survival function, being its 1-complement:

$$S(t) = 1 - F(t) \tag{19.2}$$

Values of any cumulative distribution function $F(t)$ can be calculated by integrating ('summing up' in the case of a non-continuous variable) the density distribution function values, which we will label as $f(t)$ for a lifespan value t. The value of $f(t)$ therefore expresses the probability that a randomly chosen individual will die at a particular age t. By combining the $f(t)$ and $S(t)$ values, we can define another characteristic that holds a prominent place in survival analysis, the *hazard rate* $\lambda(t)$:

$$\lambda(t) = \frac{f(t)}{S(t)} \tag{19.3}$$

So the hazard rate is defined as the probability that an individual – if it managed to survive until time t^2 – will die at that particular time. If this is difficult to grasp, we suggest you simply see the hazard rate as an immediate risk of death at a particular age. If we study various kinds of organisms throughout their full lifecycle, we can expect to find either a constant hazard rate,

---

[2] Hence the division by the $S(t)$ value, which adjusts the $f(t)$ probability so that it does not account for the proportion of individuals that already died before time t.

or their hazard rate might be increasing at older ages, or alternatively we might see the highest hazard rate in early life stages, etc. In the case of our seedlings, we can expect a constant hazard rate or an increased value of $\lambda(t)$ in the first weeks, before the replanted seedlings settle in their new environment.

We can define a cumulative function even for the hazard rate, which is labelled as $\Lambda(t)$ and defined as follows:

$$\Lambda(t) = \int_0^t \lambda(t)dt = -\ln(S(t)) \qquad (19.4)$$

The way the Λ is defined in the last part of Eq. (19.4) suggests that we might plot the $S(t)$ function on a log-transformed scale. The shape of the resulting curve can then be compared with three theoretical types of survival risk that are well known from population biology textbooks: Type I where there is an increase in mortality in later life stages; Type III where there is an increase in mortality in juvenile stages; and Type II where there is constant mortality (hazard rate), represented by a descending straight line in a graph with a log-transformed $S(t)$.

19.3 Differences in Survival Among Groups

One of the simplest questions we can ask about the survival dynamics of individuals is whether the survival curves differ between two or more groups of individuals, e.g. males and females, various population cohorts, different species as in example 1 of Section 19.1, etc. The null hypothesis being tested assumes an identical distribution of survival times across the groups being compared.

Harrington & Fleming (1982) published a set of test procedures comparing two or more $S(t)$ curves, differing in the weight given to various ages of the objects under investigation. All the test variants (chosen by selecting a value of a single, continuous parameter ρ within a range from 0 to 1) calculate the expected frequencies of deaths and compare them with observed frequencies using a χ^2 test statistic. This includes the most frequently used *log-rank test* (also known as the Mantel–Haenszel test) with ρ value set to 0.

These tests, which compare across groups, are seen as non-parametric tests, although they use a χ^2 statistic. This is because they are based on non-parametrically estimated survival curves. The tests are usually performed in a two-sided manner for a symmetrical null hypothesis, but for a dataset with just two groups we can also test a one-sided hypothesis that *the survival rate is higher in one group than in the other*.

19.4 Cox Proportional Hazard Model

Cox proportional hazard models are a major class of statistical models allowing us to examine and test the effects of one or multiple predictors on the life expectancy of an object, often an individual. Unlike methods comparing survival of two or more groups, introduced in Section 19.3, the Cox model does not refer directly to a survival curve, but to a curve describing the change in hazard rate ($\lambda(t)$, see Eq. (19.3)) with the age of an individual or object.[3]

---

[3] Note that the hazard rate curve can be calculated from an estimated survival curve, as shown in Eq. (19.3).

The Cox model assumes that there is a common hazard rate curve, usually labelled as the *baseline hazard rate curve*, $\lambda_0(t)$, which is then modified in a multiplicative way by the effect of some chosen predictors. The baseline hazard rate curve is estimated non-parametrically, similarly to the way the survival curve $S(t)$ is estimated by the Kaplan–Meier method. The systematic (non-random) part of the Cox model can be described in the following way for the i-th case:

$$\hat{\lambda}(X_i, t) = \lambda_0(t)e^{\eta_i} \tag{19.5}$$

You will recognise the *baseline hazard rate* at the right side of the equation, but the actual effect of predictors (X_i) is hidden within the η_i value. It represents the same entity seen in GLMs (Chapter 15), namely a linear combination of predictor values:

$$\eta_i = \sum_j \beta_j x_{ij} \tag{19.6}$$

The predictors affect the hazard rate value on an exponential scale, which means that the baseline hazard rate is always multiplied by a positive value which keeps the hazard rate in a sensible range. The effects of individual predictors, represented by the estimated regression coefficients β_j, can be judged either on their original scale or after the exponential transformation. On its original scale, a regression coefficient with a positive value implies an increase in the hazard rate of that case, i.e. represents an effect shortening the lifetime of the case (e.g. individual). Similarly, a negative coefficient implies a decrease in the hazard rate value and hence represents an effect increasing the chance of survival at that particular life stage (t).

When we work with exponentially transformed regression coefficients (often seen in the summaries of Cox models), the negative coefficients are changed into values smaller than 1, while the positive coefficients into values larger than 1. The $\exp(\beta_j)$ value tells you how many times the baseline hazard rate changes with a unit change of the corresponding explanatory variable. This interpretation applies directly to numerical predictors only. As an example, if a Cox model estimates the effect of an individual's weight (kg) with a regression coefficient +0.182, the exponentiated value is then 1.1996 (approximately 1.2) and so we can say that our model predicts that a 1 kg increase in the weight of an individual leads to the hazard rate increasing (approximately) 1.2 times, i.e. by +20%.

As we have seen in previous chapters, we must take into account how categorical predictors are coded in regression models, and this is true for Cox models also. By default, one factor level is taken as a reference level and the regression coefficients are estimated for the remaining factor levels. Such coefficients then express the relative change of the expected response value for individuals belonging to that level, as compared with individuals from the reference group. So if we encoded animal gender by two levels (*female* and *male*, say) and the *female* level is selected as the basis for comparison, we obtain just a single regression coefficient for the gender factor that describes how much higher (or lower) the predicted value for males is when compared with females. So if the *male* level also had a regression coefficient equal to +0.182 (and hence its exponential transformation would be 1.2 – see above), we would say that overall (across the lifespan), the males have a 20% higher hazard rate compared to the females.

Hopefully our description makes it clear that the effect of a particular numerical predictor (or of a particular non-referential factor level) is represented in a Cox proportional hazard model with a single number. This means that the position on a baseline hazard rate curve is multiplied by this effect irrespective of the time (t) value. In other words, the effects of the examined predictors are not supposed to change through the lifetime of observed individuals (or objects). This is an assumption implied by the word *proportional* in the name Cox proportional hazard models. While it simplifies model estimation, we must seriously consider whether this assumption applies to the processes we are studying. In our example 1, we can probably believe that differences among the species of our plant seedlings will affect them to the same extent throughout their lifetime. But for example 2, we might consider it rather inappropriate to assume that wearing a radio-collar has the same effect on survival in the initial stages of life (before the antelopes become accustomed to it), as it does in the later stages. At the very least, we must test the predictors for this proportionality assumption. The recommended tests and diagnostic graphs (Grambsch & Therneau, 1994) proceed by assuming that the predictor effects vary through the lifetime and estimate the corresponding time-dependent regression coefficients based on the model's partial residuals. The test of proportionality is then based on checking that there is no temporal change across each estimated time-dependent coefficient.

19.5 Example Data

Example datasets in the *Chap19* sheet correspond to the use case examples from Section 19.1. The first, regarding the survival of plant seedlings (Šmilauer & Šmilauerová, unpublished data), is in columns *A* to *D* and for each seedling describes its *species*, planting *location* and the *day* it was found dead since the start of the experiment. Only the seedlings with a value of 1 in the last column (*died*) died, the others were right-censored as they were still alive on day 70, the day the experiment ended.

The second dataset (in columns *F* to *J*) represents a (hypothetical) study of antelope survival and how it is affected by animal age and weight, but primarily by the mounting of a collar with a radio-tracking device onto some of the animals. The *time* when the animal was found dead (when the *status* column has a value of 1) is measured in days since the animal was released, animals with a *status* value of 0 have their *time* value based on the date the observation was ended or when their radio-collar (if mounted) ceased to send radio signals. Individuals with a radio-collar are distinguished by having the level *yes* in the *collar* column, and the *age* and *weight* are numerical predictors with, respectively, year and kilogram (kg) units, which were recorded at the time the animal was released.

19.6 How to Proceed in R

The methods of survival analysis introduced in this chapter are implemented within the *survival* package, which is installed alongside R by default. But we must still load it with the *library* command:

```
library( survival)
```

We start by fitting the survival function $S(t)$ for the whole set of seedlings using the *survfit* function:

```
sf.1 <- survfit( Surv( day, died) ~ +1, data=chap19a)
```

A very important practical detail relates to how the response data are specified, namely by enclosing the survival time and survival state variables into a call to the *Surv* function. As we do not distinguish any groups, the right side of the model formula (after the ~ character) simply contains a constant value of 1.

To obtain a very brief summary of the fitted survival function, we can just print the object returned by the *survfit* function:

```
sf.1

Call: survfit(formula = Surv(day, died) ~ +1, data = chap19a)
      n   events   median 0.95LCL 0.95UCL
     30       17       63      43      NA
```

The above summarisation tells you that the estimated curve is based on 30 observations and that among them, 17 deaths ('events') were observed. The *median* value 63 represents the median lifespan. This is accompanied by a 95% confidence interval, but its upper level could not be estimated, hence it is shown as a missing value.

The *summary* function, when applied to an object returned from *survfit*, is not summarising at all. Instead, it prints all the coordinates of the fitted curve, including confidence intervals for $S(t)$ at individual times:

```
summary( sf.1)

Call: survfit(formula = Surv(day, died) ~ +1, data = chap19a)
 time n.risk n.event survival std.err lower 95%CI upper 95%CI
    7     30       1    0.967  0.0328       0.905       1.000
   15     29       1    0.933  0.0455       0.848       1.000
   21     28       3    0.833  0.0680       0.710       0.978
   29     25       1    0.800  0.0730       0.669       0.957
   36     24       2    0.733  0.0807       0.591       0.910
   43     22       4    0.600  0.0894       0.448       0.804
   56     18       2    0.533  0.0911       0.382       0.745
   63     16       3    0.433  0.0905       0.288       0.652
```

Note that the $S(t)$ curve estimate (in the *survival* column) was computed using the Kaplan–Meier method (see Eq. (19.1)). So the first observed death (with one seedling dying, as given by the 1 value in the *n.event* column) happened at *time* 7 and at this time all 30 seedlings were at risk (*n.risk* column). Therefore $S(t = 7) = (30 - 1)/30 = 0.967$, as shown in the *survival* column. At day 15, another seedling died, but there were only 29 seedlings at risk. So we must, according to Eq. (19.1), multiply the present $S(t)$ value (0.967) by $(29 - 1)/29 = 0.9655$. The resulting $S(t = 15)$ is then $0.967 \times 0.9655 = 0.933$, etc.

If we are dealing with larger datasets with more event times, then it can be better to look at a visual summary. We can obtain it (see Fig. 19.1 at the beginning of this chapter) using the following command:

```
plot( sf.1, xlab="days", ylab="S(t)")
```

In Section 19.1 we mentioned that we want to know how many seedlings to plant for an experiment running for eight weeks (i.e. 56 days). When we check Fig. 19.1 (or the output of the *summary* function above), we can see that the lower level of the 95% confidence region for $S(t)$ is at about 0.38 starting at day 56, hence (averaged over both tested places and all three tested species) we should expect no more than 38% of seedlings to be alive at that time. This means that at the beginning of the experiment we need to plant about 2.6 times more seedlings than the number of living replicates required at the end of the experiment.

In Section 19.2 we stressed the advantages of plotting the survival curve values on a log-transformed scale. This can be achieved quite easily with the *log=T* argument added to the call of the *plot* function (graph not shown):

```
plot( sf.1, xlab="days", ylab="S(t)", log=T)
```

If we want to test the differences in survival curves among groups of observations, then we can use the log-rank test. Here we apply the *survdiff* function to test the difference among the three plant species:

```
survdiff( Surv( day, died) ~ species, data=chap19a)
...

             N Observed Expected (O-E)^2/E (O-E)^2/V
species=AM 10        6     5.83   0.00467   0.00776
species=HL 10        5     6.34   0.28331   0.49334
species=PL 10        6     4.82   0.28626   0.43699

 Chisq= 0.6  on 2 degrees of freedom, p= 0.7
```

Based on the resulting Type I error probability ($p = 0.7$), the survival seems largely indistinguishable among the three plant species. But doing the same test on the locations provides a significant difference:

```
survdiff( Surv( day, died) ~ location, data=chap19a)
...

              N Observed Expected (O-E)^2/E (O-E)^2/V
location=dry 15       12     7.08      3.41      6.45
location=wet 15        5     9.92      2.44      6.45

 Chisq= 6.5  on 1 degrees of freedom, p= 0.01
```

... and this is hopefully a sufficient excuse to estimate and plot the survival curves separately for both parts of the experimental site:

```
plot( sf.2, xlab="days", ylab="S(t)", lty=c(1,2))
legend( 10, 0.2, levels(chap19a$location), lty=c(1,2))
```

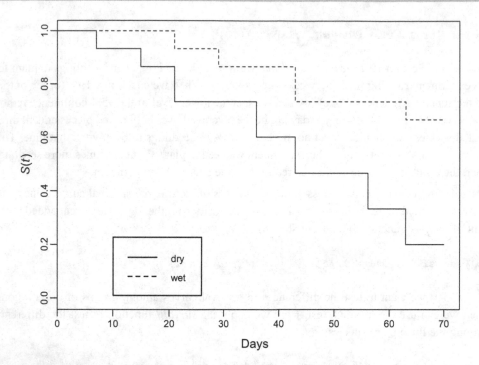

Figure 19.2 Survival curves estimated for the two locations where grassland seedlings were planted.

The second command added a key explaining the meaning of the solid and dashed lines. The resulting graph is shown in Fig. 19.2.

On this occasion the curves are plotted without confidence regions as the plot contains more than one survival curve.[4] We can see that the seedlings died more frequently at the dry location and the difference in $S(t)$ increased with time.

We will now look at the second example investigating the survival of antelopes. We mentioned in Section 19.1 that we are primarily interested in the effect of the radio-collar, but we should also eventually take into account animal weight and/or age effects. We will therefore adopt a conservative strategy and first fit a model including the weight and age as predictors. Then we will confer with the model output and see whether both predictors deserve to be retained and only then test the additional (partial) effect of the radio-collar. In other words, any variation in survival that can be accounted for by age or weight will not be attributed to a radio-collar effect.

We will fit the initial Cox proportional hazard model using the *coxph* function:

```
cox.1 <- coxph( Surv( time, status) ~ age + weight,
                data=chap19b)
```

The response variable is again defined using the *Surv* function, combining the death/right-censoring time with the *status* indicator. On the right side of the model formula we can

---

[4] However this can be overcome by adding the confidence regions with the *lines* function call (with *sf.2* as the first argument, followed by the *conf.int="only"* argument).

find the effects of *age* and *weight*. We can now judge the predictor effects using a likelihood ratio test:

```
anova( cox.1)
Analysis of Deviance Table
 Cox model: response is Surv(time, status)
Terms added sequentially (first to last)
          loglik  Chisq Df Pr(>|Chi|)
NULL    -263.73
age     -261.64 4.1692  1    0.04116 *
weight -260.70 1.8723  1    0.17121
```

Note that like the linear and generalised linear models, the *anova* function evaluates the predictor effects in a sequential manner.[5] The *age* predictor has a weak independent effect ($p = 0.041$), but there is no reliable effect of *weight* shown. We will therefore drop the second predictor from our model:

```
cox.2 <- update( cox.1, . ~ . - weight)
```

Now we can try to extend the *cox.2* model with the *collar* predictor, yielding the *cox.3* model, and then we compare these two models together, again using the likelihood ratio test. This time the *anova* function takes two Cox proportional hazard models as its arguments:

```
cox.3 <- update( cox.2, . ~ . + collar)
anova( cox.2, cox.3)
Analysis of Deviance Table
 Cox model: response is  Surv(time, status)
 Model 1: ~ age
 Model 2: ~ age + collar
   loglik Chisq Df P(>|Chi|)
1 -261.64
2 -258.81 5.671  1   0.01725 *
```

The effect of wearing a radio-collar seems to be stronger than the effect of age, but we still have no idea about the direction of either effect. For this, we use the *summary* function on the *cox.3* object:

```
summary( cox.3)
...
 n= 227, number of events= 63
```

---

[5] This implies that the reported effect of *weight* would be stronger if the right side of the formula used the *weight + age* order and the weight variable was correlated with age (as is indeed the case). So it would be prudent to check the independent effect of *weight* as well – either by omitting age from the model or by reverting the predictor order in the formula. But even under such circumstances we would see that the *weight* predictor remains non-significant.

```
              coef exp(coef)  se(coef)       z Pr(>|z|)
age        -0.13803   0.87107   0.07187  -1.921   0.0548 .
collaryes  -0.62077   0.53753   0.26448  -2.347   0.0189 *
---
Signif.codes:
             0 '***' 0.001 '**' 0.01 '*' 0.05 '.' 0.1 ' ' 1

            exp(coef)  exp(-coef)  lower .95  upper .95
age            0.8711       1.148     0.7566     1.0028
collaryes      0.5375       1.860     0.3201     0.9027


Concordance= 0.586  (se = 0.041 )
Rsquare= 0.042    (max possible= 0.902 )
Likelihood ratio test= 9.84  on 2 df,    p=0.007
Wald test            = 9.66  on 2 df,    p=0.008
Score (logrank) test = 9.92  on 2 df,    p=0.007
```

The first table with predictor regression coefficients in the *summary* function output gives the estimated coefficient values, their exponential transformation and the standard errors of the coefficient estimates, together with the corresponding tests. These tests are based on comparing the estimate and standard error ratio with a standardised normal distribution $N(0, 1)$. The exponential transformation of the regression coefficients is also at the start of the second table, with the values indicating that the effect of both predictors on antelope survival is positive. For *age*, the hazard rate (daily risk of death) decreases by 13% (i.e. $100 \times (1 - 0.87)$) with every increase of antelope age by one year. For the categorical *collar* predictor, the label used in the table indicates that the antelopes with level *yes* (wearing the collar) have about 46% lower hazard rate (i.e. the hazard rate without a collar multiplied by 0.538) than those without it. The fact that the presence of a radio-collar has a positive effect on survival rate seems surprising, but perhaps it can be explained by a change in the behaviour of those individuals which somehow reduces their exposure to predators. In the second table, the exponential transformation is supplemented with its confidence interval, allowing us to present interval estimates for the predictor effects. The alternative $\exp(-\text{coef})$ transformation enables us to compare e.g. the groups in the opposite direction (the antelopes without a collar have a hazard rate 1.86 times higher than those wearing it).

Given the non-parametrically estimated baseline hazard (and implicitly the survival) curve, it might be more informative to plot the estimated model. We will focus here on the effect of the collar, predicting the survival curves for antelopes at the median age (6 years) with the estimated Cox model. We start by plotting the common survival curve – note that the *cox.3* model must first be transformed by a call to the *survfit* function:

```
plot( survfit( cox.3), conf.int=FALSE,
      xlab="days", ylab="S(t)")
```

Next we add another two survival curves to the plot, representing the predictions for animals without and with the radio-collar, differentiated by the different line style and colour. The resulting graph is shown in Fig. 19.3.

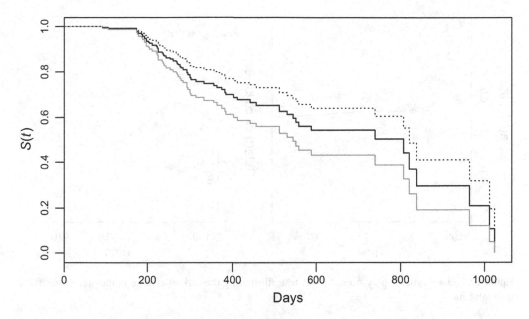

Figure 19.3 Survival curves estimated for all antelopes (black solid line), for a subset with collars (black dotted line) and for a subset without collars (grey solid line), using the median antelope age of 6 years.

```
lines( survfit( cox.3,
                newdata=list(age=c(6,6),
                             collar=c("no","yes"))),
       col=c("gray","black"), lty=c(1,3))
```

Finally, we should check the important assumption of Cox models, namely that the predictor effects do not change across the lifetime of the individuals:

```
cox.zph( cox.3)
```

```
              rho chisq      p
age        -0.110 0.873 0.350
collaryes  -0.141 1.245 0.265
GLOBAL         NA 2.225 0.329
```

There seems to be no important deviation from a constant effect of either predictor. If this were not the case, it would be important to identify the nature of the deviation using a diagnostic graph. If needed, this can be produced with the following command (the plotting area was divided into two columns because the model contains two predictors, shown here in separate plots):

```
par( mfrow=c(1,2))
plot( cox.zph( cox.3))
par( mfrow=c(1,1))
```

We can see in the left pane of Fig. 19.4 that the effect of animal age is slightly (but non-significantly) increasing in size, as the estimated curve decreases, making the coefficient even more negative.

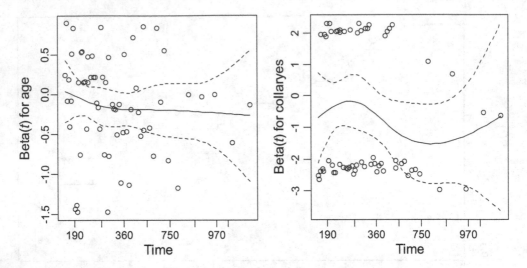

Figure 19.4 Diagnostic display from *cox.zph* test, illustrating the lack of change in the predictor effects through time.

19.7 Reporting Analyses

19.7.1 Methods

Differences in survival probabilities among the seedlings of three plant species were assessed using the log-rank test (Harrington & Fleming, 1982).

The effect of antelope weight and age, as well as the conditional effect of wearing a radio-collar, were tested by Cox proportional hazard models using likelihood ratio tests. The assumption that predictor effects do not vary across the lifespan of antelopes was verified using the test of Grambsch & Therneau (1994).

19.7.2 Results

We found no significant differences in survival probability among the three plant species ($\chi^2_2 = 0.6$, n.s.).

The increasing age of antelopes had a weak positive effect on their survival probability ($\chi^2_1 = 4.17$, $p = 0.041$). The additional effect of wearing a radio-collar was more important ($\chi^2_1 = 5.67$, $p = 0.017$): the antelopes with a radio-collar had a hazard rate that was on average 46.2% lower ($CI_{95} = (9.7\%, 68.0\%)$) than the control individuals.

19.8 Recommended Reading

P. Grambsch & T. Therneau (1994) Proportional hazard tests and diagnostics based on weighted residuals. *Biometrika*, **81**: 515–526.

D. P. Harrington & T. R. Fleming (1982) A class of rank test procedures for censored survival data. *Biometrika*, **69**: 553–566.

D. F. F. Moore (2016) *Applied Survival Analysis Using R (Use R!)*. Springer, New York, 256 pp.

T. M. Therneau & P. M. Grambsch (2001) *Modeling Survival Data: Extending the Cox Model*. Springer, New York (corrected 2nd printing, 368 pp.).

20 Classification and Regression Trees

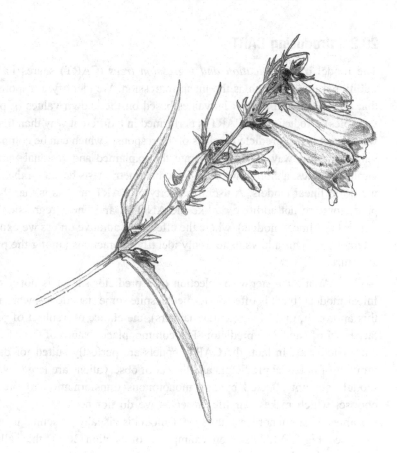

Despite its exotic name and unusual testing and presentation style, classification and regression trees are a valid member of the family of regression models: predicting values of a categorical or quantitative variable with the help of explanatory variables.

20.1 Use Case Examples

Our examples cannot be fully representative of datasets that are typically analysed with tree models, they are of limited size so their analysis is suitable for presentation in a textbook.

1. Using a dataset coming from a study of old field succession, we want to understand which functional attributes (traits) relate to plant species appearing at particular stages of old field vegetation development. Each of the 148 plant species is characterised by its successional index, roughly estimating its position on a temporal gradient of community succession, and by the values of six attributes characterising species functional properties.

2. Three plant species belonging to the genus *Melampyrum* were distinguished using molecular methods on a set of 80 specimens collected from various local populations. In addition, each plant specimen was characterised by a set of 11 morphological measures, mostly related to flowers. We want to find a set of reliable rules that can be used to determine the species identity of a new plant based on its morphological properties, as is customary in determination keys used in field work.

20.2 Introducing CART

The model of *classification and regression trees* (CART) shares its main task with more traditional models, such as the linear regression. We identify a response variable and expect that our model will predict its values based on the known values of predictors (explanatory variables). Prediction by CART is performed in a different way than that of linear models, but we still get fitted (predicted) values of the response, which can be compared with the observed values. In this way, we can separate the explained and residual variation in the response variable values, although we do not use parametric tests based on these variation fractions as we do in linear models. A useful property of CART models is that the effects of individual predictors are not additive, unlike the ANOVA and linear regression models (and also the generalised linear models), where the effects are additive unless we explicitly model predictor interactions. This allows us to easily identify interactions among the predictors from the tree structure.

While the stepwise selection of a predictor subset is not a standard part of fitting linear models (but it is often performed despite some statisticians warning users against taking this approach, given its potential dangers), the choice of a subset of predictors from a much larger set of candidate predictors is a commonplace feature of CART and is performed in an automated way. In fact, the CART models are perfectly suited for datasets where both the number of potential predictors and the set of observations are large, even huge. Further, these models are not affected by any monotonous transformation of predictors that we might choose, which makes our life easier as we do not need to worry about transforming our variables. Last but not least, the CART model is visually presented in an intuitive fashion as a tree (see Fig. 20.1, based on example 1 of Section 20.1), thus allowing it to be easily understood, at least on a basic level, even by viewers without any special knowledge of the method.

When we use a CART tree for predicting values for an observation, we must start at the tree root, which is – for a biologist somewhat counter-intuitively – at the top of the diagram. We then answer the question presented there for that particular observation. If the plant species has a leaf dry matter content (*LDMC*) value below 192.8, then we go to the left branch, otherwise we go to the right branch. We proceed similarly for the other questions that we encounter during our trip down the tree branches: if the answer is yes, we move to the left-hand branch. Finally, at the terminal branch (or *leaf*), at which we arrive based on the predictor values, we read the predicted value of the response variable. So, for a regression tree in Fig. 20.1, if a plant species has *LDMC* value 200 and the seed weight is 8.2, the predicted value of its successional index is 0.206.

Despite tree models being intuitive and easy to understand, we want our readers to grasp them more deeply, so we provide additional details on how the CART models are

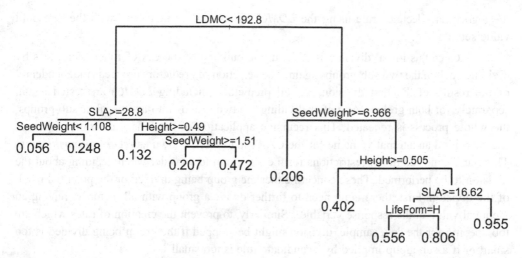

Figure 20.1 Full (overgrown) regression tree predicting the successional index of plant species based on their functional traits.

constructed. Both the *classification trees*, which predict values of a categorical response variable, and the *regression trees*, which predict values of a quantitative variable, split the set of existing observations into hierarchically arranged groups based on the predictor values. The task is to find, in the end, related groups so that each of them contains observations with very similar values of the response variable. For our above example of plant species with *LDMC* >= 192.8 and *Seed Weight* >= 6.966, we hope that all such species[1] will have their successional index value very close to 0.206, because their deviations from this fitted value contribute to the residual (unexplained) variation of the CART model and therefore might lower model quality.

The algorithm constructing a regression (or classification) tree starts by dividing the whole dataset into two groups. This division is based on a single predictor, which is used in a decision rule.[2] The form of this rule depends on the predictor type. For a numerical predictor, the algorithm attempts to find a single threshold value that maximises the differences between the two implied sub-groups in the values of the response variable. For a categorical predictor, the rule attempts to divide predictor levels into two mutually exclusive subsets that define the contents of the groups, again trying to maximise the differences between the groups in the response values. In our example 1 dataset (used in Fig. 20.1), the *LifeForm* predictor contains five levels (life forms) and the CART algorithm divided them (not in the first division) into two subsets: one containing the *H* (hemicryptophyte) level and the other containing the remaining four levels (*Ch, G, Ph, T*).

It is important to understand that, at each division, the CART algorithm tries to find the best division rule based on each of the available predictors. It then determines which of the predictors creates a division best separating the response values. For our example in Fig. 20.1,

---

[1] There were 10 such species in our dataset.

[2] The decision rule is a term borrowed from the field of artificial intelligence and simply refers to the question used to define particular dichotomous branching in the tree.

the algorithm selected a rule using the *LDMC* variable in the first split, with the threshold value set at 192.8.

Once this initial division is defined, the building of the CART model continues by dividing each of the two sub-groups again. The selection of predictors proceeds independently of the results of the first division, i.e. all predictors (including *LDMC*) are tested again, separately for both groups. And after dividing the two groups into another four sub-groups, the whole process is repeated. This recursive application of the binary division of groups stands behind an alternative name for the CART algorithm, known as *recursive partitioning*. There are some additional restrictions for the algorithm to consider when deciding about the division to be performed. These concern either the group being divided or the potential result of the division. First, there is no need to further divide a group with all members having an identical value of the response variable.[3] Similarly, to prevent the creation of rules which are too specific for the data sample, division might be stopped if the group being divided is too small or if a sub-group implied by a candidate rule is too small.[4]

Once none of the sub-groups can be further divided, the growth of a regression (or classification) tree stops. This is the state of the tree shown in Fig. 20.1 and it usually represents an overfitted ('too complex') model, which will predict the data used for its creation very well, but its general performance will be sub-optimal. We need to determine an optimum size of the tree for the prediction of response variable values from new observations, and this procedure is described in the following section.

20.3 Pruning the Tree and Crossvalidation

To reduce a fully grown regression or classification tree, we can 'snip off' its terminal branches. The tree graph in Fig. 20.1 is presented in a way that allows us to judge the importance of each division: the length of the vertical line segments reflects the drop in unexplained variation of the response variable as a result of splitting the particular sub-group. Based on this, we can identify the *SeedWeight* >= 1.51 rule (approximately in the centre of the tree) as contributing the least to our model quality. The process of removing the least effective terminal branches of a tree is traditionally called *pruning*. Starting from a fully grown tree, we can proceed with the pruning up to a state where we have no branches left. The 'stump-like' tree represents a null model corresponding to a claim that none of the considered predictors have sufficient power to predict the response variable.

We can evaluate all of the tree models, from the original one to the null model, by their predictive success, e.g. using the residual sum of squares (*RSS*) for a regression tree. But when we estimate *RSS* using the same dataset that was used for model fitting, we will inevitably obtain results indicating that the most complex model is the best, whatever dataset we analyse. We need an independent judgement about the predictive performance of our model, and this must be based on an independent dataset. But we are usually unwilling to split our precious dataset into two parts, using just one of them to construct the model and

---

[3] In fact, this 'purity' of response values does not need to be absolute, i.e. they need not be strictly identical, instead we can choose to limit the response variability by a constant somewhat larger than zero.

[4] One can intuitively expect that 'peeling off' individual observations based on their very particular values cannot create a robust model.

keeping the other one only for model evaluation. Luckily, the process of crossvalidation comes to the rescue.

The *crossvalidation* procedure starts by randomly dividing our dataset into k similarly sized parts (subsets).[5] One of the k parts is then removed from the dataset and a fully grown tree is constructed using observations in the remaining $k - 1$ parts. Based on that tree, a series of gradually pruned trees (as described in the previous paragraph) is created and the performance of each tree is evaluated using the observations of the omitted group. This process is repeated for each of the k groups, so we obtain k estimates of the predictive performance of the tree model for a particular tree size, and we can therefore estimate the standard errors of this predictive performance (see Fig. 20.2 in Section 20.6).[6]

We can use the resulting diagnostic graph to select an optimum tree size, and then apply this choice to a tree grown from the full dataset. But deciding about the best size is sometimes difficult. The graph in Fig. 20.2 shows a typical shape for a curve tracking the change of crossvalidated prediction error with increasing tree size, namely its steep drop from a null model to a minimum, followed by a much flatter growth with further increases in tree size. Although this is not the case for our dataset, the estimated values of prediction error for multiple tree sizes in the near-optimum area can form a really flat bottom of the curve, making it difficult for us to pick the minimum value.

In some cases we would recommend utilising an alternative *1 − SE rule*, particularly when we use the tree model to detect reliably supported relationships of the response to our predictors. This rule advises us to select the smallest tree size with the corresponding predictive error estimate being no more than one standard error distant from the smallest value of the crossvalidated predictive error. This rule is supported by the graph in Fig. 20.2, where the dotted line is one standard error above the smallest predictive error, corresponding to a tree with two terminal branches. While for different datasets we would apply the 1 − SE rule by selecting the leftmost point below the dotted line, in our case there is only one such tree size, representing the true minimum of the predictive error.

20.4 Competing and Surrogate Predictors

When we consider multiple predictors (explanatory variables) in any kind of statistical model, their mutual correlations bring uncertainty about the appropriate model specification. When we have a group of strongly correlated predictors, we have to select just one for our model, as the others provide similar information about the response – they 'tell a similar story'. Therefore, once we select a single predictor from the group of correlated predictors (usually the one that explains the greatest amount of variation in the response values), the other predictors of this group often cease to explain a sufficient amount of variation to justify their

---

[5] In the context of CART models, the value of k is usually small, e.g. 10, but in other applications of crossvalidation, k might be equal to the number of observations (n), so that each 'group' contains just a single observation. This leads to the 'leave-one-out' method, often used when evaluating models of discriminant analysis (see Section 22.4).

[6] Please note that the terminology is quite confusing here: what is shown by the vertical axis of Fig. 20.2 is the crossvalidated predictive error of a tree of particular size, which is further standardised – relativised by the size of this error for the original, full-size tree. But we also estimate the reliability (variability) of this estimated predictive error, in the form of the standard error (*SE*), which is then plotted as an interval. Yes, we have an error of an error here!

inclusion in the model. But their correlation with the best predictor is never perfect, and selection based on the highest value of explained variation might not be fully reliable: the relative importance of the predictors might be partly specific to our data sample.

We face similar issues even with the CART models. In each division, the model-building algorithm always selects just the strongest predictor and the other candidates are not used, even if their predictive performance is a close second to the winner. It is therefore useful to inspect information about the first few best alternative predictors that competed (by their split rules) against the one which was finally selected. Such information (a list of m best competing predictors, together with their splitting rules and an estimate of their relative performance) is provided separately for each tree branching point (node).

Another common problem with biological datasets is the presence of missing values. The CART models are capable of handling them more gracefully than most other types of statistical models. Observations with missing values for the response variable cannot be used for model creation, but missing values in a subset of candidate predictors do not require the corresponding observations to be *a priori* eliminated. Essentially such observations are ignored only when the candidate predictors containing missing values are evaluated. Additionally, the tree models might be able to predict response values even for observations where the predictors selected for one or multiple splits are missing some information. When we arrive at a split which asks about a missing predictor value, we can use either the 'majority rule' (choosing the larger – and therefore more likely – sub-group) or we can use *surrogate predictors*. The surrogate predictors (and their splitting rules) are defined at the time of model creation, with the aim of optimally reproducing the split (group membership) implied by the selected predictor.

Note that the surrogate predictors are not necessarily identical to the competing predictors discussed above, because here their quality is evaluated based on the agreement with the split definition by the primary split predictor and its rule. Often, however, the set of best surrogate predictors for a split can be rather similar to the set of competing predictors, but the corresponding rules might use different threshold values or split the factor levels differently.

When predicting response values, the algorithm 'walks' through a tree model based on the values of some selected primary split predictors, and when it encounters a split using a predictor with a missing value, it will try to use the best surrogate predictor instead (and when its value is also missing, it will use the second best surrogate predictor, etc.).

20.5 Example Data

The two example datasets are in the *Chap20* sheet of the example data file. Note that both datasets occasionally have some missing values (indicated by empty cells).

Our first example dataset, corresponding to example 1 of Section 20.1, originates from an unpublished Master's thesis of Jan Lepš (1977); the context of this study is described in Osbornová et al. (1990). We try to predict the successional preference index (*SPI*) of individual plant species using their functional traits. *SPI* values are based on the estimated cover of individual plant species in three plots representing an old field succession in Bohemian Carst: very young field (2 years after abandonment), medium-age field (8 years after abandonment) and old field (c. 50 years after abandonment). The *SPI* values are estimated as an average of 0 (for young field), 0.5 (for medium field) and 1.0 (for old field), weighted by the cover of species in the respective plots:

$$SPI = \frac{cover_{young} \times 0 + cover_{medium} \times 0.5 + cover_{old} \times 1}{cover_{young} + cover_{medium} + cover_{old}} \qquad (20.1)$$

The values 0, 0.5 and 1 were chosen (instead of the actual age in years) because succession proceeds much faster at the start. The *SPI* values consequently range from 0, for a species found only in the youngest stage, to 1, for a species found only in the oldest stage.

The *SPI* values are in column *B*, followed by six traits (*SLA, Height, SeedWeight, LDMC, Myrmecochory, LifeForm*), with their meaning explained by a comment in the first cell of the respective column. Column *I* represents the estimated total cover (number of pin hits with the point-quadrat technique, out of the total of 4000 trials). This column is used to select a sufficiently frequent plant species for the analysis.

The second example, corresponding to example 2 in Section 20.1, uses data from a study of Štech & Drábková (2005), focusing on morphological and molecular variability of plant populations of three species from the *Melampyrum sylvaticum* group. Species identity (labeled *T1, T2, T3* and based on molecular methods, and thus completely independent of the morphological data) is encoded in column *K*, while columns *L* to *V* contain 11 flower-related morphological characters all measured on a ratio scale.

20.6 How to Proceed in R

20.6.1 Regression Trees

We start with the first example, which is stored in the *chap20a* data frame. We use the *rpart* package (Therneau & Atkinson, 2018) to fit our CART models:

```
library( rpart)
rp.1 <- rpart( SPI ~ ., data=chap20a[,1:7],
               subset=(chap20a$NumHits > 5))
```

When specifying the model formula for our fitted tree, it is often good to use the notation in the above command, particularly if the number of candidate predictors is large: using a dot character at the right side of the formula, and thus specifying that all the variables in the data frame except *SPI* (already designated as a response variable) can be used in the model. But because the original data frame also contains the *NumHits* variable, which is not suitable for use as a predictor, we passed a subset of the data frame (just the first seven columns) as the *data* argument. Additionally, we also subset rows (plant species) using the *subset* argument in order to exclude very rare species, those which have too little information on their successional preference.

The *rp.1* object contains the fitted model, but the call to the *rpart* function also performed the crossvalidation and its results are stored in the object, so all we need to do is display it:[7]

```
plotcp( rp.1)
```

---

[7] Crossvalidation can be suppressed by setting the value of the *xval* argument to 0; we can use the same argument to choose a non-default number of groups (*k* in section 20.3), e.g. *xval*=5. The default value of *xval* is 10.

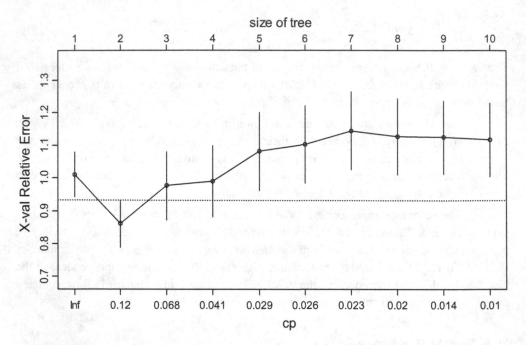

Figure 20.2 Graphical summary of the crossvalidation results for a fully grown tree. Tree size is expressed by the complexity parameter (*cp* on the bottom horizontal axis) as well as by the number of terminal branches (top horizontal axis). The vertical axis shows the crossvalidated residual sum of squares, standardised by the value for a null model fitted with all of the observations. Standardised error estimates are shown with their ±1 SE (standard error) intervals. The dotted reference line touches the top limit of the interval for the smallest error estimate, so this line can be used when applying the 1 − SE rule (see Section 20.3).

The resulting graph is shown in Fig. 20.2. We have already described its interpretation in Section 20.3, together with how it is used for choosing tree complexity. Here we just note that a tree with a single split (and hence two terminal branches) is indicated as the optimum choice.

It can also be useful to inspect the fitted tree (shown in Fig. 20.1), but note that it is overfitted and thus not quite appropriate for presenting in your research report. Rather, we should prune the tree before its presentation. We can prune the tree object *rp.1* using the *prune* function, specifying the required tree complexity. The *prune* function only accepts the complexity value on the *cp* scale, not as a tree size, so we must specify the value 0.12 for our tree:

```
rp.2 <- prune( rp.1, cp=0.12)
```

Now we can plot the reduced (parsimonious) tree. For additional flexibility, the drawing of tree branches (with the *plot* function) is separated from drawing the text (using the *text* function). A drawback of this approach is that very often the tree line segments are spread over the plotting area so liberally that there is hardly any space left for fully displaying some of the labels. We therefore need to reserve a part of the plotting area at its edges using the *marg* parameter.[8] The resulting graph is shown in Fig. 20.3A.

---

[8] The value of the *marg* argument represents the fraction of the available plotting area that is reserved at each of the four plot edges.

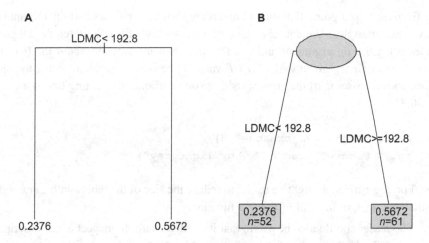

Figure 20.3 Regression tree predicting the *SPI* value using plant traits. Two graph versions are shown: (A) standard plot, (B) enhanced plot (see the code and related text for more details).

```
plot( rp.2, marg=0.05)
text( rp.2)
```

The *plot* function has multiple handy arguments, but here we mention just two. The *uniform* argument allows us to create a more compact tree by using identical heights for all branches (*uniform=T*). This is not the default behaviour however. Unless otherwise specified, branch lengths will reflect the amount of response variable variation explained by a particular split. This is quite informative in graphs like Fig. 20.1, but not so for the likes of Fig. 20.3A. The *branch* argument (with a default value of 1) changes the drawing style of branches. It takes a value between 0 and 1, and if you specify the other extreme (*branch=0*), the function draws V-shaped branches, which we know so well from phylogenetic trees. Values between 0 and 1 create intermediate forms of branching.

There are again multiple arguments on offer with the *text* function.[9] Perhaps the most important is the *pretty* argument, which can be used to improve the encoding of factor levels. We have no factor predictors in Fig. 20.3, and only a simple example of their use in Fig. 20.1. But for a factor where its splitting rule involves reference to multiple levels, listing their names above the branching node might overflow other parts of the tree. The *rpart* authors therefore resorted to a space-saving strategy where the individual factor levels are replaced (in the order shown by the *levels(data$factor)* function call) by lowercase letters of the alphabet (*a, b, c, ...*). When such encoding is not seen as an improvement, you can ask for actual level names to be shortened up to *N* characters (say *N* = 5) by using, say, the *pretty=5* argument in the *text* function call. Alternatively, you can enforce the full original level labels with the *pretty=0* argument setting.

We must also mention the *fancy* argument available in the *text* function. When specified with a *TRUE* value, the rules are shown separately alongside the two branches

---

[9] Note that both the *text* and *plot* functions are classical generic functions of R, thus they are implemented based on the first argument that is passed to the function. So most arguments discussed in this chapter only work within the context of plotted objects created by the *rpart* function.

leading from each split point, the internal nodes are shown as ellipses and the terminal nodes are shown as rectangles. We can also specify a non-default fill colour for the ellipses and rectangles using the *bg* argument and ask for additional information about the (sub-)group sizes using the *use.n* argument with a *TRUE* value. Here is an example of using the *plot* and *text* commands with some of the arguments discussed earlier, the resulting tree is then shown in Fig. 20.3B:

```
plot( rp.2, marg=0.07, branch=0.5)
text( rp.2, fancy=T, use.n=T, bg="lightgrey")
```

For larger trees, it might be useful to reduce the size of the labels with a *cex* argument value smaller than 1 in the call of the *text* function.

The reader should also be aware that it is often useful to inspect a text description of the fitted trees. To do this, we just enter the tree object's name:

```
rp.2

n= 113

node), split, n, deviance, yval
      * denotes terminal node

1) root 113 17.976210 0.4155310
  2) LDMC< 192.75 52  3.938355 0.2375962 *
  3) LDMC>=192.75 61 10.988040 0.5672131 *
```

The description starts with the total number of observations, and is followed by a short legend for tree content description. The node number is followed by the split rule, specifying the chosen predictor and its threshold value (for numerical predictors), as well as the comparison direction ($<$ or $>=$). Then comes the size of the resulting sub-group (number of observations matching the split rule), the amount of unexplained variation (group deviance) and finally the predicted value of the response variable (here *SPI*). The asterisk at the end of the last two rows in the above output indicates the terminal nodes.

In Section 20.4 we discussed competing and surrogate predictors and their use when working with tree models. They are recorded by default (up to four competing predictors and up to five surrogate predictors), but if we want to see them then we must use the *summary* function. The output is usually voluminous, but not so for our simple pruned tree (the number of decimal digits was reduced and long text lines are wrapped):

```
summary( rp.2)

Call:
rpart( formula = SuccIdx ~ ., data = chap20a[ , 1:7],
       subset = (chap20a$NumHits > 5))
  n= 113
```

```
        CP nsplit rel error    xerror        xstd
1 0.1696585      0 1.0000000 1.0102226 0.06837597
2 0.1200000      1 0.8303415 0.8615576 0.07219129


Variable importance
      LDMC        SLA   LifeForm SeedWeight       Height
        56         17         11         10            6

Node number 1: 113 observations, complexity param=0.170
  mean=0.4155, MSE=0.1591
  left son=2 (52 obs) right son=3 (61 obs)
  Primary splits:
    LDMC      < 192.75 to the left, improve=0.170,
                                    (0 missing)
    SLA       < 28.90 to the right, improve=0.116,
                                    (0 missing)
    Height    < 0.49  to the right,improve=0.085,
                                    (0 missing)
    LifeForm  splits as  RLRLR,    improve=0.046,
                                    (0 missing)
    SeedWeight< 6.54  to the right, improve=0.038,
                                    (0 missing)
Surrogate splits:
    SLA       < 28.15 to the right, agree=0.681,
                                    adj=0.308, (0 split)
    LifeForm  splits as  RLRRL,     agree=0.628,
                                    adj=0.192, (0 split)
    SeedWeight< 1.13 to the left,   agree=0.619,
                                    adj=0.173, (0 split)
    Height    < 0.25 to the left,   agree=0.593,
                                    adj=0.115, (0 split)


Node number 2: 52 observations
  mean=0.2375962, MSE=0.07573759


Node number 3: 61 observations
  mean=0.5672131, MSE=0.1801318
```

We will not explain all the technical details of the *summary* function output, but note that the list of competing predictors (labelled *Primary splits*) starts with the one that was actually selected, and the increase in the explained variation (on an R^2 scale between 0 and 1) is shown as the *improve* parameter. We can see that the second best candidate – *SLA* – had distinctly lower predictive quality than the chosen *LDMC*. In the list of surrogate predictors (*Surrogate splits*), *SLA* is again the best candidate, but it reproduces the *LDMC*-based split with just 68.1% conformity (see the *agree* field value).

20.6.2 Classification Trees

Now we illustrate the differences when fitting classification trees to our data. For this we will use the second data example, which we import into the *chap20B* data frame:

```
rpc.1 <- rpart( Taxon~., data=chap20B, minsplit=5)
```

We have added the *minsplit* argument this time, which specifies the minimum size of a (sub-)group that can still be split. This is needed for our dataset as it has a relatively small size, because otherwise the tree will not grow large enough for the crossvalidation to find an optimum tree size.[10]

We now display the crossvalidation results:

```
plotcp( rpc.1)
```

The resulting graph is shown in Fig. 20.4A. However if you repeat the fitting (with the same arguments for the *rpart* function) and plot the crossvalidation results again, you are likely to see differences in the content of the graph (as you are seeing anyway when trying the command on your own computer). In fact, the diagram in Fig. 20.4B was produced in this way.

While both graphs in Fig. 20.4 generally have similar forms, the actual estimates of prediction errors are different and the conclusions about the optimum tree size would differ as well.

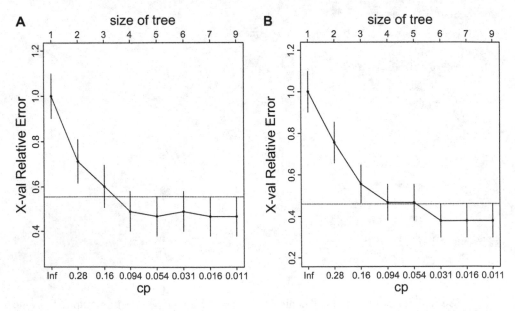

Figure 20.4 Graphical summary of the crossvalidation results for the full classification tree based on taxonomy data. The crossvalidation was performed twice, each time (A vs. B) producing somewhat different graphs and conclusions.

---

[10] When we use the default *minsplit* value of 20, the largest trees entering the crossvalidation procedure have just four terminal branches and the prediction error estimates continually decline from the simplest up to the largest tree.

This is because we rely on a random process during the crossvalidation procedure, one that creates different k groups of observations each time it is used. This is affecting the variation in the prediction error estimate when our dataset is small, as is the case in this second example. For our analysis, we will rely on the first graph produced (Fig. 20.4A), where the recommended tree size, based on the $1 - SE$ rule, would be four terminal branches, i.e. with $cp = 0.094$. This is what we will use for tree pruning:

```
rpc.2 <- prune( rpc.1, cp=0.094)
```

Let us inspect the final model first through its text description, which differs slightly from the description used for regression trees (the first command reduces the precision of the displayed values):

```
options( digits=3)
rpc.2
n= 80

node), split, n, loss, yval, (yprob)
      * denotes terminal node

 1) root 80 45 T1 (0.4375 0.2875 0.2750)
   2) CorHght>=6.05 32  1 T1 (0.9688 0.0312 0.0000) *
   3) CorHght< 6.05 48 26 T2 (0.0833 0.4583 0.4583)
     6) CorTbLen>=5.25 39 17 T2 (0.1026 0.5641 0.3333)
       12) AnthLen< 2.35 27  6 T2 (0.0000 0.7778 0.2222) *
       13) AnthLen>=2.35 12  5 T3 (0.3333 0.0833 0.5833) *
     7) CorTbLen< 5.25 9  0 T3 (0.0000 0.0000 1.0000) *
```

As we are predicting a categorical response in this model, the fitted value is the most probable category (factor level), here the taxon identity. But the output also specifies – in parentheses – the relative frequencies of individual categories within the group defined by the model. So, as an example, node 2 represents the plants with a crown height larger than 6 mm and there are 32 such specimens. Of these, one specimen (i.e. 3.12%) belonged to the $T2$ taxon, while the remaining 31 specimens belonged to the $T1$ taxon. With a sufficiently large dataset, we can interpret these relative frequencies as the probabilities of a specimen belonging to individual classes (categories), making the prediction of a classification tree model more informative.

Finally, we plot the pruned model. Here we use some of the arguments for the *plot* and *text* functions introduced with the regression tree example above. However, we add the *all* argument (which additionally labels the internal nodes) and we also illustrate (in Fig. 20.5) that the *use.n=T* argument results in a different presentation style for classification trees: observation counts are listed per individual categories.

The results in Fig. 20.5 show that the $T1$ taxon can be identified with reasonable precision using the corolla height (just one individual of $T2$ was predicted to be $T1$ and four $T1$ individuals were misclassified as $T3$). Distinguishing between the other two species was less successful.

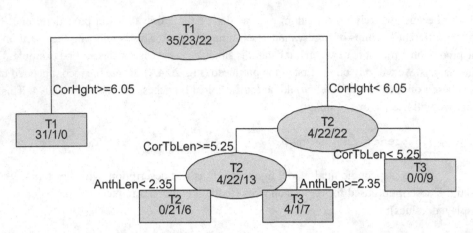

Figure 20.5 Final classification model predicting species identity based on morphological characters.

20.7 Reporting Analyses

20.7.1 Methods

The effects of plant attributes and functional traits on the successional preference index of individual species were examined using regression (*or* classification *for a categorical response*) tree models (Breiman et al., 1984) estimated using the *rpart* package (Therneau & Atkinson, 2018) within R statistical software. The optimum tree size was chosen based on crossvalidation results.

20.7.2 Results

The most parsimonious regression tree (Fig. 20.3B) shows the effect of the leaf dry-matter content (*LDMC*) trait on the successional preference of plant species in old field vegetation. Species with lower *LDMC* values tend to prefer earlier successional stages compared to those with *LDMC* above the threshold of 192.8 mg g^{-1}.

We constructed a classification tree (Fig. 20.5) clearly distinguishing the *T*1 species from the other two. The distinction between *T*2 and *T*3, based on the length of the corolla tube and the length of anthers, is less reliable.

20.8 Recommended Reading

L. Breiman, J. H. Fiedman, R. A. Olshen & C. J. Stone (1984) *Classification and Regression Trees*. Chapman & Hall/CRC, Boca Raton, FL.

J. Osbornová, M. Kovářová, J. Lepš & K. Prach (1990) *Succession in Abandoned Fields: Studies in Central Bohemia, Czechoslovakia*. Kluwer Academic, Dordrecht. Series Geobotany 15, 169 pp.

M. Štech & L. Drábková (2005) Morphometric and RAPD study of the *Melampyrum sylvaticum* group in the Sudeten, the Alps and Carpathians. *Folia Geobotanica*, **40**: 177–193.

T. Therneau & B. Atkinson (2018) *Rpart*: recursive partitioning and regression trees. R package version 4.1-13. https://cran.R-project.org/package=rpart

21 Classification

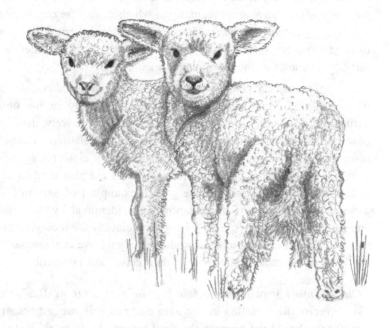

21.1 Use Case Examples

1. We have 20 records on the composition of grassland plant communities on an island. We want to identify groups of records with highly similar composition that might eventually represent more widely usable vegetation types. Similarly, we also wish to find groups of plant species that frequently occur together. These groups will presumably share similar environmental preferences and, by their occurrence (or higher abundance), can be used to characterise particular vegetation types.
2. We want to study the intraspecific variability of a plant species. We measure the morphological characteristics (length of the uppermost leaf, length of the corona tube, width of the flower lip, number of flowers per inflorescence, etc.) of several plants within multiple local populations of that species. We ask whether particular groups of populations are more mutually similar to one another than they are to other populations, i.e. whether they create clearly separated *clusters*, which may represent some lower-level taxa.

21.2 Aims and Properties of Classification

Let us consider a set of objects that represent numerous independent observations. For all objects we record a particular set of characteristics that are represented by variables in our dataset. Alternatively, we can say that each object is characterised by the measurement of a multivariate variable. The set of statistical methods focusing on the analysis of such multivariate data represents the *methods of multivariate analysis* or, more commonly, the *multivariate methods*. While the usual statistical methodology focuses on the estimation of model parameters and/or on hypothesis testing, some of the multivariate methods have a more modest aim, namely to better understand complex data and their structure.[1] We ask whether particular object types occur regularly or whether there are consistent relationships among the variables – generally speaking, we seek *repeatable patterns*. Finding such patterns then allows us to propose new research hypotheses. One useful group of methods for finding patterns in our data is known as the classification methods.

The primary task of **classification** is to place observations into groups according to their similarity. Thus a group will comprise relatively similar observations, which differ sufficiently from other groups of observations. Alternatively, these methods can find groups of variables that have strong relationships (e.g. correlations). Classification is used in many research fields, and in biology it has a particularly close relationship with taxonomy – see example 2 in Section 21.1. But these methods are also used in the classification of plant communities (phytosociology), the goal of example 1 of Section 21.1. If successful, we can assume that the groups of vegetation types identified by the classification differ in their environmental conditions. Similarly, we can classify the biological taxa (not necessarily plant species) occurring in various communities. Again, we can assume that species belonging to the same group might share some of their ecological preferences.

> Classification is primarily a tool for the first stage of data analysis, when we try to summarise the variation in our data and possibly suggest research hypotheses. These methods should not become the final target of our work, instead they provide directions for further analyses.

The methods used for finding clusters (groups) of observations or of correlated variables can be divided into two large groups: hierarchical and non-hierarchical methods. *Non-hierarchical classification* divides the dataset into several clusters on a single level. We can either specify the required number of clusters in advance or this number can be determined based on some criterion. The methods of *hierarchical classification* create clusters at different hierarchical levels: the clusters at higher levels contain the clusters of lower levels. The results of hierarchical methods are usually presented graphically as a *dendrogram* (see e.g. Fig. 21.2).

Hierarchical methods of classification are further distinguished into agglomerative vs. divisive methods. The *agglomerative methods* proceed from the 'bottom', creating cluster cores from the most similar pairs of observations (or variables), which are then further extended by additional objects or clusters. The term *cluster analysis* is often applied to the agglomerative methods. The *divisive methods* proceed from the 'top', first dividing the entire set of objects into the two most distinct parts, and then working with each part as if it were a whole, independent set, dividing it into two parts again, etc. Of these two approaches, the hierarchical agglomerative methods dominate in biological applications, thus they are the

---

[1] We should stress, however, that there are also multivariate statistical methods allowing us to test hypotheses and estimate parameters of complex models for our multivariate data. They mostly belong to *constrained ordination*, handled in Section 22.3.

primary focus of this chapter. More details about these and other classification methods can be found in chapter 8 of Legendre & Legendre (2012).

21.3 Input Data

The objects we want to classify can be characterised either by numerical (quantitative) or categorical (factor) variable values. We can take an example from bird taxonomy, where we might use both the length of the beak and the colour of the feathers in the same analysis. Quantitative data are typically described in different units (length, weight, etc.). Furthermore, variables representing e.g. different length parameters might not share the same scale. That is why numerical variables are typically standardised. In most cases, such standardisation is implemented by *z-transformation*. We estimate the mean and standard deviation for each variable (say X_j) and then calculate the standardised values as

$$z_{ij} = \frac{X_{ij} - \overline{X}_j}{SD_j} \tag{21.1}$$

The z-transformation makes all variables dimensionless, and sets their means to zero and their variance to one. This kind of standardisation is most appropriate when we can assume that individual variables have an approximate normal distribution (see Chapter 4). In addition, the individual variables are often scale-transformed before the standardisation (e.g. by a log-transformation), depending on their properties. We must be aware that the decision to standardise and/or transform a variable might substantially affect the meaning of the results we obtain.

21.4 Similarity and Distance

We have already seen that cluster analysis is used to find groups of similar objects. We must therefore precisely define the meaning of *similarity*. Many measures of similarity among objects have been proposed, often quite specific to particular research fields (or identical measures but simply referred to differently across fields). A closely related concept is the *distance* (or *dissimilarity*) among classified objects, which intuitively has a negative relationship with similarity. For a recent overview of the most frequently used similarity and distance measures in ecological research, see chapter 7 of Legendre & Legendre (2012). Here we introduce three of the simplest measures only.

When we work with categorical (qualitative) variables, perhaps the simplest similarity measure for a pair of objects is

$$\frac{\text{number of variables with identical value}}{\text{total number of variables}} \tag{21.2}$$

As is often the case for similarity measures, the value of this measure (often called the *simple-matching coefficient*) is equal to 1 for fully identical objects and 0 for objects differing in all their characteristic (variable) values. We can use the 1-complement of this value to obtain a measure of dissimilarity (distance).

In contrast, we typically use *Euclidean distance* for measuring dissimilarity of numerical (quantitative) variables. Let us label the value of the *j*-th variable on a first object as $x_{1,j}$ and on a second object as $x_{2,j}$. We can then compute the Euclidean distance between the two objects as

$$ED_{1,2} = \sqrt{\sum_j \left(x_{1,j} - x_{2,j}\right)^2} \qquad (21.3)$$

For two objects with identical variable values, the Euclidean distance is equal to 0, but its upper limit depends on the number of variables and their scale. The use of Euclidean distance is often combined with variable standardisation (see Section 21.3).

We must also quantify the similarity of variables when we attempt to classify them. For numerical variables, we often use a correlation coefficient (r). Remember, however, that the minimum r value is -1, not 0. The Pearson correlation, although the typical choice, is only appropriate for describing the relationship between two variables when it takes a linear form.

21.5 Clustering Algorithms

Here we focus on agglomerative hierarchical clustering as it represents the most frequently used method. Once we have chosen a similarity (or distance) measure to compare individual objects, we can calculate the matrix of distances among all pairs of objects. This matrix is then a starting point for one of the clustering procedures (algorithms).

Each procedure starts by finding the pair of objects with the smallest distance (i.e. the highest similarity). This pair then becomes the first cluster. Then we can calculate the distance of the remaining objects to this cluster. Each method varies in how it calculates this distance or, more generally, the distance between two clusters of objects. Three frequently used methods are illustrated in Fig. 21.1.

The *single linkage* method (representing the distance between two clusters as the distance between their most similar members) is rarely used for clustering biological objects, but sometimes used to find the shortest path connecting a set of objects (*minimum spanning tree*). The *average linkage* method takes on various forms within biological literature, however the most commonly used type is called UPGMA.[2] Beyond the algorithms illustrated in Fig. 21.1, community ecologists also frequently use Ward's method, which is based on minimising data variability within clusters, thus maximising differences among the higher-level clusters.

21.6 Displaying Results

The results of hierarchical clustering are usually shown in the form of a dendrogram (see Fig. 21.2).

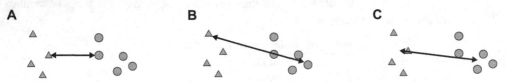

Figure 21.1 Measuring distances (dissimilarities) between two groups of objects in different agglomerative algorithms: (A) single linkage method, (B) complete linkage method, (C) average linkage method.

---

[2] The UPGMA acronym originates from 'unweighted pair group method with arithmetic mean'.

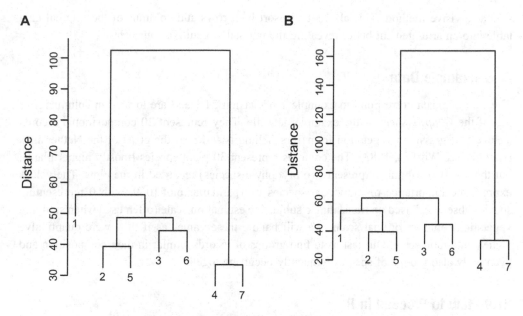

Figure 21.2 Graphical summary (dendrograms) contrasting the results of applying two different algorithms of agglomerative hierarchical clustering to the same dataset. The dendrogram in part A was produced using the average linkage method, and the dendrogram in part B used Ward's method.

The vertical axis shows the level of dissimilarity at which two objects (or two groups of objects) are merged into a cluster. We can see in both parts of Fig. 21.2 that the data sample is formed by two quite distinct groups of objects: those labelled 1–3, 5 and 6 belong to the first group, while objects 4 and 7 belong to the second group. The numbering of objects was set *a priori*, or alternatively we could use the names of locations, etc. The most similar two objects are 4 and 7, as reflected in the lowest vertical position of the horizontal part of their branch. The results of the two clustering algorithms differ only slightly (namely the (2, 5) pair are more similar to the (3, 6) pair in part A, but in part B they are more similar to object 1).

21.7 Divisive Methods

Nowadays *TWINSPAN* (*two-way indicator species analysis*) is the most widely used divisive hierarchical method for analysing biotic communities.[3] It was devised for classifying a set of vegetation records, but can equally be used to analyse communities of organisms other than higher plants. At each step, the TWINSPAN method divides the (full, then partial) set of observations into two groups. It also determines a set of variables (e.g. plant species) that characterise one or the other side of the dichotomic split at each division, and then recursively repeats the division on each of the groups until reaching a chosen minimum group size. The division is based on an algorithm from an ordination method called correspondence analysis, discussed in Chapter 22. The TWINSPAN method also classifies the species in parallel using a

---

[3] Please do not confuse the classification methods with the classification and regression trees (CART) discussed in Chapter 20. The CART method produces graphs (trees) resembling dendrograms, but differs substantially from the hierarchical clustering methods by optimising the similarity of values for *a priori* chosen response variable in the clusters, rather than optimising the overall similarity of classified objects.

similar divisive method. This allows us to sort both rows and columns of the original data table into an arrangement better revealing the internal structure of our dataset.

21.8 Example Data

The example data correspond to example 1 of Section 21.1 and are located in columns *A* to *AD* of the *Chap21* sheet of the example data file. They represent 20 compositional records (relevés) of grassland vegetation from Terschelling island near the coast of the Netherlands (Batterink & Wijffels, 1983). The columns represent 30 plant species (mostly higher plants, but the last two columns represent two bryophyte species) recorded in the plots. The values express the importance of individual species in a particular plot (0–9, with 0 representing species absence), based on translating a subjective estimation scale (often used when studying vegetation) onto an ordinal scale. We will handle these values as if they were quantitative values on a ratio scale. Our task is to find groups of records similar in their composition and eventually also groups of species frequently occurring together.

21.9 How to Proceed in R

The *cluster* library (Maechler et al., 2018) provides a rich array of algorithms for cluster analysis. The agglomerative methods are executed with the *agnes* function.

```
library( cluster)
```

We start by classifying observations (data frame rows) using Ward's clustering algorithm:

```
ag.1 <- agnes( chap21, method="ward", metric="euclidean")
```

We submitted the original data as the first argument in the *agnes* call and the function calculated a distance matrix (20 × 20) using Euclidean distances.[4] The other clustering algorithms introduced in Section 21.5 are also available, and can be applied by setting the argument *method* value to the desired option ('average', 'single', or 'complete').

We can use the following call to plot the dendrogram:

```
plot( ag.1, which.plots=2, main="", sub="",
      ylab="Euclidean distance")
```

This creates the graph shown in Fig. 21.3. Note that the argument *which.plots* suppresses an alternative graphical presentation which is otherwise shown alongside the dendrogram, while the *main* and *sub* arguments remove the excessive titles from the graph.

---

[4] The *metric* argument is redundant here, as its 'euclidean' option is implicit; the only other option available here is 'manhattan', which chooses the Manhattan distance. But note that this choice is rather lame for most applications of cluster analysis in community ecology. It is usually preferable to calculate the distance matrix separately, e.g. with the *vegan* package, using the *vegdist* function (see Section 22.6.1).

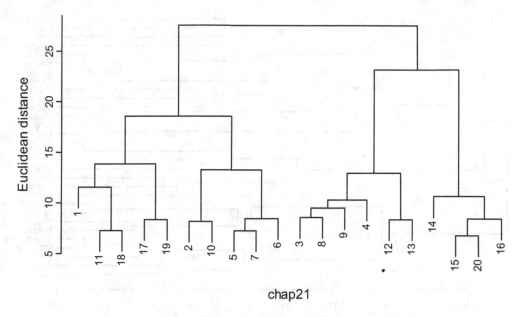

chap21

Figure 21.3 Dendrogram for the dune meadow data analysed with Ward's method of agglomerative clustering, which is based on Euclidean distances between data records.

There are two potential difficulties with plots produced in this way. First, the labels of terminal branches are plotted at different vertical positions: to change this, we can either use an optional argument *hang* = -1 (in fact, any negative value would do) or we can use the same solution we suggest for the next issue. The second issue is that this plotting function cannot rotate the dendrogram by 90 degrees, even though this would be very useful for larger datasets. We can transform the clustering results into another format in order to get around this. This format is normally produced by an alternative clustering function (*hclust*), and we transform to it using the *as.dendrogram* function. We can then plot the transformed clustering results and add the *horiz* argument. We will illustrate this procedure later when we create the species classification.

Sometimes the hierarchical nature of agglomerative clustering obstructs the recognition of distinct groups of, say, grassland communities. By examining Fig. 21.3 we can envisage anything between two and six distinct communities, depending on how high we perform the 'cut' across the dendrogram, parallel with the horizontal axis. After we make this decision, we can use the *cutree* function to specify the desired number of clusters with the *k* argument:

```
cutree( ag.1, k=4)
```
```
 [1]  1 2 3 3 2 2 2 3 3 2 1 3 3 4 4 4 1 1 1 4
```

Note that the *cutree* function returns a vector of whole numbers $(1, \dots, k)$ indicating the cluster a particular object belongs to (the objects are sorted in the same order as the rows or columns in the data frame).

We encounter a problem when we attempt to cluster species (response variables) based on their similarity: the *agnes* function provides no suitable dissimilarity measure. We therefore calculate a matrix of correlations among individual data frame variables (i.e. among

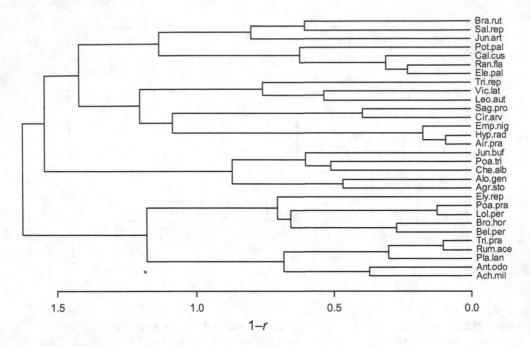

Figure 21.4 Species dendrogram for the dune meadow data, analysed by a complete linkage method of agglomerative clustering, using linear correlations among species as a measure of similarity.

the plant species) and take its 1-complement so that the distance is 0 for a perfect positive correlation, reaching a maximum of 2.0 for a perfect negative correlation. Finally, we change the general numerical matrix format into a distance matrix using the *as.dist* function. We also ask the *agnes* function to use the complete linkage algorithm:

```
ag.2 <- agnes( as.dist( 1 - cor( chap21)),
               method="complete")
```

Now we can plot the results using the alternative plotting method outlined above:

```
plot( as.dendrogram( ag.2), xlab="1-r", horiz=T)
```

The resulting graph is shown in Fig. 21.4.

If our reader has some experience with the ecological preferences of plants in temperate European grasslands, she will clearly see that the groups at the top of the dendrogram represent species occurring in quite wet conditions, while those at the bottom represent species from rather nutrient-poor and dry grasslands.

21.10 Other Software

The commercial PC-ORD program (http://www.pcord.com) is alternative software often used for performing hierarchical classification in the field of ecology. The divisive TWINSPAN method is implemented in the Twinspan for Windows software that can, at the time of publication, be downloaded for free from http://www.ceh.ac.uk/services/wintwins-version-23.

21.11 Reporting Analyses

21.11.1 Methods

Vegetation records were classified by a hierarchical agglomerative clustering algorithm using Euclidean distances among the records and Ward's method of cluster merging.

21.11.2 Results

Clustering results are summarised by the dendrogram in Fig. 21.3. We interpret three distinct clusters of observations in the dendrogram. The cluster with records 14–16 and 20 corresponds to the wettest meadows, characterised by the presence of species like ... [etc.]

21.12 Recommended Reading

Quinn & Keough (2002), pp. 488–491.

M. Batterink & G. Wijffels (1983) Een vergelijkend vegetatiekundig onderzoek naar de typologie en invloeden van het beheer van 1973 tot 1982 in de Duinweilanden op Terschelling. *Report of Agricultural University*, Department of Vegetation Science, Plant Ecology and Weed Science, Wageningen.

R. H. Jongman, C. J. F. ter Braak & O. F. R. van Tongeren (1987) *Data Analysis in Community and Landscape Ecology*. Pudoc, Wageningen.

P. Legendre & L. Legendre (2012) *Numerical Ecology*, 3rd English edn. Elsevier, Amsterdam, 990 pp.

M. Maechler, P. Rousseeuw, A. Struyf, M. Hubert & K. Hornik (2018) *cluster*: cluster analysis basics and extensions. R package version 2.0.7-1.

22 Ordination

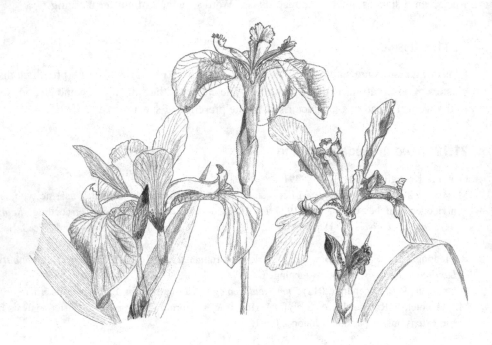

We introduce three groups of multivariate statistical models in this chapter, all of which fall under the umbrella of *ordination methods*. The common feature of these methods is that they replace the set of analysed variables with new characteristics representing axes of an *ordination space*. These axes summarise the variation of the original multivariate dataset, and in many methods allow for the prediction of data values. The key facet of ordination axes is that they are computed so that the amount of summarised variation is maximised in the first few axes. This produces a more easily understood summary of the data.

Summarising all the variation in a dataset is the primary task of *unconstrained ordination* methods, also known in ecology as methods of *indirect gradient analysis*. The same task can also be described in terms of the collected observations: we try to represent the observations by a set of points in ordination space where the distances among the points represent the dissimilarity between the observations.

The methods of *constrained ordination*[1] work with at least two sets of variables. As in the unconstrained ordination methods, constrained ordination tries to summarise the variation in one of the data tables, but focuses on the variation which can be explained by

---

[1] Also called *canonical ordination* or *direct gradient analysis*, although the latter term is sometimes used in a different context within the literature.

the variables from the other set. In this respect, their aims and use are quite similar to the methods of multiple regression and ANOVA.

We will also introduce the methods of *discriminant analysis* in this chapter. Although it can be seen as a special case of constrained ordination, we treat it separately and focus on its most frequently used form, linear discriminant analysis (LDA). This method is appropriate for a set of observations (objects) which are characterised by multiple variables, but are additionally classified into several mutually exclusive groups. Discriminant analysis tries to find classification rules – based on the measured variables – that enable us to predict membership of objects in individual groups.

22.1 Use Case Examples

1. We have 20 records describing the composition of grassland vegetation on Terschelling island (Batterink & Wijffels, 1983), the same dataset we used for classification in Chapter 21. Our task is to summarise the variation in community composition using a small set of independent gradients and relate those gradients of compositional change to the abundance (or presence) of individual plant species.
2. The second example extends the first, by considering a second table with variables characterising the environmental conditions and agricultural management for individual grassland sites. We want to test whether the vegetation composition changes in relation to environmental properties or management types, quantify the amount of community composition variation that can be explained by the environmental and management descriptors, and finally try to relate species to particular environmental effects.
3. To illustrate discriminant analysis, we use a classical dataset of R. A. Fisher, originally collected by Anderson (1936). This is a set of four morphological measurements on the flowers of 150 specimens belonging to three iris species (with 50 specimens for each species). We want to use the floral characters to define discriminant axes that allow us to predict which iris species a new specimen belongs to.

22.2 Unconstrained Ordination Methods

In unconstrained ordination methods, the data arrangement is similar to that of cluster analysis, discussed in Chapter 21. We have a set of observations (objects), with each observation characterised by multiple variables, which are usually cross-correlated to various degrees. A typical example might be data on the composition of biotic communities, where the individual observed taxa are the variables and the observations are e.g. vegetation plots, soil cores, soil traps or water samples in which the organisms were recorded. As another example, we can have multiple specimens of one or several species, with each specimen being characterised by multiple morphological or functional characteristics. We then want to identify patterns (structures) of variation in our data.

> Unconstrained ordination methods attempt to replace original variables by a smaller set of composed variables, which are mutually uncorrelated and sufficiently explain the structure within the dataset. We call the new variables *ordination axes* and in a graphical presentation of ordination results (an ordination diagram) they are indeed used as diagram axes.

The following four unconstrained ordination methods are all widely used in the field of biology: *principal component analysis* (PCA), *correspondence analysis* (CA),[2] *principal coordinate analysis* (PCoA) and *non-metric multidimensional scaling* (NMS or NMDS). We can usually describe the task of an unconstrained ordination in multiple ways. The simplest idea starts by representing our observations as points in m-dimensional space, where m is the number of variables (such as the total number of species in our plant community example) and the point position on an axis represents the value of the corresponding variable (e.g. plant species). The unconstrained ordination then tries to project this m-dimensional arrangement of points into an ordination space of fewer dimensions (we typically focus on the first two or three dimensions), and aims to arrange the original points with minimum spatial distortion. In other words, the variability of the analysed data, which is summarised on the first few ordination axes, is maximised.[3] The projection of observation points is usually complemented by the projection of the original variables into the ordination space, but not all unconstrained methods can do this (namely PCoA and NMS are unable to perform the appropriate variable projection).

More generally, we can formulate the preceding definition of an unconstrained ordination by saying that it arranges points in a low-dimensional ordination space so that the distances between the points match the dissimilarities among the observations as best as possible. Another definition of the aim of unconstrained ordination is the replacement of observed variables (usually numerous and mutually correlated) with a smaller set of new, mathematically constructed variables, which are not correlated and are defined as linear combinations or weighted averages of the original variables.

It can be demonstrated, after fulfilling certain assumptions, that we arrive at the same solution for the different tasks specified above, i.e. that a particular method of unconstrained ordination matches, in some way, all the definitions.

As with the classification methods, the unconstrained ordination is popular in taxonomy and when researchers seek repeatable types of biotic communities. If we work with community data, then we assume that the composition of the communities is determined by some environmental gradients (such as soil moisture or river depth), along which the community composition varies. We then expect that the ordination axes, arrived upon by the unconstrained ordination, will correspond to these environmental gradients. The methods of unconstrained ordination usually have some assumptions (such as a linear relationship among variables in PCA) or expect us to make data-specific choices (e.g. choosing a particular distance measure for PCoA or NMS), and we should be careful to respect such requirements and make these choices based on a firm understanding of their consequences in how we ultimately interpret our data.

Figure 22.1 illustrates the use of unconstrained ordination in community ecology. The ordination diagram (based on correspondence analysis) with cases – plots (grey circles) and plant species (triangles with abbreviated species names) – portrays more than 45% of the

---

[2] In community ecology, a pragmatic modification of correspondence analysis, referred to as *detrended correspondence analysis* (DCA), is typically used more frequently than CA itself.

[3] Typically, the first ordination axis tries to account for the maximum amount of variation that can be extracted from the original data; the second axis then tries to account for the maximum amount of variation that was not accounted for by the first axis, etc. This is not the case for ordination space using the NMS method, however, at least not before it is *post-hoc* rotated.

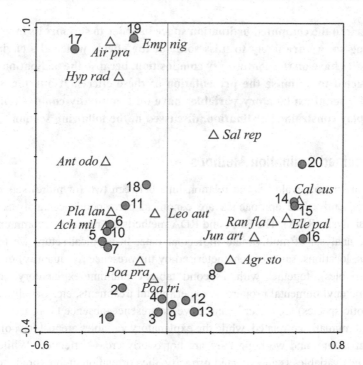

Figure 22.1 Ordination diagram of a correspondence analysis (CA) for the Terschelling island dataset characterising dune grassland composition. The first (horizontal) axis explains 27.0% of the total variation in the data, the second (vertical) axis explains another 18.3%. Vegetation plots are shown as grey circles, plant species as triangles.

compositional variation within the set of 20 grassland plant community plots recorded on Terschelling island. The CA method assumes that there are environmental gradients which determine community composition and that the individual species (together forming the community) have their optima somewhere along these gradients. We can identify groups of plots in the diagram which have similar community composition (e.g. the group of plots with numbers 5–7 and 10 represents records with very similar composition). The species are characterised by their estimated optima.[4] We can identify the horizontal (first CA) axis as a gradient of changing soil moisture based on an *a priori* knowledge of ecological preferences for plotted plant species. The species growing in moist conditions (*Ranunculus flammula, Juncus articulatus, Eleocharis palustris*) are located at the right side of the ordination diagram, while the species preferring more dry conditions (*Achillea millefolium, Plantago lanceolata, Anthoxanthum odoratum*) occupy its left side.

As the positions (scores) of the plots on the ordination axes define the compositional gradients, in many instances we can interpret these gradients more formally by relating the scores to known values of environmental characteristics measured at individual plots, e.g. using a linear regression. In this way, we can project a second set

---

[4] Unlike the PCA method: an alternative method which assumes a linear change of species abundances along the gradients (ordination axes), so that each species is plotted as an arrow.

of variables into the computed ordination space in order to support its interpretation. But in doing so, we are likely to miss some of the effects which the environmental characteristics have on the community composition, because the ordination axes were not constructed to optimise the presentation of these effects. If our focus is on the effects that a set of explanatory variables have on community composition, then we should employ constrained ordination, discussed in the following section.

22.3 Constrained Ordination Methods

Constrained ordination evaluates the relationships between two (or more) sets of variables. The most frequently used approaches are canonical correspondence analysis (CCA) and redundancy analysis (RDA). The CCA and RDA methods are popular in community ecology, including the analysis of multivariate molecular data. In a typical setup, we have a set of records (plots, locations, samples) characterised by the presence (or quantity) of a set of taxa (response variables), together with a second table containing explanatory variables that represent some environmental properties, experimental treatments, etc. Usually, the response variables (biotic species) are either quantitative or presence–absence (1–0) data and they are numerous and mutually correlated, while the explanatory variables are just few, of quantitative or categorical nature, and we hope they are not overly cross-correlated. While correlation among response variables is an expected property, the correlation among predictors (unfortunately also frequently present) is a nuisance, and we must address it in a similar fashion to when this issue arises in regression models. Constrained ordination methods are able to evaluate the strength, as well as the significance, of the relationship between the response data and the predictors. Akin to the role of partial correlation and partial regression coefficients, we can apply *partial constrained ordination* to evaluate the partial effects of one set of explanatory variables, observed in addition to the effects of another set of *covariates*.

While the methods of unconstrained (traditional) ordination (discussed in Section 22.2) provide the tools for exploratory data analysis, often generating hypotheses we can test, the methods of constrained ordination are effective tools for testing existing hypotheses related to multivariate data. They are therefore well suited to evaluate the results of experiments on the level of biotic communities. We use Monte Carlo permutation tests to carry out our hypothesis testing. We can test data coming from various experimental designs, e.g. complete randomised blocks, by using an appropriate form of the testing procedure. The analysis of data from complete randomised blocks design is illustrated by an example analysis presented in the ordination diagram in Fig. 22.2.

In the corresponding study (Špačková et al., 1998), the individual plots were exposed to one of four experimental treatments: removal of the dominant grass species (*Nardus stricta*), of plant litter, or of plant litter together with the moss layer, and finally a control treatment. The abundance and species composition of emerging seedlings was monitored in the individual plots. The data were analysed using redundancy analysis, with the identity of experimental blocks specified as a covariate to account for the experimental design. The permutation test identified significant differences among individual treatments. The first (horizontal) axis of the diagram in Fig. 22.2 shows the strongest difference in the plots where both the plant litter and moss layer were removed (at the right side of the diagram). This treatment increased the occurrence of *Cirsium palustre*, *Potentilla erecta* and *Ranunculus sp.*

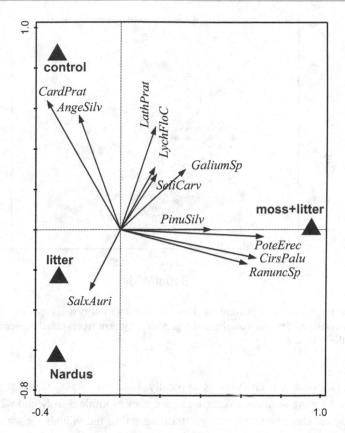

Figure 22.2 Ordination diagram for a redundancy analysis (RDA). The first two axes summarise the results of a field experiment which examined the effects of the removal of a dominant species (*Nardus*), the removal of plant litter (*litter*) and the removal of both plant litter and moss layer (*moss + litter*) on the abundance of grassland plant seedlings. The identity of experimental blocks was used as a covariate (so the method would be more appropriately referred to as a partial RDA). The two axes summarise about 38% of the variation in seedling abundance (after accounting for the differences among the blocks).

seedlings, but limited the abundance of those species which have arrows pointing in the opposite direction (to the left).

Both constrained and unconstrained ordination methods are very much common-place in the field of ecology, and are dealt with in more detail in the books of Šmilauer & Lepš (2014) or Jongman et al. (1987). A very detailed treatment of these methods is provided by Legendre & Legendre (2012).

22.4 Discriminant Analysis

In discriminant analysis (more precisely called *linear discriminant analysis*, LDA, or also *canonical variate analysis*, CVA), our observations (often biological objects) are character-ised by a set of variables describing their properties, but they are also classified using an independent criterion (i.e. the classification cannot be derived from the descriptor variables we use in the analysis). Our task is to find a classification rule (defined as a linear combination of the descriptor variables), or more often multiple rules, which predict the classification of

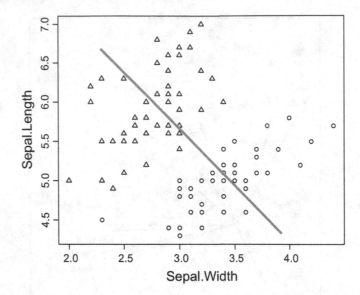

Figure 22.3 Sepal lengths and widths were measured on specimens of two iris species, which are plotted with different symbols (circles and triangles). The grey line segment represents the discriminant function best separating the two taxa.

observations. Discriminant analysis is typically used in biology when attempting to distinguish two or more similar-looking taxa (see also example 3 in Section 22.1) based on their morphological characteristics, using a 'training set' of individuals for which the classification was reliably (but expensively) determined using molecular methods. The principles of discriminant analysis are summarised in Fig. 22.3 for the simplest possible case where distinctions are made between just two classes.

Figure 22.3 is based on a simplification of an ancient dataset collected by Anderson (1936) and popularised by R. A. Fisher. We try to distinguish the two iris species using two morphological features of their flowers. Neither of the characteristics (X_1 or X_2) on its own can reliably distinguish the two species. We can, however, construct a linear function $Z = b_1X_1 + b_2X_2$ so that the specimens of one species will have low values of Z and the specimens of the second species will have high values. This *discriminant function Z* can then be used to distinguish the two species. The discriminant function is illustrated by the grey line in Fig. 22.3, where the perpendicular projections[5] of specimen symbols onto the grey line correspond to estimated Z values. If we need to distinguish three classes, then this generally requires two independent discriminant functions (axes), and for k classes we typically need $k - 1$ axes.

Discriminant analysis has much in common with multiple regression, but also with constrained ordination. Similar to multiple regression, we can also select an effective subset of predictors (e.g. morphological parameters) from a more numerous set of candidates.

---

[5] *Perpendicular projection* of a symbol means drawing a line from that symbol to the projection line, so that the two lines meet at a right angle (90°).

22.5 Example Data

The example data are divided into three tables. The first two tables correspond to example 2 (but include example 1 also) and we use them to illustrate both the unconstrained and constrained ordination. The third table represents the data for example 3.

The first table can be found in columns *A* to *AD*, representing 30 plant species recorded in 20 plots, with their abundances recorded on an ordinal estimation scale (values 0–9). The second table is in columns *AF* to *AI*, representing the thickness of the upper soil horizon (*A1Horiz*), approximate soil moisture (*Moisture*), type of management (*Mngmnt: SF* is standard farming, *BF* is biodynamic farming, *HF* is hobby farming, *NM* is nature protection management) and approximate amount of applied manure (*Manure*, with values 0–4).

The third table is in columns *AK* to *AO* and represents the dimensions of flower parts (length and width of sepals and petals) for 3×50 specimens of three iris species (taxonomic identity is encoded in the last column, *Species*).

We import (for the example code in Section 22.6) the three tables into three data frames – *chap22a*, *chap22b* and *chap22c*, respectively.

22.6 How to Proceed in R

We will use the *vegan* package (Oksanen et al., 2018) to perform our ordination analyses. Beyond the online help, an accessible introduction to its use can be found in Borcard et al. (2018).

22.6.1 Unconstrained Ordination

We start with an example of computing PCA with the data in the *chap22a* data frame:

```
library( vegan)
pca.1 <- rda( chap22a, scale=FALSE)
summary( pca.1)

...
Partitioning of variance:
              Inertia Proportion
Total            84.1          1
Unconstrained    84.1          1
Eigenvalues, and their contribution to the variance
Importance of components:
                        PC1    PC2     PC3    PC4     PC5
Eigenvalue            24.795 18.147 7.6291 7.153 5.6950
Proportion Explained   0.295  0.216 0.0907 0.085 0.0677
Cumulative Proportion  0.295  0.510 0.6012 0.686 0.7539
                        PC6    PC7    PC8    PC9   PC10
Eigenvalue            4.3333 3.199 2.7819 2.4820 1.854
Proportion Explained  0.0515 0.038 0.0331 0.0295 0.022
Cumulative Proportion 0.8054 0.843 0.8765 0.9060 0.928
```

```
                       PC11   PC12   PC13   PC14   PC15
Eigenvalue             1.7471 1.3136 0.9905 0.6378 0.5508
Proportion Explained   0.0208 0.0156 0.0118 0.0076 0.0066
Cumulative Proportion  0.9488 0.9644 0.9762 0.9838 0.9903
                       PC16    PC17    PC18    PC19
Eigenvalue             0.35058 0.19956 0.14880 0.11575
Proportion Explained   0.00417 0.00237 0.00177 0.00138
Cumulative Proportion  0.99448 0.99686 0.99862 1.00000


Scaling 2 for species and site scores
* Species are scaled proportional to eigenvalues
* Sites are unscaled: weighted dispersion equal on all
  dimensions
* General scaling constant of scores:  6.32


Species scores

             PC1      PC2      PC3      PC4      PC5      PC6
Ach.mil -0.6038   0.1239  0.00846  0.15957   0.4087   0.1279
Agr.sto  1.3740  -0.9640  0.16691  0.26647  -0.0877   0.0474
...
Bra.rut  0.1486   0.4769 -0.16876  0.50918  -0.9631   0.0295
Cal.cus  0.5385   0.1796  0.17509  0.23888   0.2553   0.1692


Site scores (weighted sums of species scores)
          PC1      PC2     PC3     PC4     PC5      PC6
sit1  -0.85678  -0.172   2.608  -1.130   0.4507  -2.4911
sit2  -1.64477  -1.230   0.887  -0.986   2.0346   1.8106
sit3  -0.44010  -2.383   0.930  -0.460  -1.0278  -0.0518
...
sit19  0.28094   2.190  -1.987  -3.234  -0.4576  -0.0239
sit20  2.34069   1.299   0.903   0.718  -0.0757  -0.9691
```

To compute an unconstrained PCA, we use (quite illogically) a function called *rda*. This function is normally used to compute a constrained RDA, but when we do not specify explanatory data, an unconstrained PCA is computed instead. The choice of the *scale=FALSE* argument is needed to compute the PCA from the variance–covariance matrix, rather than from a matrix of correlations (which we would get with *scale=TRUE*): individual variables will not be standardised to a unit variance, as standardisation is not required for a set of variables measured on the same scale. All 19 existing axes of the PCA were computed.[6]

---

[6] The maximum number of computed axes depends on the size of the data table – its number of rows (n) and its number of columns (m). The number of axes that can be computed is $\min(n - 1, m)$ for a linear ordination method (like PCA or RDA) or $\min(n - 1, m - 1)$ for a unimodal ordination method (like CA or CCA). So for our dataset, we have $\min(19, 30) = 19$ principal components (PCA axes).

The multiple rows labelled *Proportion Explained* specify the amount of variation individual axes explain (these values are on a scale from 0 to 1, rather than from 0 to 100). Similar information, but calculated cumulatively, is also shown in the *Cumulative Proportion* rows. We can therefore see that the first two PCA axes together explain 51.0% of the total variation (the first axis explains 29.5%). Obviously, the importance of axes gradually declines from the first to the last.

The description of the PCA results continues with the species (response variable) scores and then the site (observation) scores, both specified for the first six PCA axes. But instead of inspecting the scores, it is much better to plot those objects to obtain a summary overview:

```
plot( pca.1)
```

The resulting ordination diagram is shown in Fig. 22.4 without any modifications (except the colour of species labels was changed from red to grey).

The species (response variables) should be represented by arrows in the diagram, but the *plot* function obviously simplifies the presentation to reduce overall clutter in the graph. From the diagram in Fig. 22.4 we can see that e.g. plots 5, 7 and 10 have a high mutual similarity in terms of their species composition, whereas plot 16 differs substantially. By comparing the locations of plots and plant species, we can judge which species are responsible for the differences among the vegetation types.

We now demonstrate the calculation of non-metric multidimensional scaling for the same dataset. In contrast to the PCA method, here we must explicitly choose the distance (dissimilarity) measure and use it to calculate a matrix of distances among the plots. The *vegan* library offers the various types of distance measures most frequently used in

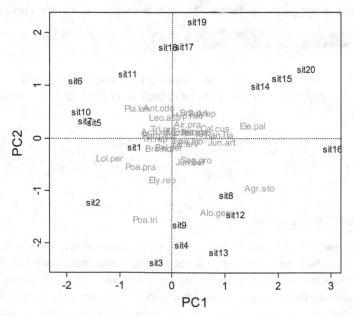

Figure 22.4 PCA ordination diagram computed for the dune meadow dataset from Terschelling island.

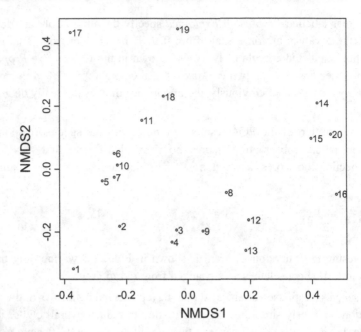

Figure 22.5 Ordination diagram of the NMS analysis for the dune meadow data, using Bray–Curtis distances.

community ecology. One popular measure is the Bray–Curtis distance, and we can calculate the corresponding matrix in this way:

```
dist.1 <- vegdist( chap22a, method="bray")
```

Subsequently, we compute the NMS solution with two *a priori* chosen axes:

```
nms.1 <- metaMDS( dist.1, k=2)
```

The resulting ordination diagram (showing plots only, as the position of species can only be roughly approximated using this method) is created in the following way and presented in Fig. 22.5:

```
plot( nms.1)
text( nms.1, adj=0)
```

22.6.2 Constrained Ordination

We continue our use of the *vegan* package to demonstrate constrained ordination methods. We have two functions available for unimodal and linear constrained ordination – *cca* and *rda*, respectively. In our simple example, we compute RDA to explain the dune meadow community data (*chap22a*) with the help of four explanatory variables from the *chap22b* data frame:

```
rda.1<-rda( chap22a ~ AlHoriz+Moisture+Mngmnt+Manure,
            data=chap22b)
summary( rda.1)
```
...
Partitioning of variance:

	Inertia	Proportion
Total	84.1	1.00
Constrained	47.1	0.56
Unconstrained	37.0	0.44

Eigenvalues, and their contribution to the variance
Importance of components:

	RDA1	RDA2	RDA3	RDA4	RDA5
Eigenvalue	21.496	13.564	5.4983	3.115	1.8755
Proportion Explained	0.256	0.161	0.0654	0.037	0.0223
Cumulative Proportion	0.256	0.417	0.4821	0.519	0.5415

	RDA6	PC1	PC2	PC3	PC4
Eigenvalue	1.5647	8.943	6.5039	4.963	3.9790
Proportion Explained	0.0186	0.106	0.0773	0.059	0.0473
Cumulative Proportion	0.5601	0.666	0.7437	0.803	0.8500

	PC5	PC6	PC7	PC8	PC9
Eigenvalue	3.0377	2.6603	1.8740	1.6339	1.3133
Proportion Explained	0.0361	0.0316	0.0223	0.0194	0.0156
Cumulative Proportion	0.8861	0.9177	0.9400	0.9594	0.9750

	PC10	PC11	PC12	PC13
Eigenvalue	0.74748	0.68804	0.38945	0.2772
Proportion Explained	0.00889	0.00818	0.00463	0.0033
Cumulative Proportion	0.98390	0.99207	0.99670	1.0000

...

Scaling 2 for species and site scores
* Species are scaled proportional to eigenvalues
* Sites are unscaled: weighted dispersion equal on
    all dimensions
* General scaling constant of scores: 6.32

Species scores

	RDA1	RDA2	RDA3	RDA4	RDA5
Ach.mil	0.56586	0.0898	-0.104041	-0.13878	-0.116919
Agr.sto	-1.24956	-0.8714	-0.098877	-0.03250	0.183643
...					
Bra.rut	0.01693	0.2741	0.449472	0.09511	-0.097305
Cal.cus	-0.43733	0.1211	-0.071342	-0.08752	-0.000697

...

```
Site scores (weighted sums of species scores)
          RDA1      RDA2      RDA3     RDA4     RDA5     RDA6
row1    1.0319  -0.2309  -1.95700   2.209    3.329    1.1547
row2    1.6663  -1.0668  -2.28141  -1.642   -2.122   -1.3173
...
row19  -0.5342   2.8416  -0.07779   2.822   -3.548    0.9314
row20  -2.3188   1.5328  -0.18693  -0.324    1.694    3.7466


Site constraints (linear combinations of constraining
                                          variables)
          RDA1      RDA2      RDA3     RDA4     RDA5      RDA6
row1    0.7689  -1.2497  -1.0890   2.2061   1.3923  -0.03880
row2    1.8877   0.0511  -2.7315  -1.4767  -0.8345  -0.48234
...
row19  -1.6361   1.7738  -0.6763   0.9612  -1.0200   1.68193
row20  -1.6297   1.7896  -0.6963   1.0625  -1.1003   1.77063


Biplot scores for constraining variables
           RDA1      RDA2      RDA3      RDA4      RDA5       RDA6
AlHoriz  -0.537   0.1029   0.2045  -0.5387   0.4102  -0.44756
Moisture -0.933  -0.0388   0.0663  -0.2328  -0.1914   0.18128
MngmntHF  0.404  -0.1688   0.6328  -0.3168   0.0514   0.55225
MngmntNM -0.470   0.8502  -0.0675   0.0532   0.2209   0.00658
MngmntSF -0.293  -0.7475  -0.1385   0.4815   0.1631  -0.27898
Manure    0.221  -0.9010  -0.1519   0.1767   0.2555   0.14009


Centroids for factor constraints
           RDA1     RDA2     RDA3     RDA4     RDA5      RDA6
MngmntBF  1.648   0.246  -1.693  -1.017  -1.869  -1.0774
MngmntHF  0.989  -0.413   1.550  -0.776   0.126   1.3524
MngmntNM -1.015   1.836  -0.146   0.115   0.477   0.0142
MngmntSF -0.633  -1.614  -0.299   1.040   0.352  -0.6025
```

The initial part of the *summary* function output reveals that the four explanatory variables explained 56% of the total variation in the community composition dataset (see the *Proportion* column in the *Constrained* row of the *Partitioning of variance* table). There are six constrained (RDA) axes that summarise the explained component of the data,[7] and they are followed by another 13 unconstrained axes that summarise the residual (unexplained) variation.

The final part of the *summary* function output again presents the scores of species and plots in the ordination space, but here this information is extended by additional types of ordination scores (particularly for predictors, but also for plots). We will not discuss the various score types here – please check one of the recommended textbooks dealing with multivariate analysis for more information on these.

---

[7] When we use purely numerical explanatory variables (predictors), the number of constrained axes usually matches the count of predictors. But here one of the predictors is a factor with four levels, so it contributes three degrees of freedom to the complexity of the constrained ordination.

The next step in a constrained ordination should be to test whether the chosen predictors are significantly related to the community composition (i.e. the response data). This can be done in the following way:

```
anova( rda.1, step=1000)
Permutation test for rda under reduced model
Permutation: free
Number of permutations: 999

Model: rda(formula = chap22a ~ A1Horiz + Moisture +
              Mngmnt + Manure, data = chap22b)
          Df Variance     F Pr(>F)
Model      6     47.1  2.76  0.001 ***
Residual  13     37.0
```

The test results support the conclusion that there is a significant relationship between the community and the explanatory variables.[8] The *step* argument specified (roughly speaking) the number of permutations used during the test.

Finally, we plot the constrained ordination results (see the resulting graph in Fig. 22.6):

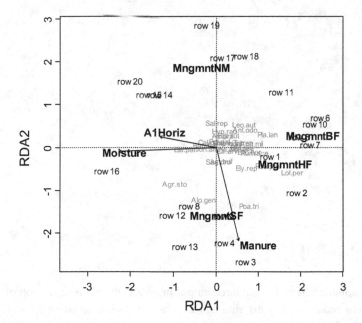

Figure 22.6 Ordination diagram (triplot) for the redundancy analysis (RDA) carried out on the dune meadow dataset, where all of the available predictors were used as constraining variables. The first two axes (those displayed) explain 41.7% of the total variation in the community composition data.

---

[8] This conclusion does not necessarily imply that the plant community has a significant relationship with every chosen predictor: for that we would need to test each predictor separately and also consider possible overlaps in their explanatory power (as we do in multiple regression models).

```
plot( rda.1)
```

Even for such a small dataset, the default ordination diagram is difficult to read due to the numerous plot elements.

22.6.3 Discriminant Analysis

We can compute linear discriminant analysis using the *lda* function in the *MASS* library (Venables & Ripley, 2002):

```
library( MASS)
lda.1 <- lda( Species ~ ., data=chap22c)
```

But this time we cannot use the *summary* function, we just print the resulting object:

```
lda.1

...
Group means:
           Sepal.Length Sepal.Width Petal.Length
setosa             5.01        3.43         1.46
versicolor         5.94        2.77         4.26
virginica          6.59        2.97         5.55
           Petal.Width
setosa           0.246
versicolor       1.326
virginica        2.026
Coefficients of linear discriminants:
                LD1      LD2
Sepal.Length  0.829   0.0241
Sepal.Width   1.534   2.1645
Petal.Length -2.201  -0.9319
Petal.Width  -2.810   2.8392


Proportion of trace:
   LD1    LD2
0.9912 0.0088
```

It is apparent from the last three output lines that the main separation of the three iris species happens along the first discriminant axis, which makes up about 99% of the variation explained by both discriminant axes together.

22.7 Alternative Software

To analyse ecological (but also other) data with ordination methods (and also by discriminant analysis), we recommend the commercial Canoco 5 software (http://www.canoco5.com), which is more user-friendly and produces plots of higher quality than the R code discussed above (compare Fig. 22.1 or 22.2 with Fig. 22.4 or 22.6). Canoco 5 offers both unconstrained (PCA, CA, DCA, PCoA, NMS) and constrained (CCA, RDA) ordination methods alongside additional, complementary methods, and it comes with a detailed user guide (ter Braak & Šmilauer, 2012). We recommend our book (Šmilauer & Lepš, 2014) for a description of how to work with this software,.

Most of the multivariate methods are also implemented in another commercial software, PCORD (http://www.pcord.com).

22.8 Reporting Analyses

22.8.1 Methods

We summarised the compositional variation in grassland vegetation communities using the principal component analysis (PCA) method, calculated from centred (but not standardised) data.

The relationship between grassland community composition and the explanatory variables, representing management regime and soil properties, was summarised using redundancy analysis (RDA) with centred response data. The significance of the relationship was tested with a Monte Carlo permutation test using 999 permutations.

22.8.2 Results

The results of the PCA are summarised in the ordination diagram in Fig. 22.4. The first two axes, those shown in the diagram, explain 51% of the total variation in community composition.

We found a significant relationship between plant community composition and the tested set of explanatory variables (pseudo-F = 2.76, p = 0.001), which explained 56% of the total compositional variation. The results of RDA are summarised by the ordination diagram in Fig. 22.6.

22.9 Recommended Reading

Quinn & Keough (2002), pp. 401–487 and pp. 491–493.

Sokal & Rohlf (2012), pp. 694–697 (discriminant analysis only).

E. Anderson (1936) The species problem in iris. *Annals of the Missouri Botanical Garden*, **23**: 457–509.

M. Batterink & G. Wijffels (1983) Een vergelijkend vegetatiekundig onderzoek naar de typologie en invloeden van het beheer van 1973 tot 1982 in de Duinweilanden op Terschelling. *Report of Agricultural University*, Department of Vegetation Science, Plant Ecology and Weed Science, Wageningen.

D. Borcard, F. Gillet & P. Legendre (2018) *Numerical Ecology with R*, 2nd edn. Springer, New York.

R. H. Jongman, C. J. F. ter Braak & O. F. R. van Tongeren (1987) *Data Analysis in Community and Landscale Ecology*. Cambridge University Press, Cambridge.

P. Legendre & L. Legendre (2012) *Numerical Ecology*, 3rd English edn. Elsevier, Amsterdam (particularly pp. 425–520 for unconstrained ordination and pp. 625–710 for constrained ordination methods, including discriminant analysis).

J. Oksanen, F. G. Blanchet, M. Friendly, R. Kindt, P. Legendre, D. McGlinn, ..., H. Wagner (2018) *Vegan*: community ecology package. R package version 2.5-3. https://cran.R-project.org/package= vegan.

P. Šmilauer & J. Lepš (2014) *Multivariate Analysis of Ecological Data Using Canoco 5*. Cambridge University Press, Cambridge.

I. Špačková, I. Kotorová & J. Lepš (1998) Sensitivity of seedling recruitment to moss, litter and dominant removal in an oligotrophic wet meadow. *Folia Geobotanica*, **33**: 17–30.

C. J. F. ter Braak & P. Šmilauer (2012) *Canoco Reference Manual and User's Guide: Software for Ordination, Version 5.10*. Microcomputer Power, Ithaca, NY, 536 pp.

W. N. Venables & B. D. Ripley (2002) *Modern Applied Statistics with S*, 4th edn. Springer, New York.

Appendix A:
First Steps with R Software

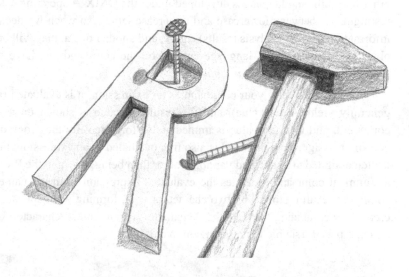

R software is a very complex beast that has a long history of development and improvement. This means that there are often alternative ways to perform a particular task and that any rules on how to use R will probably have some exceptions. In this brief introduction we will try to describe things simply, possibly at the expense of some inaccuracy.

A.1 Starting and Ending R, Command Line, Organising Data

We assume that you have already installed the R software on your computer. The details of the installation procedure depend on the operating system, on the access rights of your account and partly on the particular version of R. The essential information about installing on Microsoft Windows can be found at https://cran.r-project.org/bin/windows/base/ and for Mac OS X at https://cran.r-project.org/bin/macosx/. In the following description we will focus on using R within the MS Windows operating system, but the differences between operating systems are few, and they primarily concern handling external files.

You can start the R program from the operating system menu, e.g. by *Start | All Programs | R | R 3.5.3* (the ending depends on the program version and also on the choices made during installation). Or you can start R using a desktop icon (shown as a capital blue letter R). After R opens, it shows an application workspace mostly consisting of the *R Console* window. In this introductory guide, you will learn how to work with commands typed directly in the console window using your keyboard; the alternative ways of specifying the commands (e.g. with the RStudio add-on software) will then come as a natural, easy change.

You can find the *command prompt* in the last non-empty line of the console window, indicating the place where R software awaits your commands:

```
>
```

The R software is based around a scripting (programming) language named S, which is a functional programming language with relatively straightforward syntax rules.[1] As with other programming languages developed under the UNIX™ operating system, the S language distinguishes between lowercase and uppercase letters, so when we decide to call a piece of information (data or analysis results) e.g. **A**, and another one **a**, they will be treated as different objects. Commands in S language entered on the command line have one of two possible forms: an *expression* or an *assignment*.

If you specify your command as an expression, it is evaluated (a correct expression generally yields some value), and the resulting value is shown on a line following your command, and then the value is immediately 'forgotten' by the program. In contrast, some part of an assignment command is also first evaluated as an expression, but its resulting value is then assigned to a specified variable, rather than being shown in the R Console window. The assignment command separates the evaluated expression from the name of the variable (in which the result is stored) by two characters, $<-$, forming what appears to be an arrow, and created by combining the 'less than' character with a 'minus' character. Let us first start with an example of a simple expression command:

```
> 2 + 3
[1]  5
```

Note that to reproduce the commands we demonstrate here, you simply type the bold part shown on the first line after the '>' prompt, and then press the <Enter> key to execute the command. R evaluates this demanding arithmetic operation and confirms that its result is indeed 5. The value 1 in square brackets is a confusing little distraction, but we will explain its meaning later.

Now we will try an assignment command, naturally extending the preceding example:

```
> x <- 2 + 3
```

After you enter this command, it may seem like nothing happened, as the calculated value is not shown. But it is now stored in a variable called x that we have just created. We can confirm this by using our brand new variable as an expression:

```
> x
[1]  5
```

From now on, R will remember this value. When you close the program, R asks you about saving its workspace and if you agree with that (one of the rare occasions when you can see a dialogue box in R), the x value is stored in the workspace file and the next time you reopen that file, the x variable will be available again.

---

[1] Certainly having a knowledge of alternative programming language (e.g. C, C++ or Java) will not hurt, although their rules differ in multiple details.

Naturally, you are not learning S language to use it as a simple calculator. Rather, we want to be able to handle a typical dataset containing multiple observations for a particular variable, so we use sets of numbers (or categorical values, representing information about categories) called *vectors*. You will usually import such vectors (or an entire data table composed of multiple vectors, as we explain later) from external data, such as an Excel™ spreadsheet, but first let us illustrate how to create a simple, short vector variable with numerical values on the R command line:

```
> x <- c( 1, 4.5, 3.2, 2.8)
```

To combine four values into a single vector, we use the function *c*. It is used the same way as most other functions in S language: you specify the function name and then a list of function parameters which are enclosed in parentheses. If there are no parameters, you will input empty parentheses. If there are multiple parameters, as in our example above, then you will separate them with a comma character. You will also note that we have chosen to store our vector of four values using the same variable name (x) that we used in our earlier assignment command which stored the value 5. So what happened with the original value of x? Let us look at the contents of x again:

```
> x
[1] 1.0 4.5 3.2 2.8
```

Sadly, the value of 5 is now gone. This might come as a shock to Microsoft Windows users, where the software traditionally warns the user if she is going to perform some dangerous operation, e.g. destroy existing data. But R originates from the UNIX™ environment, where the basic philosophy is 'the computer user is the master, she knows what she is doing, so just do it'.

Now we will show another expression type of command:

```
> mean( x)
[1] 2.875
```

The *mean* function calculates an arithmetic average, but the result is not stored anywhere, just displayed and then forgotten by the software because we did not use an assignment command. The *c* and *mean* functions are already defined in S language definitions, alongside many more functions. Here are some further code examples:

```
> m <- mean( x); v <- var( x)
> sqrt( v) / m
[1] 0.5027461
```

Here we defined a new variable (and we decided to name it *m*) to store the arithmetic average of x and another variable v to store the variance. Both assignments were specified on a single line. If you put multiple statements in the same line, you must separate them with a semicolon character. Finally, we combined the information in v and m using an expression that calculates the coefficient of variation (standard deviation divided by mean). This also introduced yet another function – *sqrt*, which calculates the square root of the passed value. It also works with vectors, as we can easily illustrate with *x*-values:

```
> sqrt( x)
[1]  1.000000 2.121320 1.788854 1.673320
```

In fact, S language does not distinguish between 'single values' and vectors, an individual value is treated as a vector with a single entry. This is also the reason why the output of our first 2 + 3 expression started with the text [1]. The notation in square brackets is used to account for very long data vectors that we can sometimes find ourselves working with. When you try to display their values, they will rarely fit on a single line, so the whole number in square brackets tells you (at the beginning of each output line) which entry that particular line starts with. It also serves as a friendly reminder of the values you need to input in order to access individual entries of a vector. We will discuss this in more detail later, but for now let's just take a quick look at this by displaying the third entry of the *x* vector:

```
> x[3]
[1]  3.2
```

If you want to store some little notes explaining the purpose of individual commands with your S language script then you can use the hash character: whatever follows it is taken as a comment until the end of that line and is ignored by the R command interpreter:

```
> x[3]  # Select third entry of the x vector
[1]  3.2
```

Earlier we illustrated that two or more short commands can be placed on the same line if you separate them by semicolons. But it is definitively tidier to put each command on a separate line. An opposite issue must be solved when a command is so long that it does not fit on a single line. We can then press the <Enter> key before the command finishes (it's better that we don't do it in the middle of a function or variable name), and most of the time the R software understands that what we have entered so far cannot be a full command so it waits for additional input from you. This is reflected by a different prompt character at the start of the next command line. Instead of the usual > character, a continuation character + is shown. Let us demonstrate it with an example where we have simply pressed the <Enter> key too early:

```
> log( x
+ )
[1]  0.000000 1.504077 1.163151 1.029619
```

On the first line we started a call to function *log* which calculates (without additional parameters) natural logarithms of the values passed as its first parameter, but we pressed <Enter> before closing the *log* function call with a right-parenthesis character. R therefore displays a continuation mark and we finalise the command by typing the right parenthesis and pressing <Enter>.

The abilities of S language can be further extended by defining new functions, which are then used in exactly the same way as the functions predefined within the R software. This extensibility was probably one of the key aspects contributing to the rapid, widespread adoption of this software across the world of scientific computing. Most of the extension functions are accompanied by easily accessible online documentation and combined into specialised *packages*, also called libraries. There are hundreds of such packages, likely implementing all known statistical methods. Do you want to work with phylogenetic trees, with the data originating from animal telemetry, or with the results of an analysis of DNA chips? One or multiple packages exist for everything, as you can see for yourself by exploring the following web page: https://cran.r-project.org/web/packages/available_packages_by_name.html

Packages that are not installed as part of the standard installation procedure can be added later on from the R program itself using the *Packages | Install package(s)* command. Usually, after we select this command, the first choice concerns the depository into which we want the R program to look for available packages. The choice is yours, but we recommend the default *0-Cloud [https]* item. We can then choose one or multiple (press the <Ctrl> key when selecting additional entries) packages to install. Further, R itself can extend our choice, if the desired packages require the presence of other, not yet installed packages. To use an additional package (mostly the functions, but often also their example data), you must first open it using the *library* function. As an example, to use the *survival* library (which, as it happens, is installed automatically, but is not active until you decide so), we execute the following command:

```
> library( survival)
```

Executing such a command might lead (mostly depending on the actual chosen package) to one or a few lines of output, providing additional information about the package and its context,[2] or you might not see any output. If you have finished using the library, it is usually a good idea to close it,[3] e.g. with

```
> detach( package:survival)
```

As every object that you create with an assignment command remains available in the R workspace, you can quite quickly build a heap of trash data that you no longer need. When attempting to get rid of such data (see the next section), however, you should be careful to not delete anything you may need in the future. Better still, you might find it useful to work with your data in a more structured way, keeping non-related datasets in separate storage areas, possibly located in separate folders on your computer. The R software normally saves the data (and user-defined functions) present in your workspace into a file named *.RData* by

---

[2] Such as when you install a package created for a slightly newer version of R than you presently use.

[3] This applies particularly when working with a set of libraries providing partially overlapping functionality – it is then possible that the shared functionality is provided by functions with identical names and so you can mix up their implementation.

default. In the Windows operating system, this implies that the name of the workspace file is empty and the *RData* part is the file extension, identifying the file type. The resulting workspace file is normally stored in the current working folder of the R program. But you can name the file differently, e.g. *FieldWork2020.RData*, and you can also store it in a different place (e.g. using the *File | Save Workspace …* menu command). Consequently, when you store a data workspace from a particular research project in an *.RData* file in a separate folder, you can create a shortcut to that file on your Windows desktop. When you click on the shortcut link, Windows will open the R program with this particular workspace and whatever you add there will be stored in the same place again upon exit.

The S language has a built-in support for effectively using the language and available functions. To obtain information about a particular function, e.g. *mean*, you can use the *help* function:

```
> help( mean)
```

Alternatively, we can use a simpler form most of the time:

```
> ?mean
```

The contents of the help information (which by default displays in your web browser) includes the description of various parameters of the *mean* function and an explanation of its functionality. This is of course rather trivial for an arithmetic average, but very important for more specialised functions: all standardly available packages must have help available for the functions they implement. Another very important piece of information that you find in every online help page are examples of how you use the particular function, and these examples are located at the very end of each help page. They can support you in understanding what the parameter descriptions were really trying to tell you and also how to use the specific function in the context of related functions (this probably does not apply to *mean* so much).

We will finish our brief introduction to using the R program and S language by mentioning how to close the software. If you work in Microsoft Windows, the program contains – as any Windows program must contain – the *Exit* command in the *File* menu. But as you hopefully began to understand, the R program works around its functional language S, so to get the warm feeling of an R devotee, please close your R sessions in the following way:

```
> q()
```

But remember – you will suffer that nasty Windowsy dialogue box asking about saving your workspace, unless you choose the even funnier form, which saves the workspace without any question:

```
> q( "yes")
```

We would like to wrap up this section with a quick note on the S language examples we are using in this appendix. We use space characters liberally, simply with the aim of making the examples easier to read and understand. If you want to save some electrons (or your fingertips), you can omit most of the empty space and write, e.g. 3+2 instead of the demonstrated 3 + 2.

A.2 Managing Your Data

To list all the objects present in your workspace, you can use the *objects* function:

```
> objects()
...
```

    The list of variables shown will differ depending on how much you have worked with R before this moment. Alternatively, you can use the *ls* function. If the list of existing objects is too long, you can filter it based on their names by using the *pattern* parameter. This parameter uses so-called regular expression to describe what the object name must look like to be shown (listed). Any sufficient description of regular expression syntax would exceed the scope of this short introduction, so if you are interested in this topic we suggest you start with the *?regex* command. Here we just note that to display all data objects containing (anywhere in their name) a text sequence *lm*, you should specify the following command (the text on subsequent lines illustrates the last two lines of output shown at a particular R installation, this can vary depending on your context):

```
> objects( pattern="lm")
...
[ 55]  "lmlist.1"   "lmlist.2"   "nlme.1"    "nlme.1RE"   "nlme.2"    "nlme.2re"
[ 61]  "nlme.3"     "nlme.x1"
```

    To determine what a particular object represents, the most straightforward way is to type its name and press the <Enter> key: this effectively evaluates (and shows) the object as an expression command. But for real-world data tables with hundreds of observations (and often multiple variables), the output might be overwhelming. So to explore an unknown data object, it might be best to start with the *str* function, which works for all kinds of R objects:

```
> str( x)
num [ 1:4] 1 4.5 3.2 2.8
```

    The output of *str* tells you that *x* is a numerical vector with four entries and displays them all (because the vector is short):

```
> str( mean)
function (x, ...)
```

    This output tells you that *mean* is a function with one obligatory parameter (you cannot calculate an average without input data, right?) and some additional optional parameter(s). Let us look now at a more extensive dataset:

```
> data( faithful)
> str( faithful)
```

```
'data.frame':   272 obs. of  2 variables:
 $ eruptions: num  3.6 1.8 3.33 2.28 4.53 ...
 $ waiting  : num  79 54 74 62 85 55 88 85 51 85 ...
```

Here we have used a predefined dataset representing a data table with two columns (variables) and 272 rows (cases or observations). We first copied the predefined object into our workspace using the *data* function and then demonstrated how the *str* function handles it, describing its type and size and briefly summarising its two variables.

An alternative way to explore not just R data objects, but also objects representing the results of statistical analyses, is by using the *summary* function. It is perhaps fair to say that while the *str* function takes the stance of an external observer, primarily describing the structure of complex data objects, the *summary* function provides an insider look, having a greater understanding of the meaning of the objects being summarised. This can be illustrated with the *faithful* data frame:

```
> summary( faithful)
```

```
   eruptions          waiting
 Min.   :1.600   Min.   :43.0
 1st Qu.:2.163   1st Qu.:58.0
 Median :4.000   Median :76.0
 Mean   :3.488   Mean   :70.9
 3rd Qu.:4.454   3rd Qu.:82.0
 Max.   :5.100   Max.   :96.0
```

The summary provided for a data frame object effectively summarises individual variables present in the table in a manner that is appropriate for their data type. Both variables are numerical in our example, so we get numerical summaries which include various quantiles and the arithmetic average. The *summary* function particularly shines when used with estimated statistical models (such as the linear regression or ANOVA models).

After such extensive demonstrations of how to explore your or someone else's data, it is probably useful to note that you can move within the contents of the *R Console* window by using the scroll-bar on the right side of the window.

When R software looks up an object (data or function) that is mentioned in an expression, it not only checks your workspace (we're sure you have already realised that your workspace does not contain either the *mean* or *sqrt* function). Instead, it goes through a set of folders containing definitions for functions and/or data, which is called a *search list*. You can find the names of those folders using the *search* function:

```
> search()
```

```
[ 1] ".GlobalEnv"        "package:stats"     "package:graphics"
[ 4] "package:grDevices" "package:utils"     "package:datasets"
[ 7] "package:methods"   "Autoloads"         "package:base"
```

You can use the whole number representing the position of a particular folder as the first parameter for the *objects* (or *ls*) function to list the objects present in the folder:

```
> objects( 6)
[1] "ability.cov"          "airmiles"           "AirPassengers"
...
```

The above command shows the names of objects representing many example datasets in the R program (*package:datasets* in the above output), but additional sample datasets are also available within individual specialised packages.

The set of search folders is by no means definitive. You can define additional ones using the *attach* function and remove them again from the search list using the *detach* function. This is used primarily to provide access to the names of variables within your data frame (see the next section), namely for their use in functions that do not support the *data* parameter.[4]

To permanently delete a data object or a function from your workspace (naturally, you cannot remove anything from the folders provided by the R software itself), use the *rm* function:

```
> rm( m, v)
```

By executing the above command, you remove the *m* and *v* objects you have created earlier:

```
> m
Error: object 'm' not found
```

Be careful, though: R does not ask for your confirmation, it just executes your wish!

A.3 Data Types in R

The main data types available in the S language are vectors, arrays, lists and data frames.

The **vector** is the simplest and most essential data type: it is an ordered group of values (numbers or other value types). You can create a new vector object e.g. using the *c* function as we already illustrated in Section A.1. Here we provide another example, which uses the : operator instead:

```
> x <- 1:8
> x
[1] 1 2 3 4 5 6 7 8
```

---

[4] The *data* parameter is used by most of the functions creating (estimating) statistical models, but also by many graphing functions, and it specifies the place in which the variable names given in the model description are located.

The : operator is placed in an expression between the starting and ending values of a sequence of whole numbers, and it creates this sequence with a step of 1.[5]

Once you create a vector, you can use it in expressions such as this one in which we are calculating inverse values:

```
> 1 / x
[1]  1.0000000 0.5000000 0.3333333 0.2500000 0.2000000 0.1666667
[7]  0.1428571 0.1250000
```

When you use vectors in arithmetic expressions, the operations are usually performed on individual values, so they return new vectors of the same length as the input ones. The basic arithmetic operators include $+$, $-$, $*$, $/$ and $\wedge$ (for calculating powers). There is also a large range of additional functions, including *log, log10, exp, sin, cos, tan, sqrt, min, max, sum* or *range*. The *length* function returns the vector length passed as its parameter. Two important statistical functions are *mean*, which for a z parameter (presumably a vector with numbers) returns a value equal to the expression $sum(z)/length(z)$, i.e. the arithmetic mean, and *var*, which returns a value equal to $sum((z - mean(z))^2)/(length(z) - 1)$, i.e. the sample variance.

Besides working with numbers, we can also use two other basic data value types, namely the *text values* (more formally called *character strings*) and *logical values* (*TRUE*, *FALSE*). We can specify text values by enclosing one or multiple characters in double or single quotes (however we cannot mix them for a particular value), e.g.

```
> disturbed <- c( "yes", "yes", "no", "no", "yes")
> disturbed
[1] "yes" "yes" "no"  "no"  "yes"
```

Note that most statistical models in R work with a more specialised version of variables with non-numerical values. These are called *factors* and represent categorical data. You can easily create a factor variable from a vector with text values using the *as.factor* function:

```
> Dist <- as.factor( disturbed)
> Dist
[1] yes yes no  no  yes
Levels: no yes
> summary( Dist)
 no yes
  2   3
```

Logical values are most often created by comparing numerical or text values using logical operators: $==$ (two equal signs) tests for equivalence, $!=$ tests for difference and operators like $>$, $>=$, $<$, $<=$ can be used for comparing the order of values, including the

---

[5] If you prefer a different step size, i.e. incremental size increase, look at the *seq* function.

alphabetical ordering of text values, as we illustrate in the following examples (the last one uses alphabetical ordering):[6]

```
> disturbed == "yes"
```
```
[1]   TRUE  TRUE FALSE FALSE   TRUE
```
```
> disturbed != "yes"
```
```
[1] FALSE FALSE  TRUE   TRUE FALSE
```
```
> disturbed <= "oops"
```
```
[1] FALSE FALSE   TRUE   TRUE FALSE
```

There are finger-friendly shortcuts for the *FALSE* and *TRUE* logical values, namely *F* and *T*.

All the value types can also be combined with a special value *NA*, representing *missing* (unknown) *values*. Missing values are unfortunately quite frequent visitors to scientific datasets, but we must be careful when handling them. If you compute a sum of values, with one of them being *NA*, the result is of course *NA*. And when you try to find out (in a large set of values) which of the values are missing, you might be surprised by the result:

```
> x == NA
```
```
[1] NA NA NA NA NA NA NA NA
```

This happens because, e.g. for our *x* vector above, the first value is 1, and we simply cannot say whether it is equal to an unknown value: that answer is unknown ... The only way to get a definitive answer is to use a special function *is.na*:

```
> is.na( x)
```
```
[1] FALSE FALSE FALSE FALSE FALSE FALSE FALSE FALSE
```

We can see that there are no missing values in the *x* vector. To make our demonstration a little more sensible, we can add one *NA* value to the front of *x*:

```
> x <- c( NA, x)
```

Now we can check again:

```
> is.na( x)
```
```
[1]   TRUE FALSE FALSE FALSE FALSE FALSE FALSE FALSE FALSE
```

To access individual entries (elements) of a vector (but also of other data structures we describe later), you can use *indexing*, i.e. choose the required subset of vector elements by

---

[6] Note that the reference word 'oops' was chosen *ad hoc*, in the hope that it might tune with your feelings at this moment of learning ☺.

a specification enclosed in square brackets, which is placed after the vector name. As an example, to obtain the second and third elements of the *disturbed* vector, we can use the following expression:

```
> disturbed[ c(2,3)]
[1] "yes" "no"
```

Note that the returned value is again a vector with the same type of values as *disturbed*, but this time with just two entries based on our specification.

We can describe indexing more generally by saying that we apply – in the square brackets – an indexing vector, which might have one of the following forms:

- A vector with logical values – in this case, only the entries matching the *TRUE* values in the indexing vector will be selected. For example, the following command displays only those *x*-values which are larger than 3: *x[x>3]*.
- A vector with positive whole numbers – this is the example we illustrated earlier; the values must be between 1 and the length of the vector. We can also select individual elements, such as *x[3]*, but the value 3 still acts as an indexing vector with a single element.
- A vector with negative whole numbers – the absolute values of those numbers represent the vector entries to be omitted, rather than retained; as an example, the expression *x[−3]* returns the whole *x* vector except for its third entry.

An indexed vector can also appear at the left side of an assignment command. By doing this we apply the assignment only to selected vector entries. Here is an example:

```
> x[ is.na( x)] <- 0
```

Note that the indexing vector defined in the square brackets contains logical values: *TRUE* entries represent *x* entries with missing values, while *FALSE* entries represent all remaining values. Consequently, the missing values in *x* will be replaced with zeros, while the rest remain unchanged.

Arrays are a natural extension of vectors into two or more dimensions. The most straightforward among the arrays of varying dimensionality is a two-dimensional **matrix** with rows and columns. When indexing arrays, the indices must be provided in two or more sets, depending on the array dimensionality. To give an example, the search folder that contains sample R datasets has a matrix object with numerical values called *state.x77*, which contains various facts about individual US states:

```
> class( state.x77)
[1] "matrix"
> dim( state.x77)
[1] 50  8
```

The *class* function provides information about the data type, here for the *state.x77* object. Another very useful function is *dim*, which provides the size of an array (it does not work with vectors) – returning a vector with as many whole numbers as there are array dimensions. So for our example object, we have a matrix with 50 rows and 8 columns.

We can display the values present in the first three rows of the second column of the *state.x77* matrix using the following indexing expression:

```
> state.x77[ 1:3, 2]

 Alabama  Alaska Arizona
    3624    6315    4530
```

Note that although we display three rows of a single column, the values are shown as a vector: the indexing operator (represented by the square brackets) 'simplified' the indexed array into a vector object. There is one issue with these displayed results: we know which states are shown, but we do not know what characteristic those values represent. There is a handy function called *dimnames* that we can use for arrays to display the names assigned to entries across individual dimensions (here the row names and column names):

```
> dimnames( state.x77)
[[ 1]]
 [ 1] "Alabama"     "Alaska"    "Arizona"    "Arkansas"
...
[ 49] "Wisconsin"   "Wyoming"

[[ 2]]
[ 1] "Population" "Income"    "Illiteracy" "Life Exp"   "Murder"
[ 6] "HS Grad"    "Frost"     "Area"
```

The names are displayed as two vectors with text values (the names of US states and the names of characteristics), so we can see that the second column contains the average income in a state. To obtain the names of entries for a vector object, the *names* function must be used instead of *dimnames*. Be warned, however, that vectors you create have no names for their entries by default:

```
> names( x)
NULL
```

In the output of the *dimnames* function above, there are two strange-looking entries that have the values 1 and 2 enclosed in double squared brackets. These suggest to us that the value returned by the *dimnames* function is a list, as we can also verify for ourselves:

```
> class( dimnames( state.x77))
[ 1] "list"
```

Data objects of the **list** type represent a set of values which can be of different types and sizes. This makes lists different from the vectors and arrays introduced earlier. In our example above, both list values are vectors containing text entries, but of different length. We can create a new list object using the *list* function, such as:

```
> results.sum <- list( data=x, avg=mean(x), SD=sd(x))
```

By using the above command, we created an extremely simple summary of our results with three list elements: *data* contains the original values, *avg* represents their average and *SD* represents their variability. We can access the individual list elements using the double squared brackets we have already seen earlier,[7] e.g.

```
> results.sum[[2]]
[1] 4.5
```

But we can also access the list elements more easily using an alternative method in which we append the dollar sign to the name of the list object and then follow this with the element name:

```
> results.sum$avg
[1] 4.5
```

As with vectors, we can inquire about the names of list elements with the *names* function. If we perform calculations with many elements of a list, it might become tedious to repeat the list name (and dollar sign) before the use of each element. This is the moment we can effectively use the search list, with the aid of *attach* and *detach* functions:

```
> attach( results.sum)
> SD / avg
[1] 0.5443311
> search()
 [1] ".GlobalEnv"        "results.sum"        "package:stats"
...
[10] "package:base"
> detach( results.sum)
> SD / avg
Error: object 'SD' not found
```

Attaching your data to a system's search path has its dangers though: if using common names (such as *SD*) for the elements in your list, you can mask access to system objects of the same name. Or you might forget to detach a list when it is no longer needed and after attaching another one with the same name, you might get confused as to what data you are actually using. There is an alternative solution using the *with* function. This function attaches the list (but also a data frame, see below) only while the expression (which is its second parameter) is evaluated:

---

[7] Simple square brackets can also be used, but they return (for our example with an index value of 2) a list with just a single element, representing the second element of the original list.

```
> with( results.sum, SD / avg)
[1] 0.5443311
```

All of the operations we have done with the list objects can also be performed with **data frames**. You can look at the data frame type as a hybrid of two-dimensional matrices and lists. Similar to matrices, data frames contain variables as table columns, ensuring that each variable has the same number of entries (which are the rows). But individual columns might contain values of a different kind, which is not possible with matrices. This flexibility is, nevertheless, essential for data analysis where we often work with numerical and categorical variables recorded on the same set of objects (cases), which are represented by data frame rows. Also the alternative subscription methods (double square brackets or using the $ operator) work with data frames and you can attach them to R search paths in the same way as for lists. Given their utility for data analysis, data frames are an essential currency when importing (or exporting) data. We handle data import in the following section.

A.4 Importing Data into R

Your real-world data will hardly be borne by entering their values as parameters of the *c* function. They usually originate from external databases or spreadsheets. While R provides packages capable of reading directly from files representing various database platforms or from Microsoft Excel™ spreadsheets, the easiest way to import data is still through an intermediate form using a simple text-based format, whether stored in a file or simply placed on the operating system's Clipboard from within your spreadsheet software.

Here we describe the path which takes data from an Excel spreadsheet (such as the one providing sample datasets for this book) to a data frame object ready for analyses within the R program. The data in the spreadsheet must be stored in a tabular layout as described in the preceding section on data frames: it is a rectangular table with rows representing individual observations (cases) and columns representing variables. If a variable has a categorical nature, it is best if the categories are not represented by numbers, but rather by labels that start with a letter.[8] Usually, the data for the first case are not in the first row, but rather in the second, because the first row is reserved for variable labels. It is also possible, although less common, to have labels for individual cases (e.g. the names of geographical locations).

To bring your data into R via the Clipboard, you must first select the rectangular area covering the whole data table including column names (we will assume at this point that there are no row names) and copy it to the Clipboard. Now you can go to the R program and use the *read.table* function to import the data:

```
> new.dta <- read.table( "clipboard", sep="\t", header=TRUE)
```

The first parameter value specifies that your data are not stored in a real file, but instead are located on the Clipboard. If your data are unusually large, you can use a text file and read the data from there, replacing the 'clipboard' text with a path to that file

---

[8] So although it may feel both sensible and easy, do not label your experimental blocks as 1, 2, ... but rather use $b1$, $b2$, ... as the labels.

(e.g. *c:/my-data/proj1/table1.txt*). The second parameter informs the *read.table* function that the values of individual columns are separated in the text by <Tab> characters (Excel and other spreadsheet programs do this automatically when copying data to the Clipboard). The *header* parameter specifies that the first row contains column (variable) names, rather than the values for the first observation.

The *read.table* function implicitly assumes that numbers within your dataset will have their fractional components separated from their whole number by a dot character (e.g. 3.141592). Note, however, that if you work on a Windows platform localised to a specific language, the decimal separator might be something else, typically a comma character (i.e. 3,141592). In this event, you can import the data correctly by adding the *dec=","* parameter.

There are also two shortcut functions that essentially change the default values for multiple parameters and call the *read.table* function with them in turn. For inputs using a standard decimal separator (dot), this is the *read.delim* function, while the *read.delim2* function implies that the comma character is the decimal separator. Whether you use these two functions or the original *read.table* function, you must always explicitly specify the existence of row (case) labels if they are present in the imported data. As their typical location is in the first column, you can specify their existence using the *row.names=1* parameter setting.

Here is an example of importing the first data sheet (*Chap1*) from the file containing example data for this textbook (*biostat-data-eng.xlsx*). There are no row labels, so you must select the first three columns (*A* to *C*) and the first 25 rows in the sheet and copy the selection to the Clipboard (e.g. using the *Ctrl-C* key combination). Switching back to R, you can then import the data into a *chap1* data frame:

```
> chap1 <- read.delim( "clipboard")
```

We wish to offer the reader some advice, which will hopefully circumvent learning the hard way (as we have). However experienced you may feel with using R, you should always verify the correctness of your imports. Perhaps the easiest way is to review a brief summary of the data frame, and this can easily be produced using the *summary* function:

```
> summary( chap1)
   Seedlings        Mown        LitterCov
 Min.   :  6.00   no :12   Min.   : 0.00
 1st Qu.: 18.75   yes:12   1st Qu.: 2.00
 Median : 31.50            Median :11.50
 Mean   : 49.42            Mean   :18.58
 3rd Qu.: 75.25            3rd Qu.:35.00
 Max.   :168.00            Max.   :50.00
```

Using this approach primarily allows you to cross-check whether the variables expected to be of a numerical nature were indeed imported as numerical values,[9] and whether

---

[9] It is extremely easy to add a space between a decimal separator and the fractional part, or to type the capital letter O instead of a 0 value. Any such failure results in the corresponding column being treated as a categorical variable, because not all its entries can be represented by numerical values.

those to be treated as categorical variables were imported as such. The presentation of numerical variables in statistical summaries starts with a minimum and ends with a maximum value, while for categorical variables (factors), the first five most frequent categories (factor levels) are shown and then (for a variable with more than five levels) the count of observations in other categories is displayed. If there are missing values in your variable then this is also shown in the *summary* function output.[10]

For the next stage of data import verification, you can check the levels of factors and their frequencies[11] and the range and mean values for the numerical variables. For data which feel important to you, it might also be useful to spend additional time plotting the variables, but the appropriate choices are context-specific. Introductory information about the simplest graphing tools available in R is provided in the following section.

It is perhaps also important to note that when your spreadsheet contains a column with text values, it is not imported as a vector of text values, but directly as a *factor* type usable in statistical models.

A.5 Simple Graphics

The provision of interactive high-quality graphical tools is one of the core elements of the S language and hence of R software. In this introductory text, we briefly outline the simplest graphical functions. But in many cases, their use can be replaced by functions within more specialised packages (here we recommend either *ggplot2* or *lattice* package) that provide more effective visual presentations. But the higher quality and flexibility of those advanced tools is compensated by their higher complexity, so we do not introduce them here.

At present, the recommended style of using graphing functions is not much concerned with explicitly opening drawing 'devices', such as a graphing window that can be explicitly created with the *windows* function. This is because the newer R versions automatically open a drawing device for you whenever you use a graphing function in an R session for the first time. But it is probably useful to know that such functionality exists and allows you to target specialised graphing devices (e.g. output into metafile format or PDF files), although the present R versions are also able to do so in a more interactive way.

Perhaps the most basic graphing function is the *plot* function. The two commands in the first line just generate some data to plot: a sequence of integer values from 1 to 20 for *x* and a set of 20 random numbers in a range from 0 to 1 for *y*:

```
> x <- 1:20; y <- runif( 20)
> plot( x, y)
```

The *plot* function used in this form (with two numerical vectors of the same length, representing the horizontal and vertical coordinates) creates an *XY* scatter plot, using default choices for settings like axis ranges, axis labels, symbol type, size or colour. Some of these graphical attributes can be changed by passing additional parameters to the *plot* function

---

[10] Please note that empty cells in a spreadsheet are not treated as zeros, but as missing (*NA*) values.

[11] For our data example, we know they come from a balanced design, so it feels right that *no* and *yes* levels for the *Mown* factor both have frequencies of 12.

`plot( x, y, ...)`	*XY* scatter plot with specified *x* and *y* coordinates
`points( x, y, ...)`	adds symbols into an existing graph at specified coordinates
`lines( x, y, ...)`	adds line segments into an existing graph, connecting the passed coordinates
`text( x, y, labels, ...)`	adds text values into an existing graph; *labels* is a vector of text values (or numbers) of the same length as *x* or *y*, and the text in *labels[i]* is drawn centred at the coordinates *x[i]* and *y[i]*. If omitted, the implicit *labels* value is *1:length(x)*
`abline( h=c, ...)`	adds a horizontal line into an existing graph with specified vertical coordinate *c*
`abline( v=c, ...)`	adds a vertical line into an existing graph with specified horizontal coordinate *c*
`abline( lmobject, ...)`	adds a line segment into an existing graph representing a fitted regression line described by the model object *lmobject*, which was produced by the *lm* function
`legend( ...)`	this rather complex function allows you to add a figure legend into an existing graph, with customised contents (symbols, lines, labels) and position

(e.g. by adding the two *col= "blue"*, *pch= 16* parameters, you change the plotted symbols into blue filled circles), other parameters (concerning e.g. the graph layout) must be changed at the level of the drawing device, using the *par* function.

Above is a brief overview of basic drawing functions that either create new graphs or add some extra contents into an existing graph.[12]

A.6 Frameworks for R

For an effective data analysis based on R software, we must master working with functions, data objects and scripts (sequences of commands) using S language, or at least become sufficiently competent. R software (even without the specialised add-on packages) has a steep learning curve and if you are a researcher working in the field and analysing your data after your seasonal work, there is a good chance that you will forget a great deal between your R sessions. But there are tools available that make the task of remembering function parameters and working efficiently a little easier.

For a start, there is the R Commander (*Rcmdr*) package, which offers a style of analytical work more similar to user-friendly environments such as the Statistica™ software. After you open the *Rcmdr* package with the *library* function, it creates a standalone window in which you can use menu commands and dialogue boxes to enter or import data, test hypotheses, estimate parameters of selected model types and create basic graphs (Fig. A.1).

---

[12] After executing the *plot* example given earlier, there is no sense in continuing with the *points* function, as the symbols were already included. But you can try the following two functions, omitting the , ... part representing optional arguments. Doing so, *lines(x, y)* adds line segments connecting the plotted points in their original order, while *text(x, y)* adds the observation rank numbers to the plot.

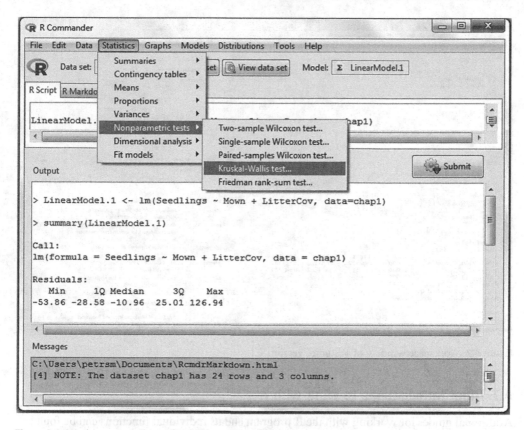

Figure A.1 Workspace window of *RCmdr*.

The R command implied by your menu/dialogue box choices is then shown in the *R Script* area, while the results are shown in the *Output* area. This way, you are still learning how to use the S language directly to achieve the same task. There are also multiple extensions (implemented as separate packages, their names starting with *RCmdrPlugin.* text) that provide extra functionality to R Commander. The R Commander library implements many of the methods described in this book, but not all of them. It is a useful, simple-to-use tool for beginners, but its simplicity is also its greatest weakness.

An alternative approach to make your work with the R program more efficient is to use the RStudio™ framework, probably suitable for a little more advanced R users. RStudio is independent software, offered by a private company (http://www.rstudio.com) both in a free version and in multiple commercial versions offering greater capabilities (particularly concerning teamwork) and prepaid support.

The philosophy of RStudio is not to shield you from typing the scripts (i.e. the S language code), but rather to make their use more efficient in terms of easy editing of multi-line commands, having a pop-up help for the parameters at your fingertips when typing a function call, providing better integration of graphic output, etc. (see Fig. A.2). It is also more straightforward to combine your data and analytical scripts into projects, stored in a structured way on your computer.

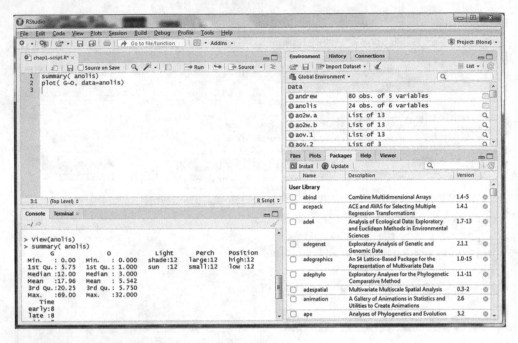

Figure A.2 Workspace window of RStudio, version 1.1.

A.7 Other Introductions to Work with R

Additional guides for working with the R program and its individual functions can be found at https://cran.r-project.org/.

The guides are located primarily on the page accessible through the *Manuals* link at the left side of the introductory web page, while the most commonly asked questions about R installation and use are addressed in a 'frequently asked question' overview, accessible through the *FAQs* link.

Beside the online guides, we heartily recommend the following textbooks:

A. Field, J. Miles & Z. Field (2012) *Discovering Statistics Using R*. Sage, Los Angeles, CA, 957 pp.

W. N. Venables & B. D. Ripley (2002) *Modern Applied Statistics with S*, 4th edn. Springer, New York, 498 pp.

Index

Page references shown in bold refer to a place with a definition or an extensive explanation of corresponding subject. The references shown in *italics* refer to R software scripts illustrating analytical approaches related to the subject.

ed in the United States
ter & Taylor Publisher Services